Aerial Nurse Corps of America

Act first, then talk
Lauretta M. Schimmoler

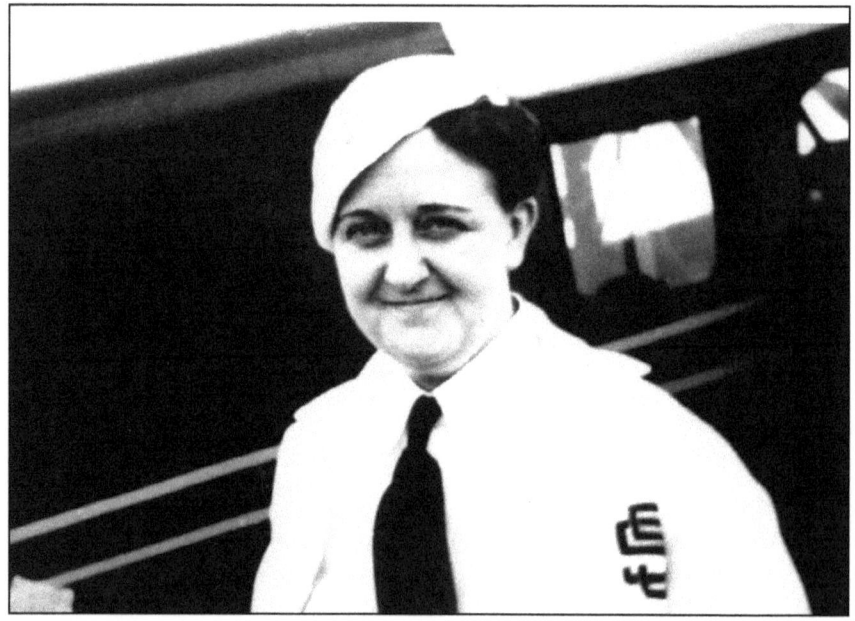

Schimmoler wearing Amelia Earhart's 99-logo designed jacket.

Aerial Nurse Corps of America

Lauretta Schimmoler and Leora Stroup
Pilot-In Air Evac

Cynthia Broze

Semper Publishing
Phoenix, Arizona

© 2023 by Cynthia Broze

All rights reserved. No part of this book may be reproduced in any manner without written permission from the publisher.

Publisher's Cataloging-in-Publication data
Broze, Cynthia, 1953-
 Aerial Nurse Corps of America: Lauretta Schimmoler and Leora Stroup Pilot-In Air Evac/Cynthia Broze
 pages 372
 Includes biographical references and index
 LCCN 2023926695
 ISBN (paperback edition) 987-0-9826509-5-0
 Published in 2023

1. Aviation nursing—United States—History—20th century. 2. Transport of sick and injured—United States—History—20th century. 3. Nurses United States—History—20th century. 4. Nurses—United States—Biography—20th century. 5. Pilots—United States—Biography—20th century. 6. Air ambulances—World—History—20th century.
 BISAC: Transportation/Aviation/History, Medical/History, Biographies
 DCC: 610.73092–dc23

Every reasonable attempt has been made to identify owners of copyrights. Errors or omissions will be corrected in subsequent printings or editions.

Published by Semper Publishing, Phoenix, Arizona
Contact: semperpublishing.com
Printed in the United States

"Illuminating...Broze deftly documents the bureaucratic obstacles."
—**Kirkus Reviews**

"A fun book and an easy read about the birth of the air ambulance. As a flight nurse for air ambulances in the 1980s, I was amazed to learn the concept began in 1936. Thanks to the pilots and nurses whose ingenuity, fortitude, and determination paved the way. Thanks for honoring these brave women and bringing their stories to life."
—**Marci Smith, RN**, CCRN, CEN, ATLS, ACLS, Flight Nurse, Ret.

"A realistic picture of the fortitude required to become a female aviator and nurse in a society that was suspicious of any woman who did not function as a dutiful housewife. It greatly enhanced my understanding of Air Rescue and Transport in an area I was completely unfamiliar with. I found the book fascinating. I give it my highest recommendation."
—**Jeffrey W. Gaver, MD,** FACEP, Aeromedical Physician, Ret., and author of *Epilogue: Aeromedical Flight Tales.*

"A Masterwork. Filled with historical photos that support the text. These women demonstrate the importance of persistence and hard work to achieve a goal. Without Broze's years of dogged research, much of these revelations would be lost."
—**Judy Olausen, BS,** Author/Photographer of the *New York Times* best selling book, *Mother.* Once named to Hasselblad's list of the top ten photographers in the world.

"Outstanding stories about flight nurses, pilots, and wild air races. Great photos of the old airplanes from those years."
—**Eduardo Barreto, RN,** Pediatric/PICU Nurse, Airplane enthusiast and RC pilot.

Also by Cynthia Broze

Nurses of Los Angeles: Uncapping the Mystery

Contents

Acknowledgements and Forward .... x-xi

Preface and Introduction .... xii-xiii

Chapter 1 - Lauretta Schimmoler 1

Chapter 2 - ANCOA 39

Chapter 3 - The World War II Effect 109

Chapter 4 - Leora Stroup 151

Chapter 5 - The Companies 189

Chapter 6 - Commanders, Nurse-Pilots, and Flight Nurses 235

> Merle McGriff McAfee, Edith Corns Lloyd, Ruth G. Mitchell, Matilda Grinevich, Genevieve Waples Smith, Florence F. Fintak, Florence Haering Boswell, Fay McWhorter Mayes, Wanda Fill, Carol Landis, Ellen Church Marshall, Margaret Gudobba Killen, Mary Eileen Newbeck Christian

Chapter 7 - Air Ambulance Histories 303

> The United States in WWI, The British in WWI, Marie Marvingt, Australian Inland Mission Aerial Medical Service (Royal Flying Doctors Service), Robin Miller, Nancy-Bird Walton, American Nurses Aviation Service, Ruth Nichols/Relief Wings, Beryl Markham, Individuals with Air Ambulances, Organized Air Ambulance Service

Notes 319

Bibliography 341

Index 343

About the Author 357

Acknowledgements

Several individuals helped me obtain information. I could not have written this book without their assistance. Linda Blicke of the Bucyrus Historical Society trusted me with Schimmoler's collection; the entire BHS group were so kind during my days in the charming town of Bucyrus—I'm glad I could visit.

Judith Johnson went beyond where most people who hold precious photos would go. The book would have been less complete without her contribution. Her mother's scrapbooks gave me such joy when I received them.

Carlos Alvarado, the helpful archivist at the Army Medical Education Department, guided me to Stroup's papers and assisted me in scanning. Robert Skinner graciously donated his papers posthumously and allowed researchers to use them—his writings inspired me and informed this book.

I'm grateful to my advanced readers for their time and opinions: Marci Smith, Judy Olausen, Eduardo Barreto, and Jeffrey Gaver for his forward. Your enthusiasm towards my book helped propel me forward when I reached the stage of wondering if anyone would enjoy it.

Thanks to Bev Williams, an RN, a pilot, a member of the Ninety-Nines, and a native of Bucyrus. She spent hours discussing with me the joys of flying and building planes, and the camaraderie among pilots. If the ANCOA had existed during her nurse and pilot years I'll bet she would have joined.

I appreciate all the archivists who found photos and items for me, including several who worked during the challenging Covid pandemic years: Sherry Severson, Amber Watts, and Samantha Harper at the Forsyth Library Archives; Katherine Behnke & Sara Fisher of the International Women's Air & Space Museum; Bill Stolz at Special Collections & Archives, Wright State University; and Lee Dobratz at the Ellis County Historical Society.

Other individuals returned my calls or emails and sent me a photo or two. Many people do not reply to an unrecognized name; it is a pleasant surprise when they do. Thank you Ellen Boeding, Ken LaRock, Judy Wieging, Kenneth Miller, Danny Burns, Lynnea St. John, Mary Ellen Vachata, Barbara Prochaska, and Clair Pecinovsky.

Forward

Like many medical professionals who served in the aeromedical transport system, I took for granted most of the technology and innovation stemmed from MASH units in the 1950s Korean War.

While military units deserve many compliments for their contributions to our present-day system, in reading this book I came to appreciate the time and activity the Aerial Nurse Corps of America expended in this area prior to WWII. The ANCOA significantly impacted the development of air evacuation and transport of sick and injured patients.

These women overcame several barriers, especially as they lived in a society reluctant to accept women aviators and physician extender providers. Interacting with their male colleagues and conservative organizations required a special blend of personal skill, communication, tact, and finesse.

The photographic collection presents their mission and enhances the text, including sections on pins and badges. The bibliography and ancillary information greatly aids the documentation—an excellent reference for the history of Air Transport and Rescue.

This book covers a wide range of interests and should appeal to a diverse cross-section of people. Although it can stand as a history of Air Ambulance Rescue, it also features biographical accounts of ANCOA members. It serves as encouragement for future generations of aeromedical transport professionals, regardless of their gender. You will enjoy this book.

                              Jeffrey W. Gaver, MD, FACEP, Aeromedical Physician, Ret.

Preface

History is like a compost pile—someone must continue turning it over to remain viable. The Aerial Nurse Corps of America (ANCOA) enjoyed relative fame in the U.S. from 1936-1944: various newspapers and well-read magazines featured them. But the world soon forgot.

Then, while researching for his 1954 book *Medical Support of the Army Air Forces in WWII,* historian Hubert Coleman found the military's rejection letters to Schimmoler and included the story of her struggles in his book. Flight Nurses re-discovered the ANCOA when they honored Schimmoler's contribution in 1966. Aviation journals published a few articles about them in the 1980s. Still, these mentions did not show the complete picture.

I discovered the ANCOA while writing my book, *Nurses of Los Angeles: Uncapping the Mystery.* Why did this unique organization, with more than 600 members, recess into history with no eponymous book to remember them by? Since Schimmoler established the first company in Los Angeles, I expected libraries and archives around Los Angeles County would contain much of their history. I was wrong.

I visited ten archives in six states, read hundreds of newspaper clippings, and spoke to numerous people. Many important photos I found were degraded clippings—I had to colorize some just to make them readable. While I've attempted to make this book a definitive compilation, hidden family scrapbooks and photo boxes must hold additional knowledge. And, unfortunately, much has been discarded.

Since no ANCOA members are alive, I've gleaned their lives through published interviews, activities, and biographical sketches of the prominent members. When possible, I've used their own words to tell how they began, what they did, and their ideas about the specialty they created.

I've discussed the airplanes they used, the famous pilots they knew, and the air races they staffed. Air races in the 1930s were huge—unlike any airplane demonstrations we could attend today. And the ANCOA nurses were always waiting in the first aid tents with their medical kits, ready to help.

Why did I decide to write this book? Certainly to document the history, but mainly because it's a good story. With a great ending.

Introduction

We expect a skilled nurse will assist us if we are sick and require air transport. Before 1936 this was far from reality. Air transportation of critically ill patients began sporadically during World War I, but they crammed the wounded behind the pilot's area with no one to attend to them—the sick and dying patients had to fend for themselves.

Lauretta Schimmoler realized this and sought to change it. She thought nurses trained in the aspects of air ambulance transport would be valuable for society. She hoped it could also benefit the military.

She found nurses who believed in her cause. Some were pilots or became pilots, although nurses didn't usually fly the planes. Dedicated nurses like Leora Stroup championed the idea when others doubted its relevance.

Schimmoler understood airport management, flight school operations, aircraft manufacturing, first aid, chemical warfare, air mail transport, weather, and flight recorders. She even designed special medical equipment to fit inside small airplanes. But the various ranks scrutinized her actions because she wasn't a nurse.

Schimmoler and Stroup were born, spent their childhoods, and were buried within 120 miles of each other in Ohio. Both became pilots and early members of the Ninety-Nines club. Stroup had also thought nurses should train for aerial duty even before she met Schimmoler. And Stroup had an edge on Schimmoler—she was a nurse—but Schimmoler barreled ahead despite lacking those credentials.

Schimmoler expected people would see the value and appreciate what she and the nurses wanted to accomplish with this specialty they were trying to create. She was wrong. She hadn't realized one essential detail when developing her idea: nursing administration groups and the military didn't accept proposals from outsiders. Thus, she would spend her air ambulance life trying to work with them, through them, or around them.

Chapter One
Lauretta M. Schimmoler

National Commander; Licensed Pilot

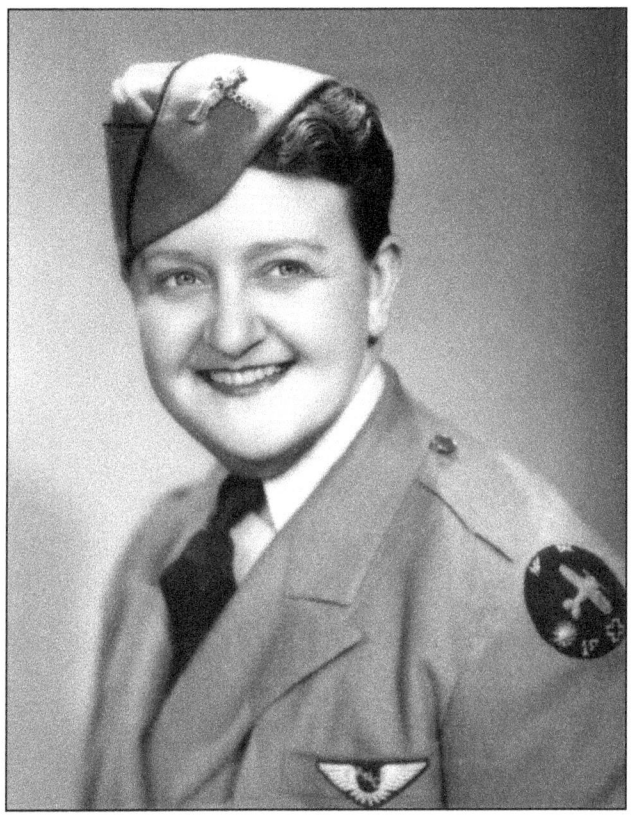

Figure 01.01. Schimmoler's official ANCOA photograph, 1938. She wears a commander patch on her pocket, a 1st Division patch on her arm, and an ANCOA pin on her cap. Bucyrus Historical Society Collection (BHS).

Lauretta M. Schimmoler wouldn't be stopped. We know few facts about the voracity of her childhood, but as an adult she proceeded at full force. Her independent nature grew into a fierce drive to succeed. Airplanes fired her blood and it didn't cool. She spent her life chasing firsts in the aviation field; however, she made her most significant accomplishment on the ground rather than in the air. Regardless of the altitude, she accomplished something no person in the United States had even tried to do.

Chapter One

Schimmoler was born in Fort Jennings, Ohio, on 17 September 1900, to Louis and Josephine Schimmoeler (nee Stevens). Her father made harnesses and later repaired shoes. She attended public schools in Delphos, Ottawa, and Crestline.[1] Born the second of eight, her sisters Cecelia (deceased at age 10), Eulalia Georgia, Lucille Marie, Jeanette Julia, and her brother Gilman Ferdinand were also born in Fort Jennings. When Schimmoeler turned eleven, the family moved.

Lauretta sent a postcard to her grandfather, on 9 October 1911, to update him about her family's move to Plymouth, Ohio. "The potatoes and apples are fine. This is a pretty place." She signed it, Lauretta Schimmoeler. Her signature confirms the family initially spelled their name with an additional E after the O. Later in life she deleted the E—it made her name easier to pronounce.[2]

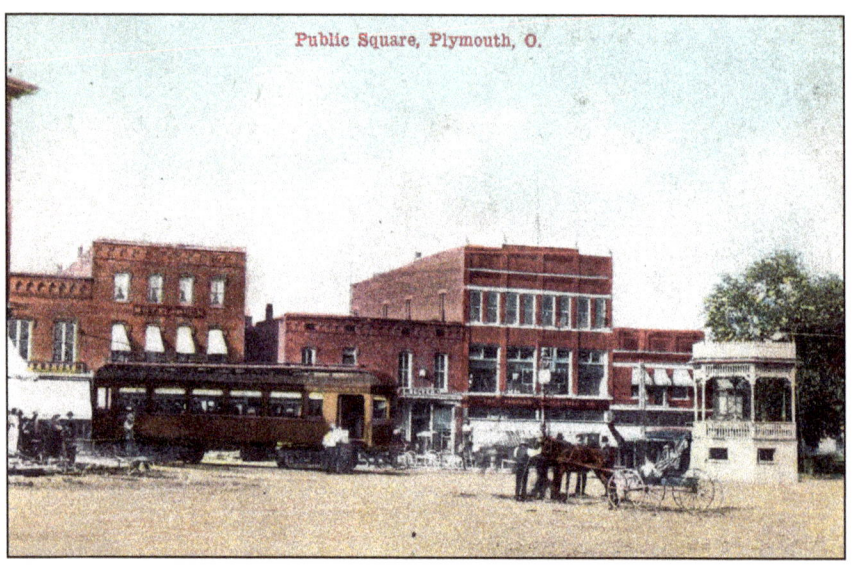

Figure 01.02. Public Square, Plymouth, Ohio, 1911. Courtesy of Judy Wieging, Fort Jennings, Ohio.

At some point, all or part of the family moved to Bucyrus, Ohio. The 1929 Bucyrus Directory lists Alberta, Lauretta, and her mother living at 412 River Street, the house Schimmoler started her chicken business. The Historical Society documents her father residing at 412 River Street then; the 1929 Bucyrus Directory lists her mother as "the widow of Louis." His obituary couldn't be located to confirm it, but the women were probably on their own.

Schimmoler had married Bellevue native Charles Henry Rudge, on 28 August 1919, in Bucyrus. Records list his occupation as a molder.[3] Their marriage did not last; they divorced in early 1920.[4]

But she experienced a more defining event in 1919 than her marriage—a day that would alter the course of her life—even if she didn't realize it. She'd traveled to Dayton to visit friends. They drove to old McCook Army Air Field to watch Lieutenant John Macready attempt his world altitude record.

During the flight, Macready lost consciousness and plunged five miles before he regained his senses and took control of the plane. Schimmoler said she was scared while watching it but, "What a thrill." [5]

One point to note, although Schimmoler told this story in 1940 and undoubtedly repeated it many times, Macready did not earn his world record in 1919; he achieved it in 1921. Captain Rudolph Schroeder, another altitude-test pilot at McCook, achieved the world record in 1919, not Macready. Macready replaced Schroeder in 1920 after Schroeder made a third world record on 7 February 1920.

The story Schimmoler told sounded more like Schroeder's 1920 event—he removed his foggy goggles, and his eyeballs froze. He lost consciousness from lack of oxygen and carbon monoxide poisoning; he plummeted six miles in two minutes before regaining consciousness, landing his plane while blinded. [6] Because of this freezing injury to his eyesight, Macready replaced him. Schimmoler either forgot the exact year she witnessed her seminal viewing event, or she misremembered the pilot's name.

On 13 May 1920, she married again—to Bucyrian native Thomas Ignatious Long. [7] That year, she moved to Liberal, Kansas, and became an assistant manager with the Tri-State Adjusting Association, an insurance business. Perhaps the job was too tame; she stayed only two years.

She left Kansas for Columbus, Ohio, to attend the Bliss Business School in the fall of 1922. She graduated with honors in 1923. [8] It's unknown if Long moved with her to Kansas, Columbus, or back to Bucyrus. They divorced that same year. Whether it was the impact of two divorces or her ambitious future goals, she did not try marriage again.

Crawford County Courts hired her as Assistant to the Court Stenographer. [9] As a member of the Order of Gregg Artists, she was well qualified for the job. Gregg Shorthand Artists were a select group of shorthand scribes who demonstrated unquestionable artistic merit.

After a series of shorthand tests where the applicant precisely demonstrated script and phonography, they would grant membership into the order. The participants often had to test several times before acceptance. [10] Pen stenography based its form on elliptical figures and lines that bisected; Gregg shorthand became the most popular form of pen stenography.

Chapter One

Speed was critical. Court reporters transcribed testimony at 200 words per minute. Although Schimmoler excelled, one can barely imagine she'd feel content to transcribe dictation for years. During this same time, she studied law under Judge J.W. Schwenck. Her stenography position and law study lasted only two years; both ventures must have been intertwined. Schwenck's letter of recommendation stated Schimmoler was "a very efficient employee…absolutely honest and reliable. She left the office, which was for no fault of hers." The unexpected lay-off led to another job which became her life's work for many years. [11-12]

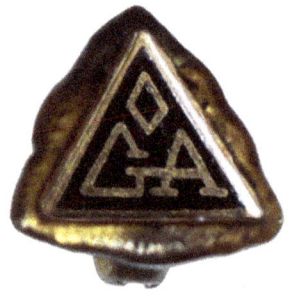

Figure 01.03. Schimmoler's pin for the Order of Gregg Artists. Author photographed at BHS.

She quickly secured a job as a bookkeeper at the Bucyrus Hatchery Company. With her business knowledge, she thought she could run a chicken business better so she decided to start her own and breed fancy chickens. [13] She opened the Riverview Leghorn Farm, specializing in White Leghorn Chickens, at 412 River Street in Bucyrus. She continued to work as a bookkeeper at the Bucyrus Hatchery Company and managed her own business for nine years. [14]

On 26 September 1928, she took her first plane ride in the 90-horsepower Waco 10 biplane of Gene F. Foster from Crestline, Ohio. [15] Foster was a barnstormer who charged passengers five dollars for a fifteen-minute ride. Later he became a test pilot, a World War II pilot, and worked with the Martin Marietta Corporation on airplanes and missiles for forty-five years. [16] Schimmoler had chosen a future world-class pilot for her inaugural flight—even if by chance.

That first ride cemented her desire to learn to fly; she applied for a student pilot permit. The Aeronautics Branch of the Department of Commerce granted her permit #24288 on 10 August 1929. Apparently, few women applied because her acceptance letter began, "Dear Sir." [17]

She quickly enrolled in the nearest flight school, Sycamore Aviation College, about eighteen miles from Bucyrus—the only female student in the class of twenty-five. She must have impressed the school owners because they hired her immediately as the advertising manager. [18]

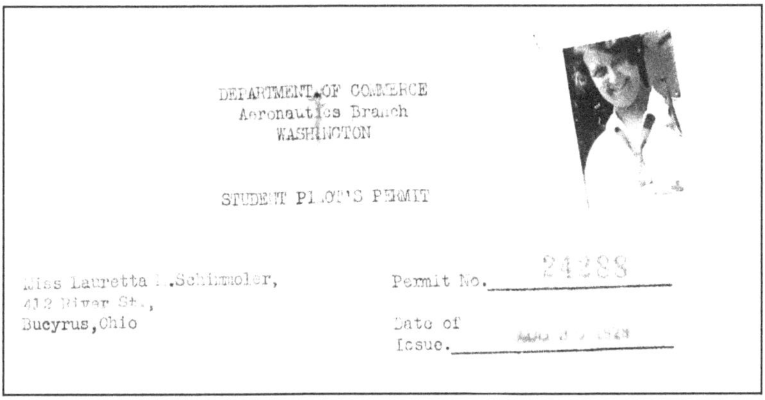

Figure 01.04. Shimmoler's student pilot permit, 1929. BHS Collection.

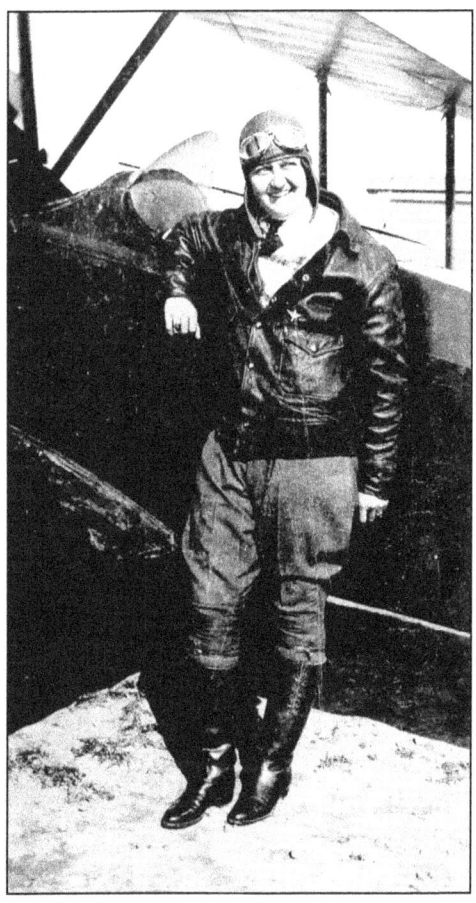

Figure 01.05. Shimmoler standing next to her training plane, a Swallow TP, in a forty-acre field in Sycamore, Ohio, 1929. BHS.

Chapter One

Although she didn't record it in her Pilots Log Book, she later wrote on the inside cover that she took the controls of an airplane for the first time, for fifteen minutes, on 31 July 1929, with her instructor O.E. Hollenbaugh, in a Swallow TP (Training Plane) in Sycamore. [19-20]

The TP was a simple yet rugged biplane with room for an instructor and a student in tandem open cockpits. The fuselage was a welded steel tubing covered with fabric. The wings were typical for the period: spruce spars with spruce and plywood ribs covered in cloth.

The Commerce Department regulated flying schools and licenses. They required eighteen hours in the air, eight dual flights, ten solo flights, two rights, and two left tail spins to obtain a pilot's license. She completed her first solo flight on 9 October 1929. [21] She said of her first solo:

> It was great, and I'm thrilled. But it was a funny feeling to know there was no one along to get me out of trouble. If I had to set the plane down by myself. [22]

Sycamore had an airfield, but the area was less populated than Bucyrus. She reasoned Bucyrus would be a much better place for a flying school—the central location would increase the business. She discussed her idea with the flight school's owner that he should move it to Bucyrus. He agreed. But first, Bucyrus needed an airfield. [23]

As Chairman of Bucyrus' Chamber of Commerce Boosters, Schimmoler encouraged the city to purchase sixty-four acres of farmland on Winchester Road from the owner Peter Metzger and establish a municipal airport and a flying school. [24] The site already contained a wooden hangar. The Rotary Club circulated a petition to place the vote on the November 1929 ballot. Voters approved a $40,000 bond by a large majority to purchase and equip the airport. [25]

Mayor Arthur Shuler opposed the purchase. He vetoed the money transfer from the bank, placing the airport purchase on hold. Schimmoler did not wait. She secured the backing of eleven local businessmen and leased the land from Metzger, for $448 per year, on 14 April 1930. Schimmoler established an airport in Ohio even before she had completed her pilot's training. [26]

Publications have long touted Schimmoler as the first woman in the U. S. to establish and manage an airport. Sites on the internet state it as fact. The Ohio Woman's Hall of Fame and *Kanes Famous First Facts* list it. [27] Some writings claim the Guinness Book of Records certified her as the first female airport manager in the U.S. (unverified). [28] This assertion, however, is not correct. She was the first woman in Ohio, but the first in the U.S. was in California.

In March 1930, Margaret Perry Cooper, a charter member of the Ninety-Nines, leased an abandoned airport in Culver City, California—three weeks before Schimmoler leased the Bucyrus field. Perry's airport and flying school opened on 9 May 1930, a year before Schimmoler officially opened Port Bucyrus.[29] But "the first woman" doesn't go to either Schimmoler or Perry Cooper. Twyla Kelly established Kelly Airport and Flying School in Hawthorne in July 1927. Kelly was a businesswoman, not a pilot, who understood airplane mechanics and airport operations.[30] Was she the first?

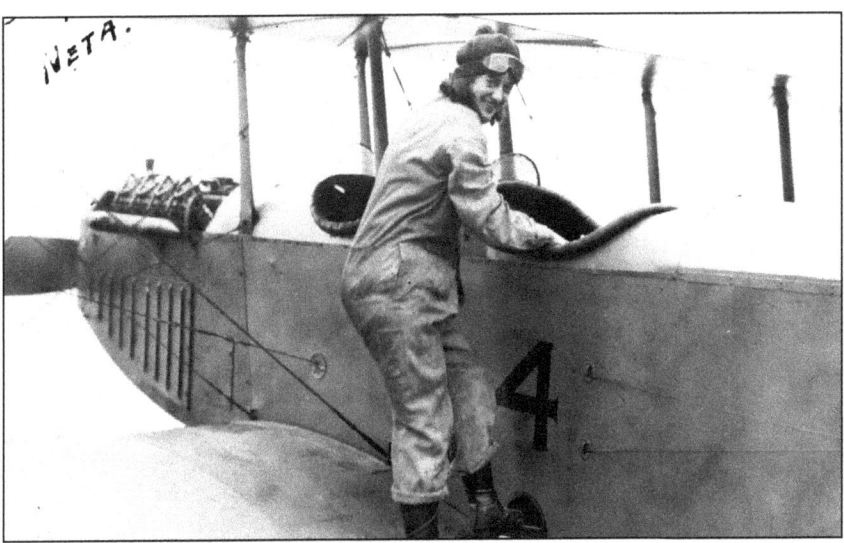

Figure 01.06. Neta Snook and her Canuck, a Canadian version of the JN-4 Jenny airplane, 1920. She bought it wrecked, had it shipped, and rebuilt it.

Neta Snook achieved a long list of aviation firsts, but she is best known as the woman who taught Amelia Earhart to fly in 1921. Born in Illinois and raised in Iowa, Snook learned to fly in 1917 at age 21. She decided to move to Los Angeles in 1920 because of its perfect flying climate.

Bert Kinner, the creator of Kinner airplanes, had recently constructed the second commercial air field in Los Angeles at Long Beach Blvd and Tweedy Road. Snook needed a job. Her background in plane mechanics and flight instruction made her invaluable so he hired her. She stayed two years.

In her book, *I Taught Amelia Earhart to Fly*, she said "…I tested the planes, did the aerial advertising, carried passengers, and taught students." Later she mentioned twice she "operated Kinner Airport," but didn't specify her duties. She never said Kinner managed it or stopped—what she meant isn't clear. Ames Historical Society (AHS) named her as the first woman to manage a commercial airport but gives no references.[31] Internet posts cite AHS.

Chapter One

Schimmoler knew she wasn't the first woman. A newspaper clipping from her archive mentions a woman in California was the first woman to manage an airport, although it doesn't mention her name.[32]

Schimmoler never used the phrase "first woman to manage an airport." But when Vi-Air-Ways promoted her to Vice-President, she did say she was the first woman to operate, promote, manage, and supervise the building of a commercial airport. This statement is probably true. Establish, manage, or operate is a matter of semantics. Whoever it was Schimmoler wasn't alone.

Schimmoler passed her pilot's exam on 4 August 1930 at the Municipal Airport in Akron. She flew a guest passenger during her first cross-country flight from Akron to Cleveland on 7 August. Her application stated she weighed 160 pounds and was 5'6" with brown hair and blue eyes. She received license #15907 on 8 September.[33]

On 8 August, she took off from an airfield in Akron, en route to Lorain, with her instructor Hugh C. Robbins. She'd just purchased a Waco OX 90 biplane from him with egg money and the sale of advanced tickets to people she planned to fly over Bucyrus. Before he turned over the ownership, he wanted to be confident she knew the operating functions of the plane. She detailed that flight:

> It was a beautiful day, the air was smooth. As I approached what I thought was Lorain, I didn't recognize the city from the air, so I signaled my passenger for information. All I got from him was a negative shake of the head. For a second, I pondered... could it be it meant he wouldn't help me, as he had said, or was it that I had not reached Lorain? This must be it, I thought as I began to look around, hoping I might recognize something down there. Then I saw the old beach house that a tornado had wrecked in the late 20s, still unrepaired. I knew then my calculation was correct.
>
> My next worry was to find the airport. In the distance to my left, I saw what appeared to be two shiny buildings that looked like hangars, and I headed my plane in that direction, by this time feeling quite elated that I had flown the course I had charted.
>
> It was at the airport that I was about to land. My passenger gave me a frantic signal not to land but to circle the airport again. Following his instructions, I finally landed, but to my surprise, in the opposite direction of my original approach. Before getting out of the plane, he knelt on the seat in front

of the cockpit and gave me a lecture I never forgot. In rapid succession, it went like this: 'What are you trying to do, commit suicide? Didn't you see that smoke downtown? Didn't you see that sock on the hangar? It's your airplane… if you want to crack it up, that's alright, but I don't want to be in it.'

Obviously, my face must have been one of surprise, for he followed with this question… 'Don't you know what you were doing?'

My answer was 'No.' Then he told me I was about to make a down-wind landing, which meant a crack-up. All the pride I had in myself a few moments ago was entirely shattered. I had failed to put into practice the training I received as a student pilot. I sat there for some time, thinking of the serious mistake I had made. About an hour later, he returned and asked me, 'Do you think you can fly me back to Akron?'

'I think I can,' was my reply. [34]

With this purchase, Schimmoler became the first Bucyrian to own a plane and Bucyrus' only pilot. [35] On 10 August, she licensed the plane, flew from Akron to Bucyrus, and parked it in the wooden hangar. [36] In addition to her plane, flyer L.H. McBride, from the nearby town of Bloomfield, had leased space in the hangar for his Swallow TP. [37]

The Battle of Port Bucyrus Began

The battle over the voter-approved airport purchase began at the council meeting on 19 August 1930, when the City Council read the ordinance. Mayor Shuler said he would veto it again if it passed. Councilmen John Quaintance and William Relnemeyer voted no. [38] The airport purchase remained on hold.

That same night, and only nine days after Schimmoler parked her plane, a highly suspicious fire destroyed the hangar and both planes inside. Columbus Deputy Fire Marshall, Jack Sheckler, arrived the next day and started an investigation. Sheckler said, "No power runs through airplanes when not in operation. They cannot ignite themselves. All power to the airport had been cut off at the entrance, as is customary. No power would flow through the electric wires during the night." He also reported an automobile "had been seen leaving the airport shortly after 10 p.m." They set the loss at $7,100. Insurance covered Metzger's $3,300 hangar and McBride's $1,000 Swallow TP. Schimmoler's $3,200 Waco OX90 wasn't covered. She was not dissuaded. Instead, she doubled her efforts to rebuild.[39]

The City Council continued to meet resistance in selecting the airport site. At their meeting in December 1930, Councilmen George Ryan and Chris Gaa voted "no" to the motion to direct the purchase of the chosen site. The Mayor pointed out:

> The price is quite exorbitant for the 64-acre farm when the tax duplicate showed the land appraised at $85 an acre. The Council should expect me to veto if it passes.[40]

Finally, on 19 May 1931, the Council adopted the ordinance authorizing the service director to purchase the tract of land for $15,000. Again Mayor Schuler maintained the price for a landing field was exorbitant because the land had been reduced in value on the tax duplicate from $5,379 to $3,970.

> The fact that you were authorized by the majority vote of the electors of the city to purchase an airport still does not warrant wasteful expenditure of public funds.

In his final plea, the Mayor urged the Council to transfer the $15,000 to the poor fund for the next winter and threatened a popular referendum. It did not work. For the first time in eight years, the city council unanimously voted to override an executive veto. They ordered Clarence Cober, the City Service Director, to purchase Port Bucyrus.[41-42]

The Council made preparations, but the owner could not furnish the deed because it was currently under lease to Schimmoler. The Council called her, and she agreed to give up her renewal rights when the contract ended. The Council immediately adopted the amended ordinance authorizing the purchase of the tract.

Schimmoler told the Council she would submit her bid to lease the Port next year when the city advertised bids. The Port would continue operating under Schimmoler's ownership until her lease expired in April 1932.[43]

With the Port's purchase confirmed, the Chamber of Commerce negotiated with two airplane manufacturing companies: one for standard airplanes and one for power gliders. They planned to start the new factories with potential employment for fifty men.[44] Warmer weather arrived, and Schimmoler sprang into action to complete the airport.

She built an all-steel "practically fireproof" hangar, large enough for four planes, on the old hangar's foundation. They removed fences, hauled away the tall grass, and installed the gasoline tanks. Grading machines leveled the furrows. Workers fenced off areas for parking. She planned for a workshop, an office, and classrooms. Planes landed, and the business progressed. The secretary of the Crawford County Automobile Club, M.B. Morisey, landed from a trip in Philadelphia, stored his airship overnight, and fueled it with 100 gallons of gas. Gene Foster planned to light later in the week to visit his family in Crestline. [45-47]

Schimmoler chose the name Port Bucyrus for the airport. The City Council approved it in compliance with a state law, which required the approval of a council body to name an airport for a city. Schimmoler started her flying school, the Bucyrus Institute of Aviation, and advertised: LEARN TO FLY $10 per hour dual, $5 per hour solo. Special for two weeks. Ground Course Free. Plans called for the airport to be open by 1 May. [48-49]

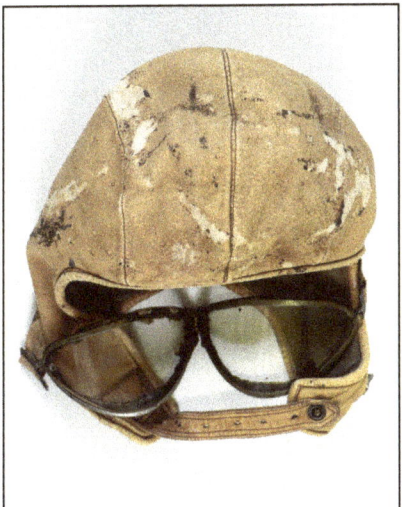
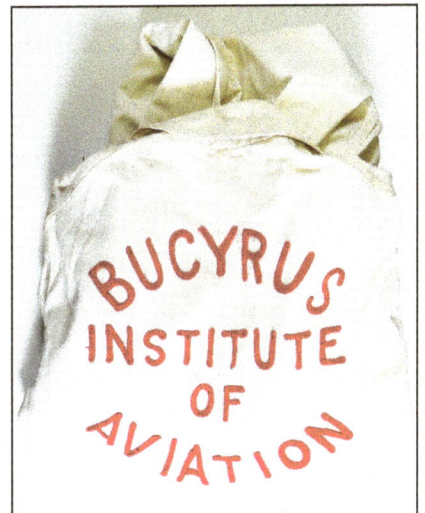

Figures 01.07., 01.08., and 01.09. Schimmoler's leather helmet and goggles, her Bucyrus Institute of Aviation flying overalls, and her altimeter (altitude meter), c. 1930. Author photographed at BHS.

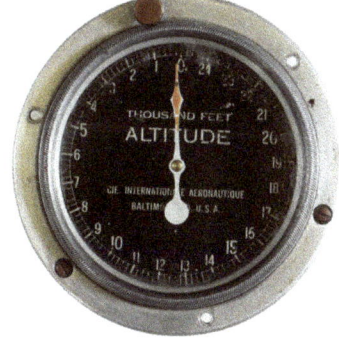

Chapter One

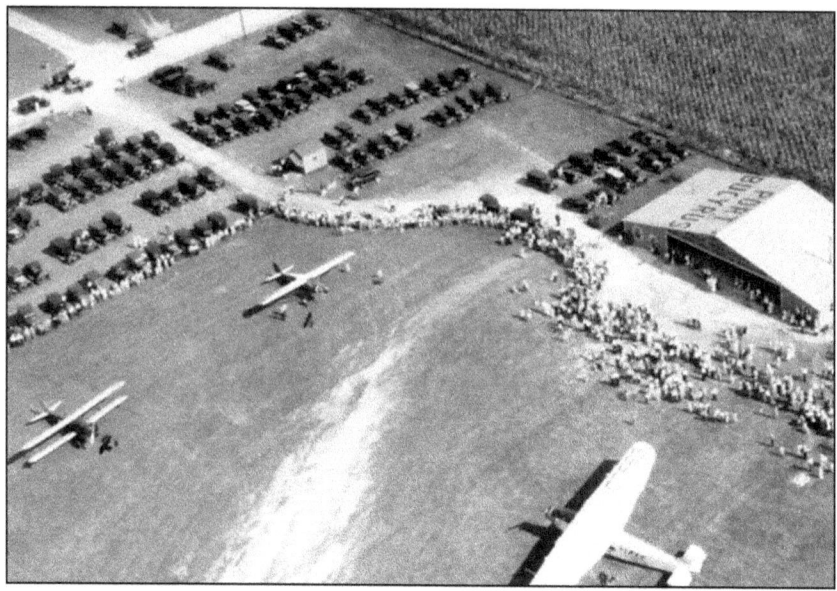

Figure 01.10. Aerial view of the Port Bucyrus dedication 19 July 1931. Note the Port Bucyrus air marker on the roof. BHS.

In early May, twenty-seven members of the Crestline Glider Club moved various aerial equipment to Port Bucyrus and established their headquarters at the field for its advantages, including the open county surrounding. The available field size in Crestline was considered too small for safety and provided no hangar—they had to knock down their hangar and store it in a garage between flights—they leased space in Port Bucyrus for the glider. [50]

Schimmoler secured space for several planes: a Curtiss Wright Junior pusher-plane, a neighboring manufacturer owned, and her Waco 90. She leased a New Standard Kinner K-5 for student training and long-distance taxi/passenger service, well-suited because of its maneuverability. [51-52]

The National Air Transport airline, bought by Boeing in 1930, had recently established two lines of operation that followed the Pennsylvania Railroad and they had considered crossing the lines at Port Bucyrus. They'd already made trial flights. She signed a contract with Chicago & Eastern Airways to use the Port on a regular stop for their future Chicago-Pittsburgh lines. [53-54]

Finally, the work was completed at a reported cost of $10,000. Two runways stretched 2,100 feet from southeast to northeast, and 2,500 feet from northeast to southwest. The Port contained hangar facilities, gas and oil supplies, and light repair aids. The hangar cost $13,000. They set the official dedication for 19 July 1931. [55-56]

More than 2,000 cars jammed the highways as Ohio pilots and friends flocked to the new field. The whir of propellers filled the air—twenty-plus planes flew in. Pilots prepared to win races for prizes and honors. Before the start of the aerial program, more than 175 pilots, members of the Chamber of Commerce, the Rotary Club, and other city officials attended a luncheon in the hangar. [57]

Carol Johnson, a Cleveland test pilot, won the twenty-five-mile race. Jerry Nettleton, from Toledo, secured the four-mile free-for-all event in five and one-half minutes. Shirley Ertzel and Harry Sanders of Cleveland won the dead stick landing events. Elmer Palmer, a Plymouth aviator, won the balloon-bursting contest when he downed five bags from his plane in thirty seconds at an altitude of 500 feet. [58]

She featured prominent guests among the pilots and patrons: Frank McKee, the State Aeronautical Director; Dr. William J. Gorey, State Examiner; O.V. Overholser, State Aeronautical Association; and George W. Lumm, Toledo Standard Oil Division. Mary E. VonMarch, transport pilot on the Michigan Goodwill Tour, attended as a special guest of Schimmoler. J. Howard Pry, the official pilot for the Mansfield Air Races scheduled in late July, presented the awards. [59]

During the twenty-five-mile race, a broken water pump forced down Julian Miller of Castilia—he landed safely in a hay field. Howard Fry from Ashland lost part of his landing gear when a coupling broke off. No major accidents marred the festivities, and the dedication succeeded. [60]

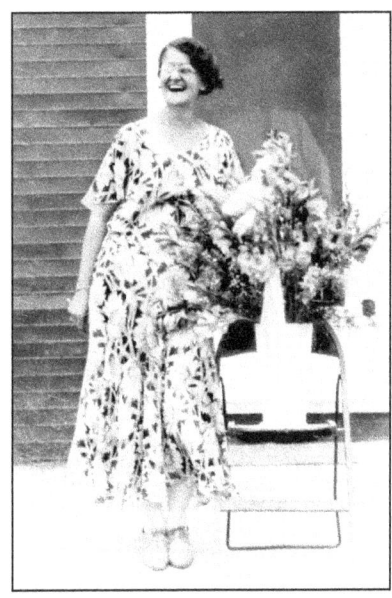

Figure 01.11. Schimmoler enjoying the Port Bucyrus opening on its dedication day, 19 July 1931.

Chapter One

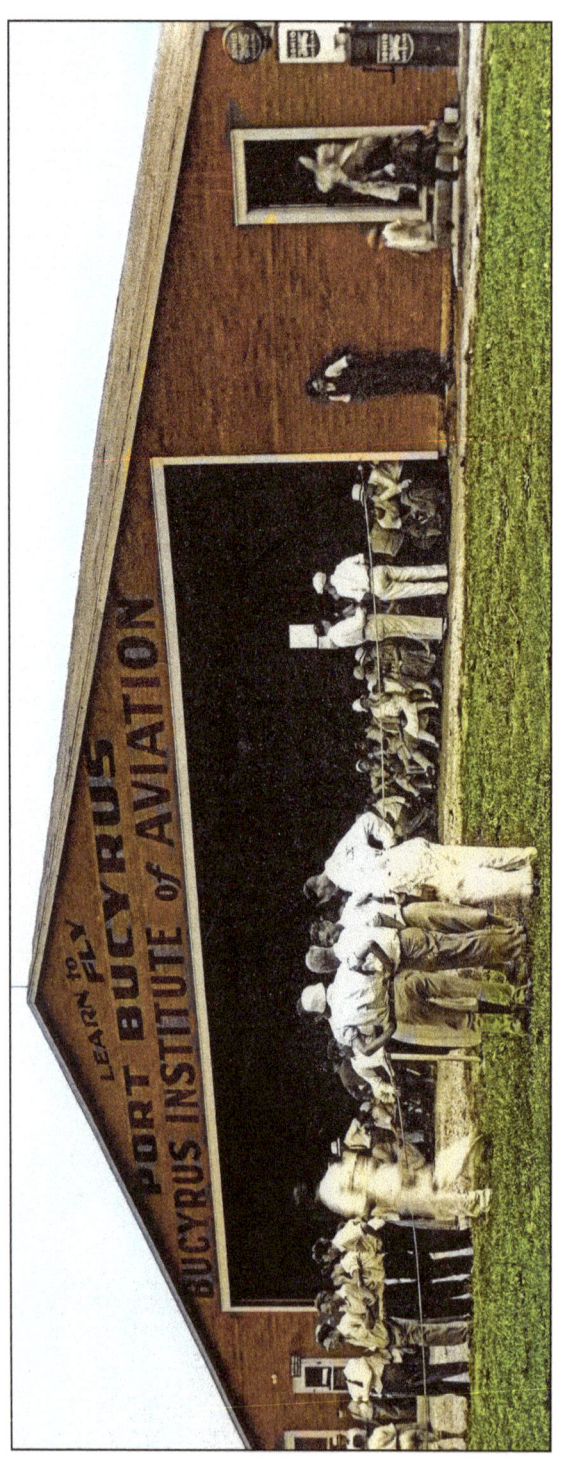

Figure 01.12. Port Bucyrus official dedication 19 July 1931. Colorized photo, BHS.

Figure 01.12. The Port Bucyrus official dedication 19 July 1931. Port Bucyrus and Schimmoler's flying school, the Bucyrus Institute of Aviation, included a runway stretching 2,100 feet from southeast to northeast and a 2,500-foot runway from northeast to southwest. Note the Sohio fuel pump. Sohio was a contraction for Standard Oil Company. John D. Rockefeller, among the wealthiest men in modern history, incorporated the company in 1870 with headquarters in Cleveland, Ohio. Colorized by Fred Fischer.

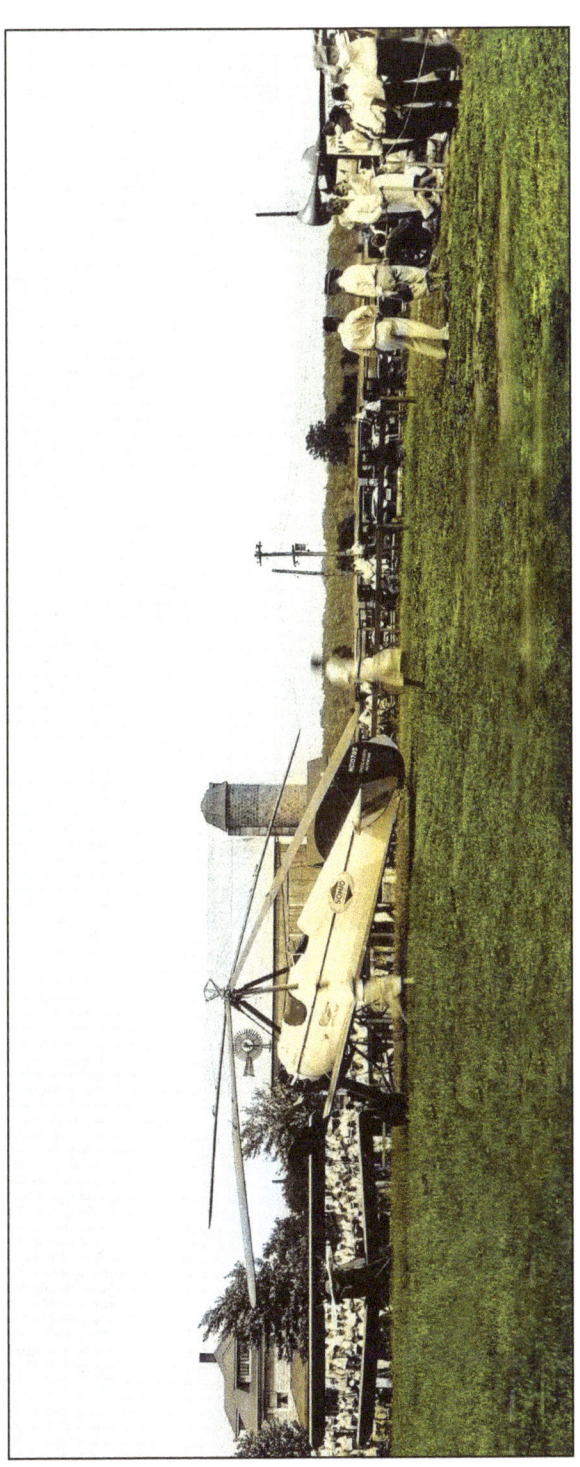

Figure 01.13. Blanche Noyes' Pitcairn PCA-2 Autogyro at the Port Bucyrus dedication 19 July 1931. Colorized photo, BHS.

Blanche Wilcox Noyes arrived from Cleveland in the highly anticipated plane—a Pitcairn PCA-2 Autogyro. It contained an airplane-like fuselage, two open-style cockpits in tandem, and a single engine mounted tractor-fashion in the nose. The lift, by the four-blade main rotor, was augmented by stubby, low-set monoplane wings that also carried the control surfaces.[61] An aerial salute opened the event at 2 p.m.[62] Noyes flew the Pitcairn PCA-2 autogyro, NC10785, S/N B-14, during the years she worked for Sohio. Colorized by Fred Fischer.

Chapter One

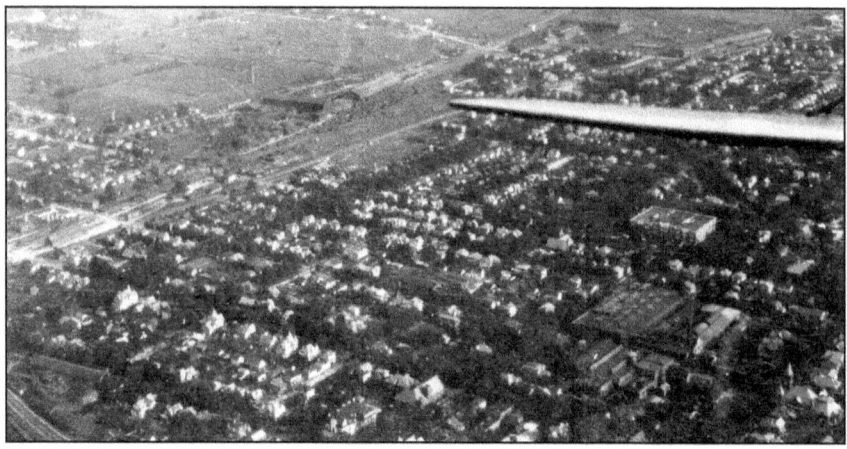

Figure 01.14. Schimmoler flying over Bucyrus. BHS Collection.

Following her airport's opening, officials placed Schimmoler in charge of the women's events at the Mansfield Airport Races, thirty miles from Bucyrus, on 24 July. That would be Schimmoler's first air race.[63]

En route to Mansfield she cracked-up her plane and arrived late. They immediately ushered her to another plane and told her to get going—they needed a third woman for an event. She took off in the unfamiliar loaner, which "bounced like a grasshopper before taking off." Suddenly it tacked to the right and cut across the bows of two other entrants. She felt guilty and meandered in the sky before landing.

Of course, she didn't win. When she landed, she rushed to apologize to the other pilots for cutting them off. They assured her, "You didn't cut us off. You were keeping your course all right." But the ragged start had jarred her and spoiled her first air meet.[64]

Crestline Glider Club made good use of Port Bucyrus. Nine members used the Bucyrus Institute of Aviation for flying lessons. On 26 July 1931, W. N. Roberts, Department of Commerce Inspector, tested eight glider flyers for licenses. Seven passed, including Richard Snyder, a sixteen-year-old who was the youngest glider pilot in Ohio, and seventeen-year-old Gretchen Reighard, the only female glider pilot within 100 miles.

To complete the test, the pilots had to demonstrate four hours of continuous flying. Each pilot rode the glider 500 feet into the air, making a complete circle before landing. They needed to pass three of these flights to succeed in the test. Schimmoler used the day to obtain a limited commercial pilot license during the inspector's visit.[65]

Schimmoler

In August 1931, Schimmoler persuaded the Riddell Company (a clay-working machinery manufacturer) to airmark the roof of its Bucyrus plant in fifteen-foot tall letters. She said she expected several other businesses to co-operate in placing markers. In 1929, the Bucyrus high school building had set markers, but they had since become unreadable. [66]

Early in the twentieth century, few pilots had radio navigation; while flying, they would look at the ground for landmarks to determine their location and to find a landing strip. In 1926 the U.S. Government began to promote airmarkers—the painted name of a town or local airport on a rooftop, often with an arrow pointing towards the airport. Federal aviation agencies regulated their size and appearance: ten to thirty-feet tall and the color Chrome Yellow Number Four on a black background. The goal was to have a marker every fifteen miles. The government did not undertake the painting of the markers. Instead, they enlisted volunteer groups, including the Ninety-Nines, an organization of women pilots. [67]

With the passage of General Code Section 6310-44 on 25 June 1929, Ohio instituted the world's first mandatory municipal air marking law. Municipalities had to mark buildings for aeronautical purposes, with costs paid from the general fund. The code required the letters to be twenty-feet tall. They often incorporated airport pointers; the pointers created problems because sometimes the installers didn't remove them when the airports changed locations. Surface markers, plowed or painted in fields and on concrete, were acceptable if no suitable roof was available.

The Department of Commerce determined the best location would be the south side of hip roofs because, in the northern hemisphere, a pilot would view the markings with his back toward the sun, making them more readable. And the snow melted off the southern roofs more quickly than the northern sides. Markers should face the outskirts of the municipalities so a passing pilot could read them without the need to fly over the downtown area. [68]

In August 1932, Schimmoler received a commendation from John Groves, Chief of the Airways Bulletin section of the Department of Commerce, for her success placing the Bucyrus Marker and told her a notice would appear in a future printing of the Department's Air Commerce Bulletin. She had sent a letter requesting markers on routes four and five near Bucyrus. He advised her that Ohio had already assigned 143 markers and they would consider additional local markers at the next assignment. [69]

Approximately 30,000 airmarkers were active during this time. But on 17 January 1942, the war department decided to remove all markers within 150 miles of the Atlantic and Pacific coasts to foil possible air invaders who might use them as convenient targets. Cities could not construct new markers.

Chapter One

The Secretary of War, Henry Stimson, allowed markers only within fifty miles of airfields conducting flight training. [70]

In 1942, two army offices were involved in an airmarker hoax. They claimed someone had marked the location of an airplane factory to lead the enemy. They provided aerial photos. An "overzealous Army press agent" released the information to newspapers before anyone had examined it. The subsequent investigation revealed the alleged markers were bags of fertilizer on the ground of a farm. The Army removed the officers from their posts. [71-72]

Before the war began, famous aviator Blanche Noyes organized campaigns to inspect the airmarkers. The lack of maintenance during the war had weathered many remaining. Now, she started a campaign to re-establish the markers. Congress appropriated $100,000 for the project in 1947, but the money was insufficient to repaint them. The government encouraged the Ninety-Nines and other civic groups, such as the Boy Scouts, to repaint the markers until they allotted more money. The government never did pay up, but States continued to install markers. Even into the mid-fifties, Ohio made plans to mark more cities. [73-75]

Schimmoler's Leghorn chicken business continued to flourish. She supplied the luxurious Pennsylvania Dining Car system with choice eggs. [76] Having a pilot's license and a nearby airport opened new opportunities. She decided to deliver chickens by plane. On 16 May 1932, she prepared to deliver her first air shipment for her Bucyrus Hatchery—a large order of Barred Rock chicks to Mrs. O.C. Busch, eighty-five miles away in McClure, Ohio.

She swaddled the chicks in red flannel and tucked them at her heels, hoping the strong wind and altitude wouldn't affect the sensitive birds. Periodically a chick would stick its head out to investigate. She had to bend down while still piloting and re-tuck them. She landed her plane in a large pasture near the Busch's home, the chicks chirping in good health. [77-78]

Schimmoler's Port Bucyrus lease she'd signed before the city bought it, expired on 14 April 1932. The City Council had previously indicated they planned to lease it to her, and she had said she planned to submit a bid when they offered it. But she didn't. The city warned if they received no bids within one week, they would padlock the airport doors and nail boards across the windows to prevent entrance or its destruction. They had not yet decided the fate of the buildings and grounds. [79-80]

To prevent the Port from being padlocked, a group of businessmen organized to discuss the options. "Names of the leaders in the movement have been withheld for the present," the local newspaper stated. The week for submitting bids expired. No one, including Schimmoler, submitted a proposal.

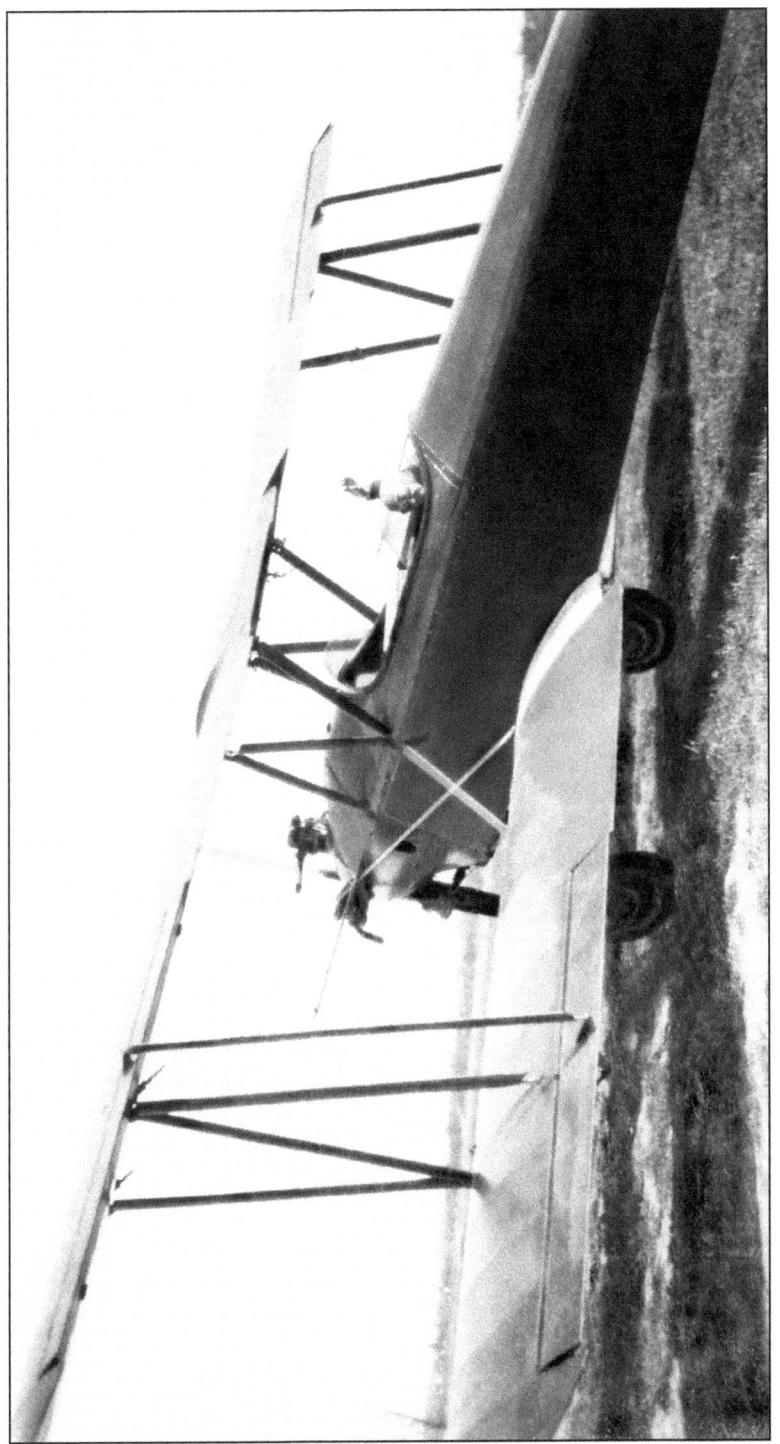

Figure 01.15. Schimmoler waving from the helm of her Waco 90 biplane she used to deliver the chicks, c. 1930s. BHS.

Chapter One

> Port Bucyrus closed its doors on Saturday, 20 April 1932. They locked the hangar, and a city official took possession of the keys. [81]

The council hoped to re-advertise and extend the bidding period. In the interim, they'd allow summer planting of potatoes in part of the airport's acreage. "Enough ground will be left, however, for landing purposes." [82] Oddly, the newspapers did not mention Schimmoler when writing about this unfortunate event. Previously they had named her in all articles about the Port. Mayor Schuler continued his same financial cries:

> The Port should be leased for no less than five hundred dollars at approximately eight dollars per acre. The present lessee pays seven dollars an acre. [83]

The present lessee was, of course, Schimmoler. While the newspaper didn't state why she had not submitted a bid, the increase in cost could have been a factor. Was she attempting a stand-off? Indeed. She knew few others would submit a bid—everyone had expected her to continue to manage the Port. Was she making other plans? One local newspaper said Schimmoler was considering an offer from Delaware Flying Field. [84]

The news quickly reached Fred L. Smith, State Director of Aeronautics. He arrived at Bucyrus the following Wednesday for a conference with the Mayor. Smith offered Mayor Schuler any state assistance aside from financial. The Mayor assured him financial was the only aid the airport needed. [85]

The city allowed Schimmoler to keep her plane and other equipment in the hangar for one more week. Bucyrus Institute of Aviation closed its doors. Pilots could still land on the field, but the buildings were locked. Mayor Schuler said the city did not have funds for operating an airport. The newly-organized Bucyrus Aero Club called a meeting, asking all interested persons to attend. [86]

Two days later, the City Council again advertised for leasing bids but refused to re-open the airport. Prosecutor J. D. Sears served as a spokesman for the Bucyrus Aero Club. He told the city council that as "servants of the people," they should follow the mandate. They should appoint any manager and open the airport as it "served as a refuge for pilots during a storm." [87]

Sears assured the council someone would submit a bid that would at least cover the Port's operating expenses. The city had received enough advertisement from the Port to warrant the expenditure. F.L. Hopley from the group said a prolonged closure would harm Bucyrus. The former Mayor, E.F. Songer, also spoke on behalf of the Bucyrus Aero Club.

On 22 April, City Solicitor C. F. Schaber prepared a short supplemental lease. Schimmoler signed it, and Port Bucyrus re-opened.[88] At least until 1 June. Schimmoler submitted a bid for $510.00 on 28 May. The board accepted, and she signed a one-year lease starting on 2 June.[89] Schimmoler began her first official lease from the city two years after she had initially leased the land.[90]

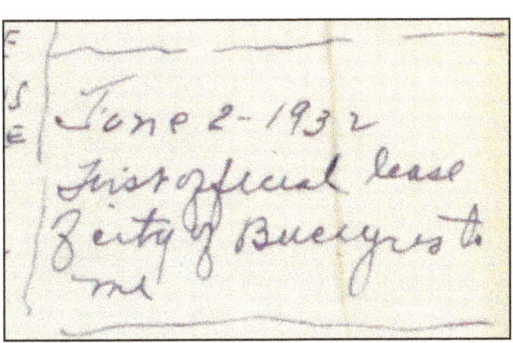

Figure 01.16. Schimmoler's notation, written on the inside cover of her Pilot's Log, about leasing Port Bucyrus: "June 2-1932, First official lease of city of Bucyrus to me." BHS.

She re-opened Bucyrus Aviation Institute. She hired pilot Richard McDougal as a ground instructor and Merle Foltz, a licensed engine and airplane mechanic.[91] Schimmoler told a *Plain Dealer* reporter:

> I get as great a thrill from helping the mechanics overhaul motors as I do at the controls of a speeding plane. I don't mind the grease on my hands and clothes.

"Schimmoler eats, sleeps, and works at aviation. She knows airplanes from engine to empennage," the reporter said. In the early days of flying, pilots needed to be mechanics; qualified repairmen were few and far between.[92-93]

Schimmoler met with her good friend Amelia Earhart while preparing for the National Air Races in Cleveland, scheduled for 27 August – 7 September. She needed to arrange sleeping quarters for female pilots from the Ninety-Nines and the Betsey Ross Flying Corps at the Westlake Hotel. Many Ninety-Nine pilots were members of both organizations.[94-95]

Two newspaper clippings in Schimmoler's archive state she belonged to the Betsey Ross Flying Corps.[96] But it contained no ephemera, no mention of her membership, or any activities with the group. Fellow Ninety-Niner pilot, Opal Kunz, had formed the Betsey Ross Flying Corps in 1931 as a semi-military unit to support the Army Air Corps and to assist in national emergencies such as floods, earthquakes, and other disasters.[97]

Chapter One

Schimmoler continued to promote the Port. She flew to Akron in June 1932 to discuss their upcoming Glider Meet.[98] On 7 August 1932, she hosted Ohio's first Glider Meet. Around 4,500 people attended from different areas and out of state. Four gliders participated in the events for precision landings and flight duration. Three gliders from Camp Perry, a National Guard training facility on Lake Erie in northern Ohio, attended and demonstrated formations and military maneuvers under the guidance of State Director of Aeronautics, Captain Fred L. Smith.[99]

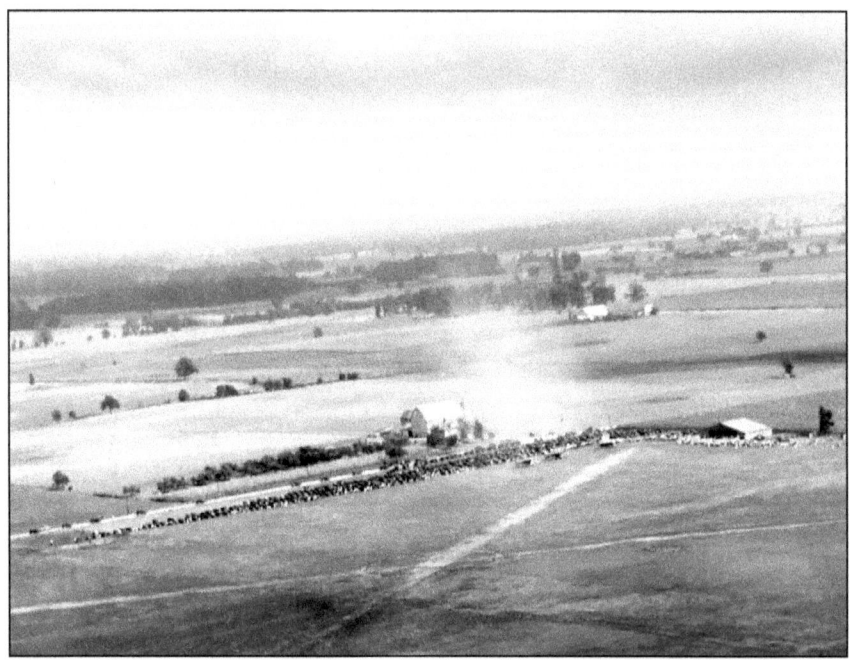

Figure 01.17. Ohio's first glider meet at Port Bucyrus 7 August 1932. BHS.

Pilots from the University of Michigan and Crestline won top honors. Akron pilots Bill Bodenlos, Dick Randolph, Pratt Jones, and Joseph Funk participated. A Goodyear Zeppelin Company pilot/researcher, Dr. Wolfgang Klemperer, demonstrated a car towing a plane for its take-off. Mr. Marshall, a University of Michigan pilot, won the endurance contest with a flight of two and one-half minutes in a glider designed and constructed by mechanical engineering professor R.E. Franklin. He and his brother Wallace Franklin had begun producing their gliders in 1928 before any domestic manufacturers existed.[100]

During the spot landing contest, most pilots overshot the goal by 100 feet. Gretchen Reighart of Crestline looked destined to win; she made the required turns but stopped within twenty-three feet of the goal. The only remaining contestant, Mr. Bullock of Crestline, landed seven feet from the finish line. Jerry Westling ended the program with a rousing parachute jump from 2,500 feet. [101-102]

In August 1932, Universal Flyers sent a tri-motor Ford plane to Mansfield Airport. Schimmoler cruised over Mansfield with the famous aviator Ray Loomis who had stayed in the vicinity after attending the Glider Meet in Bucyrus. A graduate of the U.S. aviation schools at Brooks and Kelly Fields in San Antonio, Texas, Loomis had gained fame, having established an unsurpassed record for his ability and safety in the air. He carried more than 250,000 airplane passengers, without accident, for eleven years—more than any other airman. [103]

After the flight, Schimmoler told Loomis she admired flyers Frances Harrell Marsalis and Louise Thaden, who had recently broken the women's endurance record over Long Island in their "Flying Boudoir," a nickname given by the press for cosmetics the pilots used on board. They kept their aircraft aloft for eight days, four hours, and five minutes in 1932. They refueled mid-air by having a fueling plane drop a gas hose. Marsalis and Thaden took turns operating the gas nozzle while they hung on to the wing.

Outdoor Girl Cosmetics sponsored a supply plane that lowered food into a basket for the flyers—they perched on the wing, held on with one hand, and caught the basket with the other. [104] Schimmoler said about the flight:

> Although they are my friends, and I rejoice with them in their successful aerial adventure, my secret ambition has long been to attempt an endurance flight. Someday I hope to do it. [105]

Schimmoler met Earhart and other pilots at the 1932 Cleveland National Air Races. She encouraged them to attend the second annual Bucyrus Air Show in September. [106] Port Bucyrus was fortunate to have Salesman Schimmoler.

The headliners for the air show included Frances Marsalis, without Thaden, in the "Flying Boudoir." Marsalis barnstormed and raced. She traveled the popular air show circuits demonstrating "The Spin of Death," an act she developed that thrilled the crowds. [107]

Viola Gentry, a celebrity female aviator, also attended the meet. In 1928 Gentry set the first non-refueling record for women when she flew eight hours, six minutes, and thirty-seven seconds straight. In 1924, she became the first woman in North Carolina to receive a government-issued pilot's license. The press dubbed Gentry "The Flying Cashier" because of her day job in a New York restaurant. [108-109]

Chapter One

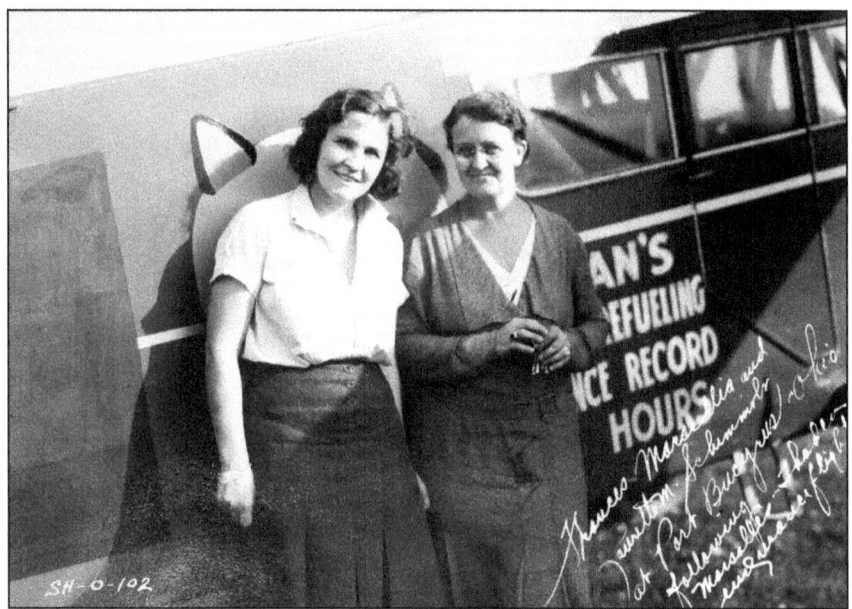

Figure 01.18. Frances Marsalis, left, and her "Flying Boudoir" airplane, (the Thrush J NC9142, I.J. Fox prototype) with Lauretta Schimmoler, right, at the Port Bucyrus Second Air Meet, 11 September 1932. BHS.

The American Glider Pilot Champion, Jack O'Mara, arrived in his Chanute Glider. Also attending was J.E. Herndon of Kansas, the second-place winner at the recent National Air Races in Cleveland. Other participants included Calvin Johnson of the Curtis-Wright Air Corporation, Walter Carr, and Glen Shomate. Fred Smith, the State Director of Aeronautics, and Howard Rough, the Department of Commerce Supervising Inspector, had permitted participants to fly below the regulation of 500 feet but not less than 300 feet. Parachute jumps closed the program on both days. Mr. W.B. White of the Curtiss-Wright Aerial Exhibition Company in Long Island managed the Bucyrus event. [110-111]

Because of the successes of the air meets, the flying school, and the multiple business contracts, the State Director of Aeronautics for Ohio named Port Bucyrus the best and busiest small airport in Ohio for the year 1932.[112] The Port now consumed all Schimmoler's time and its management forced her to give up her eleven-year hatchery business as the airport duties kept her too busy. "It was," Schimmoler said, "this lovely job which I gave up for flying. I don't regret it."[113]

On 2 November 1929, twenty-six women gathered at Curtis Field in New York to establish a female pilots' organization to coordinate the interests of women in aviation. They named the new club the Ninety-Nines, chosen to represent the number of original charter members. They elected Amelia Earhart as the President and Louise Thaden as the Secretary. [114] Although not a charter member, Schimmoler joined the Ninety-Nines in 1932 and became active in the group. That year the members elected her as the second Secretary-Treasurer (a combined title) and later as the first stand-alone-title of Treasurer. She held the office until 1934.

When Schimmoler joined the Ninety-Nines, the Cleveland area didn't have a chapter, so she helped organize one. The group elected her in 1932, by unanimous vote, to Governor of the North Central Section—the largest group of 99s pilots, which included women in Ohio, Wisconsin, Michigan, Indiana, Illinois, and Kansas. [115-116]

Later that year, Schimmoler started a movement to establish the Ninety-Nines National Headquarters at Cleveland Municipal Airport. She had criticized the lack of facilities for female pilots at Cleveland Airport and demanded a presence there. [117]

Airport officials quickly met her demands. In November, she inaugurated the first quarters for members of the Ninety-Nines at Cleveland Airport, located in the United States Airline hangar. Schimmoler established the Woman's Division charter service and flying school, at Vi-Air-Ways, as Vice President of the Women's Division. [118]

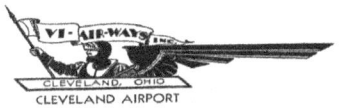

Figure 01.19. The announcement for the Women's Division opening, at Vi-Air-Ways, Inc., at the Cleveland Airport, and Schimmoler's appointment in 1932. BHS.

CLEVELAND AIRPORT

We are pleased to announce the opening of a
WOMEN'S DIVISION
under the supervision of
MISS LAURETTA M. SCHIMMOLER

Miss Schimmoler having had many years of experience qualifies her for this position. Miss Schimmoler is the first woman in the U. S. to operate a commercial airport, having promoted, supervised the building, and managed Port Bucyrus.

The NINETY-NINE CLUB, a national organization of Women Pilots, will make their headquarters in our offices. Amelia Earhart is president of the Ninety-Nine Club, and Lauretta Schimmoler is secretary-treasurer.

VI-AIR-WAYS offers to all Women Pilots and women interested in aviation very desirable and comfortable quarters on the second floor of the United States Air Lines Hangar.

It is our sincere desire to give to women the opportunity they have not had in the past.

We cordially invite you to visit our offices and lounge, and to make them your headquarters when at the Cleveland Airport.

VI-AIR-WAYS, INC.

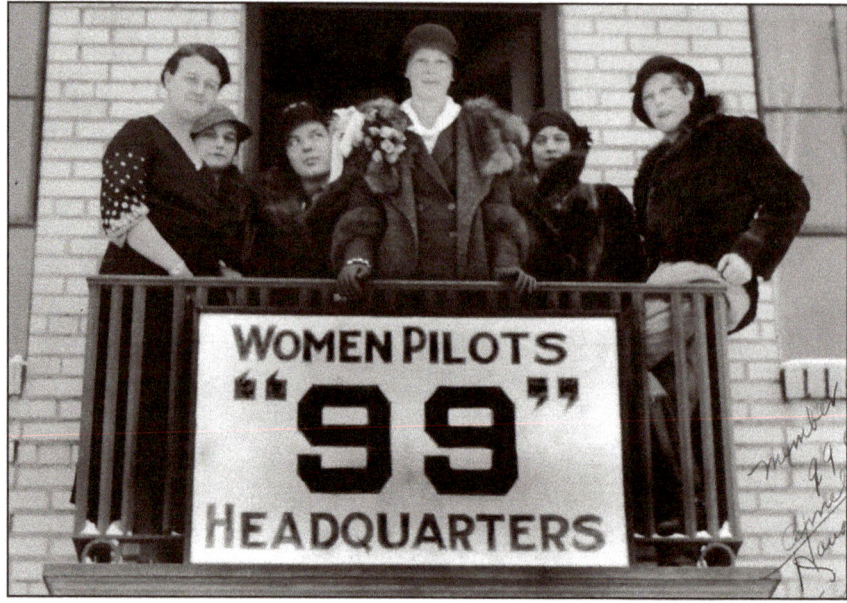

Figure 01.20. Ninety-Nine club members at its headquarters on the balcony outside of the Vi-Air-Ways' offices. Lauretta Schimmoler, left, Amelia Earhart, center, 11 December 1932. Schimmoler's handwritten note on the lower right corner states: "Member of the 99 Club met Amelia Earhart. Hanging of the first 99 Emblem on any airport in the U.S., United States Airlines Hangar. Cleveland winter of 1932." BHS.

Figure 01.21. Schimmoler's 99s membership pin, an interlocking 99 design, complete with a rotating propeller, c. 1939. Author photographed at BHS.

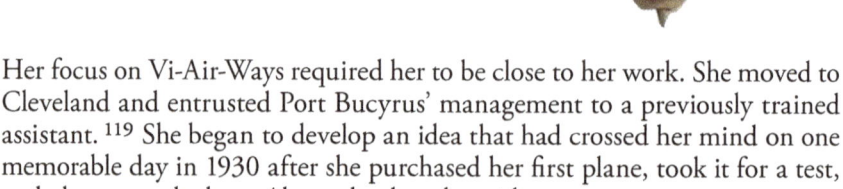

Her focus on Vi-Air-Ways required her to be close to her work. She moved to Cleveland and entrusted Port Bucyrus' management to a previously trained assistant.[119] She began to develop an idea that had crossed her mind on one memorable day in 1930 after she purchased her first plane, took it for a test, and almost cracked-up. About the day, she said:

> After taking off, I circled over Lorain taking a last look at the remaining scars left by the tornado, then headed my plane toward Akron. While cruising along, my thoughts wandered back to the hectic hours and days that followed the tornado…

buildings off their foundations, trees uprooted, debris blocking streets… destruction in all directions, making it difficult for emergency equipment to work.

Being so enthusiastic about flying, it occurred to me, 'Gee! If nurses had been trained in aviation, they could have flown in and rendered aid so much more rapidly.' This was a turning point in my career.

Up to now, my plans had been to develop an airport at home and operate a flying school. This inspiration struck me so forcefully that I decided I would complete my original plans and then devote my time and efforts to training nurses for aviation. I believed that through educational methods, I could expel the fear of flying that generally existed. [120]

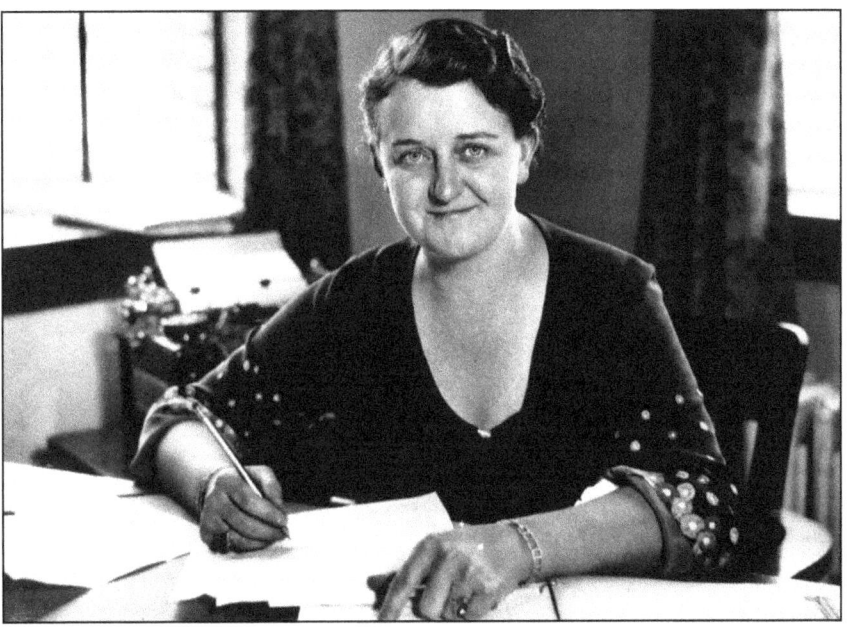

Figure 01.22. Schimmoler at her desk in Vi-Air-Ways, Cleveland Airport, 11 December 1932. BHS Collection.

She had successfully developed an airport and flying school; now, she could focus on her ultimate plan—Aerial Nurses. In December 1932, she coined a name for them: the Emergency Flight Corps. [121]

She wrote to the Army Nursing Service, "If I were to interest nurses and train them for air duty, would I be rendering my country a service?" The reply stated

Chapter One

in part, "I don't think nurses will ever need to fly, and if they do, they will fly in government airplanes and won't need any special training." [122]

Schimmoler knew about airplanes but was quite naive in her knowledge of the professional nursing organizations—both military and non-military. Nursing had a lengthy history as a closed group; they did not accept new ideas from non-nurses. And the military surrounded itself with a deeper level of protection. It's surprising anyone even took the time to answer her inquiries on the issue. The reply didn't dissuade her. Perhaps her naiveté on this issue served her well because if she had known, she might have realized the near-impossible task she had chosen.

In January 1933, she met with a group of nurses in Cleveland to discuss her idea of Aerial Nurses and air ambulances. She said, "The response that followed left no doubt about the ultimate success of the plan." She charged them to develop the idea. [123]

The more she thought about the plan, the more she realized she lacked knowledge about the technical problems; she could not intelligently discuss the concepts with various officials she would need to meet. She decided to learn more before starting. [124]

Schimmoler's mother died on 31 March 1933. Her two-year lease for Port Bucyrus would end in June. She must have stayed in Cleveland, at least through July, because when she attended the first National Meeting of the Ninety-Nines on 3 July 1933, in Santa Monica, California, she listed her residence as Cleveland. [125]

The Ninety-Nines' meeting coincided with the National Air Races, 1-4 July, at Mines Field in Los Angeles. The 99's float traveled from the downtown City Hall to the Municipal Airport. Their float—an airplane mounted high above a trailer that carried pilot Edna Crumrine—won first prize. Dressed in white flying togs, women pilots followed in six automobiles. Thousands of spectators cheered along the entire parade route. [126]

Schimmoler said her mother's recent death, and conversations at the national races with several Ninety-Nines pilots, spurred her decision to pack up her idea and move to California. She would start the Aerial Nurse plan in Los Angeles, not Cleveland. Her manuscript simply stated: "Later, in 1933, I went to the west coast." She immersed herself in the various air meets Southern California offered while preparing to launch the Aerial Nurse Corps of America. [127]

She probably sold her planes before she moved to Los Angeles; her 1935 re-application to the Ninety-Nines states she only owned a partial interest in a

Kinner Fleet. But the Ohio skies had taught her well: on the application, she listed she'd flown 210 miles in the following airplanes (the manufacturers' designation is noted after the dash). [128-129]

Swallow TP–Swallow TP	Swallow Axelson–Swallow HA
OX5 Bird–Bird	Kinner Bird–Bird BK
OX Waco–Waco Te	Kinner Waco–Waco Kinner
Waco 90–Waco 90	Waco F–Waco F
Waco C–Waco C	Arrow Sport–Arrow Sport
OX5-Bird–Bird A	Challenger Robin–Challenger Robin
Great Lakes–Great Lake	Kinner New Standard–Kinner Standard
Waco Cabin–Waco Cabin	Warner Monocoupe—Monocoupe Warner
Stinson S–Stinson S	Lambert Monocoupe—Monocoupe 90
Bull-Pup–Bull Pup	Lycoming Stinson–Lycoming Engines
NB-8–NB-8	Aeronca C–Aeronca C
Davis–Davis	Leblond Davis–Davis D1-L
	Ford Tri-Motor–Ford Tri-Motor

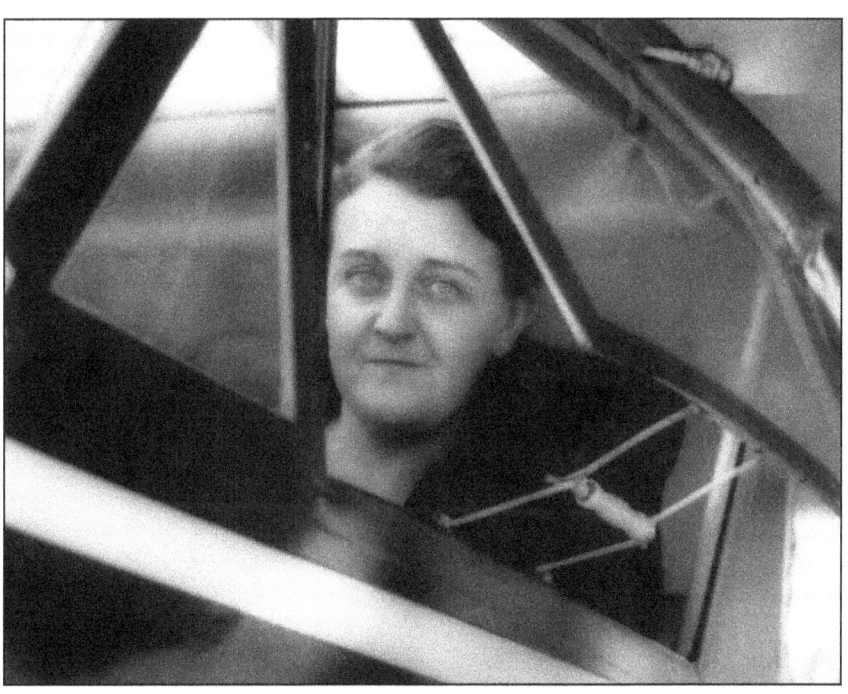

Figure 01.23. "In my monocoupe one wintry day in Cleveland," 1932.

Chapter One

By August 1933, she was living in Los Angeles, was the Ninety-Nines' Secretary-Treasurer, and had joined the Southwestern Chapter. Los Angeles was a solid choice of residence for aviators. California, and particularly Los Angeles, was well known for aviation activities. Ruth Elder, the 1929 Powder Puff Derby fourth-place finisher and a Ninety-Nines charter member, said Los Angeles was "the aviation center of America." 130-132

Races flew from Los Angeles to Cleveland: they hosted the National Air Races in 1928, 1933, and 1936. Poncho Barnes, the first female stunt pilot, lived there. Earhart, and many other well-known pilots, lived in Los Angeles or moved there later. Southern California's temperate climate made it ideal for year-round flying. Schimmoler settled in the Glendale area and began to formulate her Aerial Nurse plan.

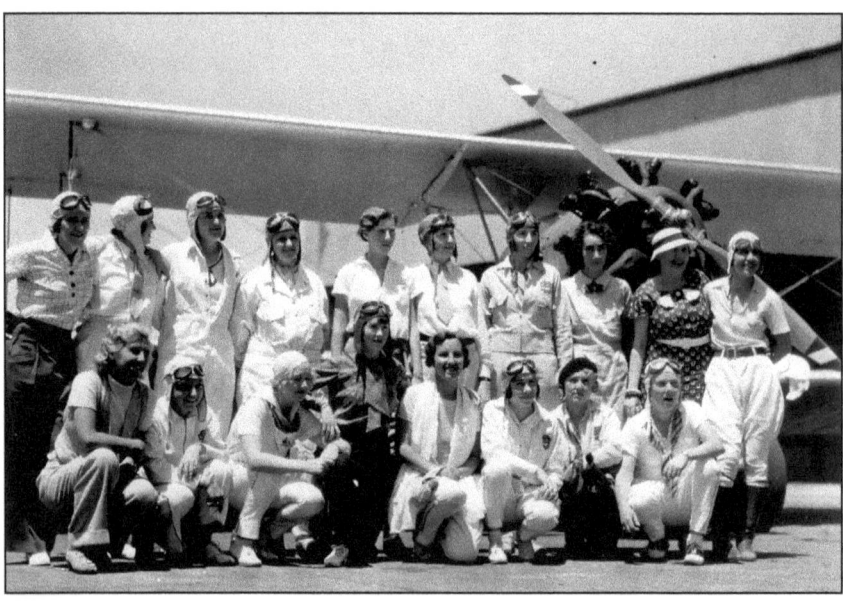

Figure 01.24. Kern County Air Meet, Bakersfield, California, 6 May 1934. Members of the 99 Club. Standing, left to right: Janet Knight, Elliot Roberts, Gladys O'Donnell, Lauretta Schimmoler, Kay Case, Pansey Bowen, Dorothy Kinsman, Clema Granger, Esther Johnson, Peggy Gauslin. Kneeling: Henrietta Lantz, Hilda Jarmuth, Esther Jones, Ardette Caldwalder, Edna Crumrine, Melba Beard, Ethel Sheehey, and Kay Van Doozer. BSH Collection.

She'd already realized her first required step: to intelligently discuss her air ambulance plan with various officials. She also needed employment to pay the bills. She hearkened back to her stenography skills and obtained a position with the Army Air Corps Mail Operations, Route 4, at the Union Air Terminal in Burbank, as Secretary to General Ira C. Esker.

The military headed this postal division as the Army Air Corps had recently begun to deliver all air mail. She was pleased to have a job, but she had no idea this stenography position would put her in the middle of one the biggest scandals of that time.[133]

The 1930 McNary-Watres Air Mail Act gave President Hover's postmaster general, Walter Brown, authority to consolidate mail routes in the public's best interest. Brown awarded contracts to only three air transport companies and forced out smaller competitors that had previously been delivering the air mail. These exclusive contracts created a scandal called the Spoils Conferences. Some of the contracted air transport companies filed legal actions to no avail. When President Roosevelt took office in 1933, he appointed a committee to investigate Brown's contract awards.[134]

Roosevelt canceled all of Brown's domestic contracts on 19 February 1934. He asked the Chief of the Army Air Corps, Major General Benjamin Foulois, if the Army could deliver all of the air mail. Foulois thought they could. The Army brass hoped delivering mail would promote the importance of the Army Air Corps during peacetime. Foulois had ten days to prepare.

He directed aircraft to be equipped with directional gyros, artificial horizons, and radios—even though he knew they didn't have enough for all the planes. They incorrectly installed some flight instrumentation. Regardless of the equipment shortages, the Army Air Corps Mail Operations (AACMO) began to deliver the mail.

The Army Air Corps had said it would use its best pilots with the most experience in night-time flying. That did not happen. More than half of the 260 pilots assigned were Reserve Junior Officers with less than two years of flying experience and fewer hours of experience flying at night or during inclement weather.

Airmail pilots flew mostly at night with extreme turbulence, snowstorms, and in fog. These young men wanted to prove to the Army Air Corps they could do the job, so they often cleared themselves for a flight. No system of checks and balances.[135]

The Air Corps pilots took the oath as postal employees but struggled to implement operations. Even before delivery began, three pilots died on test flights: ten pilots died during a million flight miles. Sixty-six crashes occurred. The unreliable radios had a short-range capability—too short. The lack of funds, the shortage of spare parts, and a winter of "the worst and most prolonged history of bad flying weather in many years," created AACMO's ultimate failure.

President Roosevelt halted the AACMO's delivery service 11 March 1934, less than a month after it had begun. He restored service contracts to the air transport companies by 1 June 1934. On 12 June 1934, Congress nullified the 1930 law and passed a new air mail act.

They enacted punitive measures against the executives who had conspired at the Spoils Conferences. The Air Corps moved on to focus its attention on improving its organization, equipment, and training.[136]

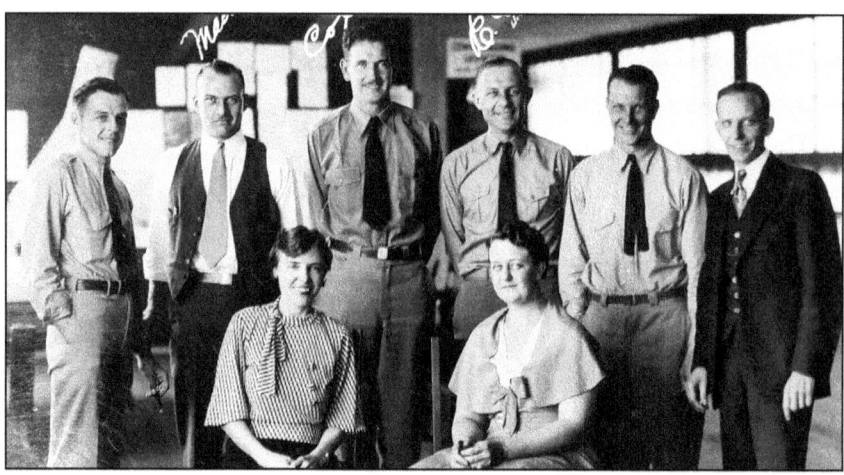

Figure 01.25. Civilian and Military office personnel who worked on U.S. Army Air Mail Operations, A.M. Route 4, at United Airport. Schimmoler is sitting at the right, 1934. Her note on the photograph says, "General Ira C. Eaker was our Commanding Officer." BHS Collection.

Schimmoler had unwittingly participated in this historical fiasco, and when AACMO disbanded, she lost her stenographer position. Her boss, General Ira C. Eaker, gave her a glowing letter of recommendation. He said:

> I am not unaware of the fact that you worked long hours beyond those your hours of employment specified and that you did this because there was work to be done and because you had a high sense of duty and loyalty to the project. You proved efficient, thorough, alert, and quick to learn new work and showed initiative of the highest order.
>
> If the Army is again faced with a similar responsibility, it can have no better luck than to find you available for similar duty. I personally would ask for you if you were at all available and any similar undertaking, or one requiring personnel, should ever arise again.[137]

In 1935 Schimmoler joined the Woman's Air Reserve (WAR) to organize their first aid facilities.[138] Pilot Poncho Barnes started the organization in 1931 with the idea that pilots would fly doctors and nurses to earthquakes, floods, and other disaster areas to render medical assistance.

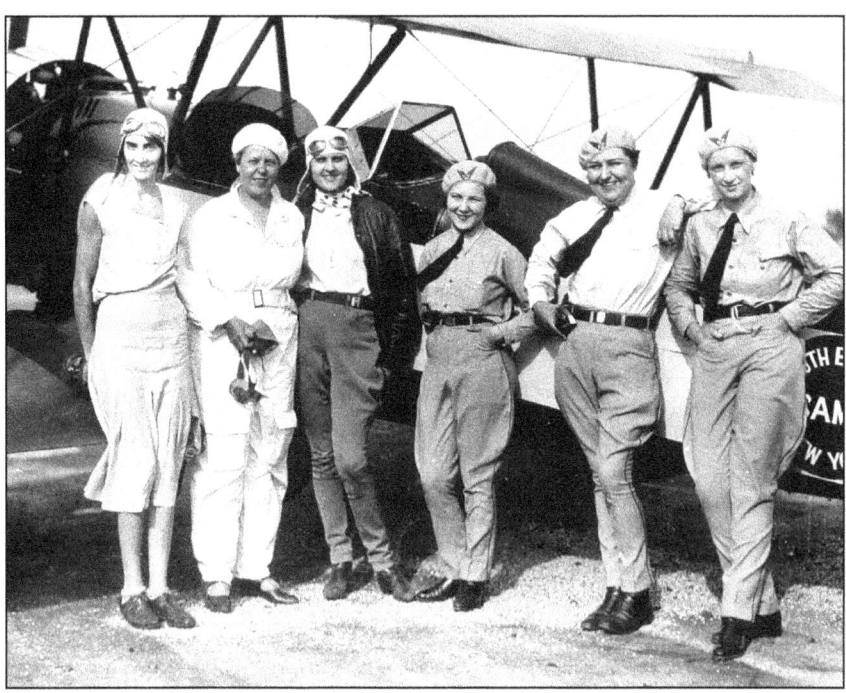

Figure 01.26. Clema Granger, Mary Charles, Gladys O'Donnell, Ruth Elder, Pancho Barnes, and an unnamed flyer, with Ruth Elder's plane, at the 1933 National Air Races in Cleveland, The three women at the right, with Barnes in the middle, wear the Women's Air Reserve uniforms. BHS Collection.

This concept sounds similar to Schimmoler's idea of the Aerial Nurse Corps except she didn't include volunteer doctors in her Corps. Perhaps she applied WAR experiences to developing the Aerial Nurse Corps. Although she didn't mention it, her organizational knowledge of WAR's first aid facilities would be a logical expression.

WAR might not have fulfilled all of Barnes' good intentions. The group lacks many documented activities. The year 1935 holds their most recorded tasks: staged practice disasters, guests-of-honor attendances at a few events in their showy military-styled uniforms, and staffing first aid tents at an occasional air show or airport opening. Military-styled uniforms and staffing first aid tents at air shows would become the hallmark of the Aerial Nurse Corps of America.[139-141]

Chapter One

With her business skills and references, she obtained a more secure position at Lockheed Aircraft Corporation in accounts payable. Now she could pay her bills and develop her ultimate plan for the nurse-staffed air ambulances.

She continued her membership in the Los Angeles aviation community. Schimmoler had a reputation as a dedicated worker. She arranged meetings and dinners. Because of her various business and advertising experience, the Ninety-Nines quickly appointed her as the advertising committee chairman of the Southwest Division, including the areas in Arizona, California, Nevada, and Utah. The Southwest Chapter rented the clubrooms at the Clark Hotel on South Street in downtown Los Angeles; her nearby location in Glendale made her involvement easier. [142-143]

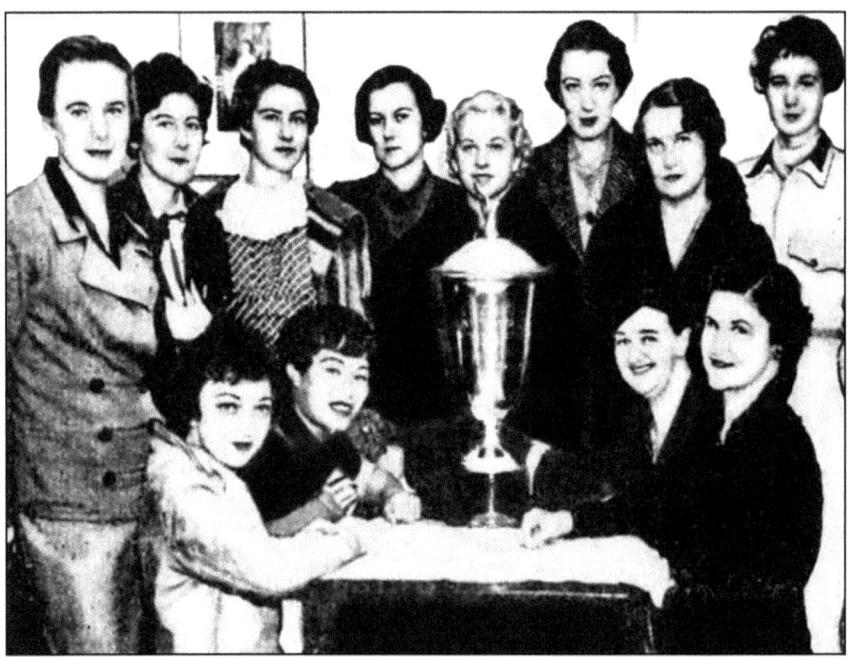

Figure 01.27. Flyers in the California Pacific International Exposition Race at National Air Aviation Week, 1935. Standing: Kay Van Doozer, Peggy Gauslin, Evelyn Hudson, Yolanda Spirito, La Verne Wolfram, Onita Thorley, Betty Furman, Cecile Hamilton. Sitting: Hilda Jarmuth, Katherine Cheung, Lauretta Schimmoler and Grace Prescott. The winner, Bessie Owen, is not pictured in this pre-race photo. BHS Collection.

Schimmoler continued to enter local flying races. The San Diego Chamber of Commerce sponsored the California Pacific International Exposition efficiency race during the 1935 National Air Aviation Week. Schimmoler entered the October 20th race, which started at the Grand Central Air

Terminal in Glendale and ended at Lindberg Field in San Diego. The race wasn't a speed dash but one of precision flying: they gave pilots a specific compass course and altitude they were required to follow.

Before the race began, each entrant stated their ground speed. Officials calculated the time each pilot would need for the race. They charged a pilot with errors, measured in minutes, if she veered off the course or failed to maintain the stated speed and required altitude. Santa Barbara flyer, Bessie Owen, won with an error rate of only seven and one-half seconds. Grace Prescott of San Diego came in second with forty-five seconds, and Cecile Hamilton of Los Angeles at third with fifty-nine seconds of error. [144-145]

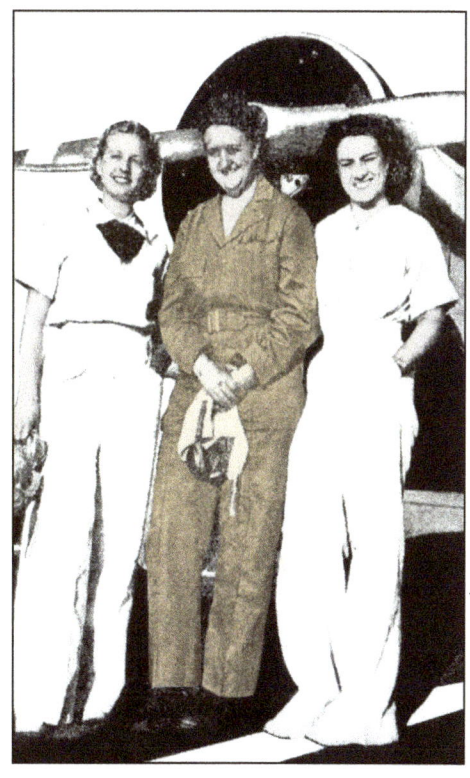

Figure 01.28. LaVerne Wolfram, Lauretta Shimmoler, and Evelyn Hudson after the Grand Central Air Terminal Air Show, 5 July 1936. Colorized clipping, BHS.

On 5 July 1936, Schimmoler flew in formation with fliers LaVerne Wolfram and Evelyn Hudson at the Grand Central Air Terminal during a two-day air show. Hudson had recently moved to Los Angeles from Hawaii, where she had become the first woman granted a private pilot's license in that state. [146]

Ten thousand people attended the show, which included bomb dropping with sacks of flour. Stunt flier Tex Rankin ended with an inverted power dive from a 2,000-foot altitude, straightening out his plane within a few feet of the ground. [147]

Schimmoler never said she worked on the Spitz Flight Recorder, but this photo states, "personnel working on the Spitz Flight Recorder at Union Air Terminal." She might have worked there briefly or just visited.

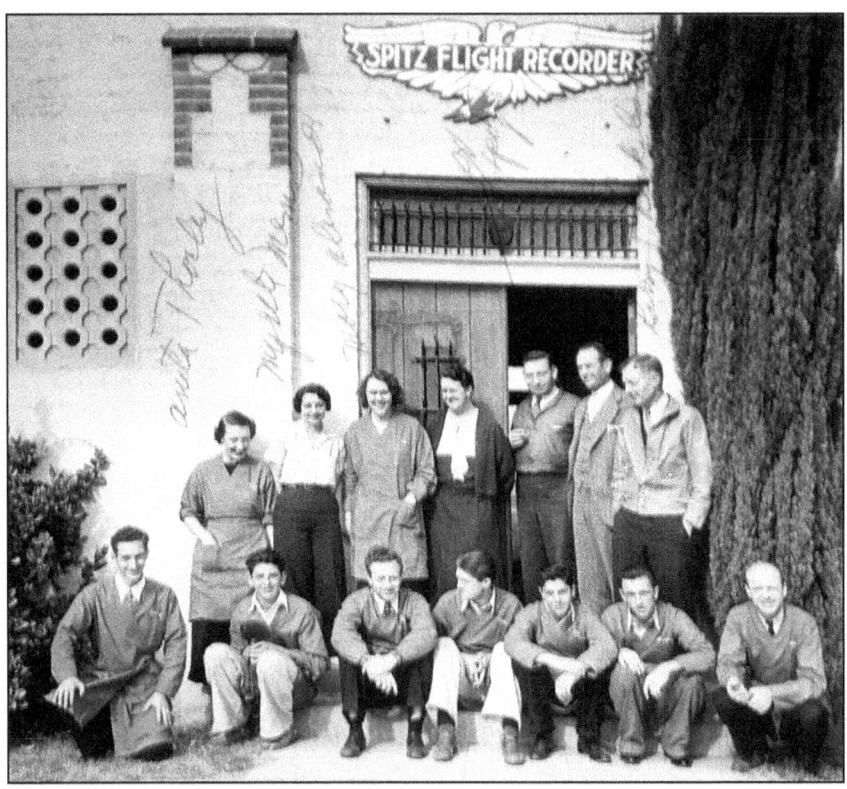

Figure 01.29. Personnel working on the Spitz Flight Recorder at the Union Air Terminal, 2 February 1935. Schimmoler stands in the middle. BHS.

Dr. Samuel Spitz of Los Angeles invented the Spitz Flight Recorder in 1935, often called the "mirror in the sky." Actuated by short-wave radio impulses, a small light moved across a strip of map of the plane's route to trace its movements. Two microphones installed on the aircraft picked up the sound of the propellers through the plane's radio transmitter. The sound allowed the Spitz to determine if the plane had landed safely or, if not, to help locate a downed plane—finally, a solution to a long-lamented problem.[148]

While working at Lockheed, she took advantage to learn everything she could about aircraft construction and manufacturing. She left Lockheed for a three-month "special assignment" with the U.S. Weather Bureau in 1936.[149] Schimmoler left no clues about her resignation from Lockheed. What new grand plans had she formulated to begin now?

She asked for and received a letter of recommendation from Fred Smith, Director of Aeronautics in Columbus, Ohio, in June 1936. He said, "Port Bucyrus has finally found an active operator to manage the airfield…Things have been very quiet since you left." He wished her luck that she would get the position she wanted, but didn't mention the type of position she had applied for. [150] She might have changed her mind about the job because she doesn't list any employers on her resume between the years 1936 to 1943.

Still pursuing various flying interests, Schimmoler joined the fraternity Alpha Eta Rho (AHP). The founders organized the International Aviation Fraternity at the University of Southern California campus on 10 April 1929. [151] The AHP Greek letters translate to the word "air."

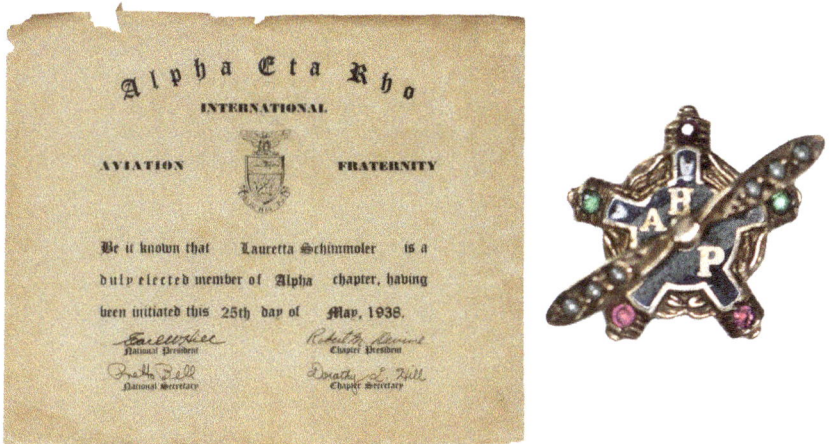

Figures 01.30. and 01.31. Schimmoler's Alpha Eta Rho certificate and pin.

Schimmoler had integrated herself into the fascinating life of a flyer in Los Angeles. But she put her piloting on a back burner to accomplish the most unusual and historically significant years of her life. This achievement would come to fruition in the coming months.

Chapter Two
Aerial Nurse Corps of America (ANCOA)

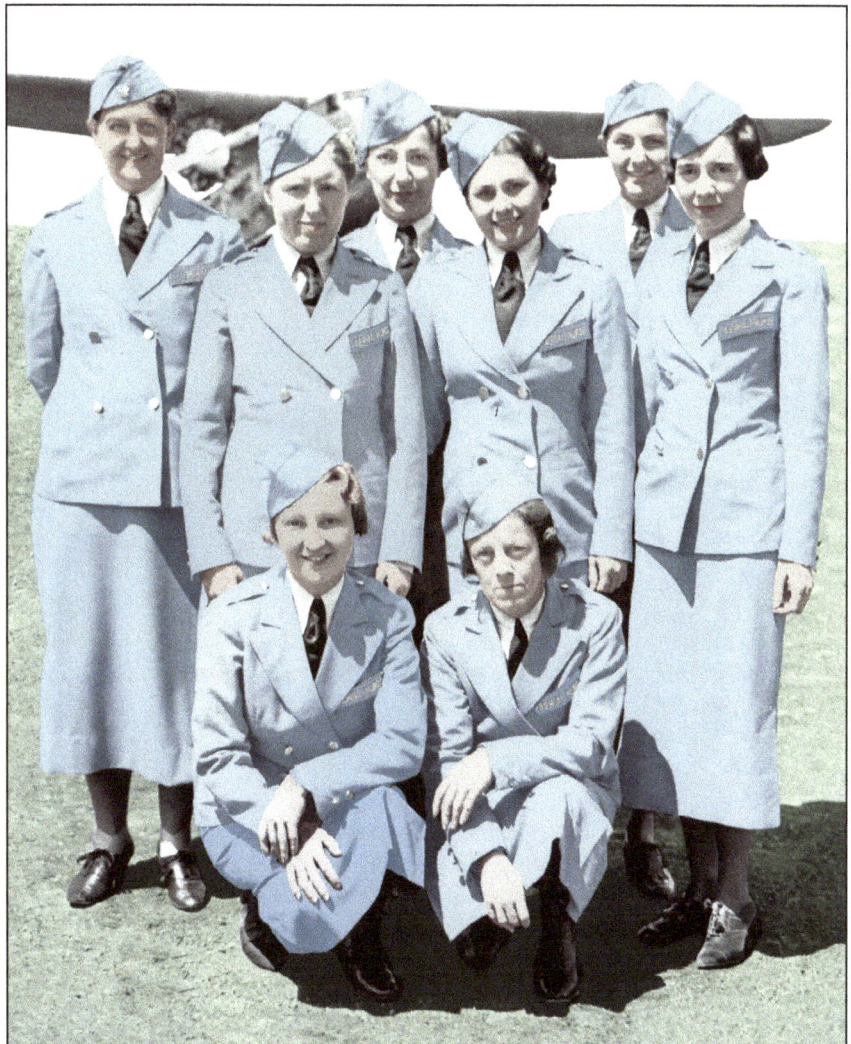

Figure 02. 01. The first official photo of the ANCOA on duty at the National Air Races in Los Angeles, their inaugural post, 4 September 1936. BHS.

Seven of the original ten nurses and Lauretta Schimmoler on the first official day of the ANCOA. Kneeling, left to right, Cecelia Getsfred, Edna Yarnell. Second row: Velma Cook, Rose Marie Cumming, Edwardine Malone. Third row: Lauretta Schimmoler, Emma Koenig, and Ora Brook.

Chapter Two

Schimmoler understood airport management and flight school operations. She'd learned about aircraft manufacturing at Lockheed and gained additional learning at the U.S. Weather Bureau. She possessed enough knowledge to discuss technical aspects of an air ambulance program with the officials she would encounter. She was ready.

Schimmoler hoped to improve the problems concerning the early days of air ambulance flights. Transport was crude. The pilot often functioned as both nurse and pilot with no one to attend the patient during the flight. The plane's low ceiling and small interiors weren't designed for patient transport.

The pilot usually propped up a stretcher, suspended it over the seats, or placed it on the floor. No safety belt secured the patient, so Schimmoler designed one. For the Aerial Nurse Corps air ambulances, Schimmoler invented a stretcher that would fit better through the narrow doorways and inside the small planes. Now she needed to find and train qualified nurses.

Although no U.S. organization had trained nurses to accompany patients on planes, commercial airlines employed nurses to assist passengers on their flights. In 1929 Ellen Church, a registered nurse who later joined the ANCOA, convinced the Traffic Manager at Boeing Air Transport of the value of nurses' skills in the air.

The slow air speeds and low altitudes of early air flights made the ride bumpy. Passengers often became airsick. Nurses understood sick people. Boeing successfully implemented Church's idea in 1930, and soon the other airlines followed the trend. [1]

Schimmoler's records do not say the impetus for her first move or if anyone helped her begin. An article in *Pilot* magazine said an association with the McLaglen Air Corps led, in part, to the ANCOA's beginning. A *99 News Letter* said the ANCOA belonged to Victor McLaglen's Division. [2]

Whatever the kick-start, in August 1936, Schimmoler selected ten registered nurses from Los Angeles County whom she viewed as sincere and dedicated. She changed the name from the original Emergency Flight Corps to the Aerial Nurse Corps of America.

The Hollywood Uniform Company in Los Angeles manufactured their blue military-styled uniforms. Nurses wore the uniform in their first photograph but didn't have the official cap pins, badges, or patches. They donned an embroidered tag with Aerial Nurse. Schimmoler's said Pilot. She also wore an oak leaf pin on her cap, like the Army used for the rank of Lieutenant Colonel or Major. Initially, she used the rank of Major. Later they would call her the Colonel.

She secured a choice first assignment: the field hospitals at the 1936 National Air Races in Los Angeles, 4-7 September. Although she would later write regulation manuals and design patches and pins, she must have hurried to train the initial group. She had less than a month to prepare.

The race was a perfect beginning for Schimmoler—she'd attended several National Air Races and helped Pancho Barnes' WAR group set up their first aid stations. She knew what to expect. She presumed people would see the value and appreciate what she and the nurses were trying to create to benefit the public: a new specialty called the Aerial Nurse.

The National Aeronautics Association had given a five-year option to Hopkins Airport in Cleveland for the National Air Races, but Hopkins was under construction in 1936 and couldn't host the meet. [3] The races moved to the Municipal Airport at Mines Field in Los Angeles, the current Los Angeles International Airport site.

The *Los Angeles Times* began to hype the race weeks before the date, with good reason: the event promised to be spectacular. Most airplanes in the 1930s flew 70-200 miles per hour; Roscoe Turner, who held many speed records, was developing the largest radial engine with the power to fly more than 355 miles per hour. The previous year, multimillionaire Howard Hughes had set the world and transcontinental speed records of 352 mph in a one-off plane the H-1 Racer. Hughes groomed his planes and constructed at least six new flying bullets with in-line engines for the Los Angeles meet.

Officials built a mile-long grandstand to seat 60,000 spectators and a $14,000 security fence around the airport ($307,304 in 2023 inflation dollars). [4] Two hundred fifteen security and police officers camped at the airport in thirty-four tents. Twelve trucks provided transportation for 200 military police. [5] The Hollywood Chamber of Commerce planned a gala luncheon for aerial celebrities at the Hollywood Roosevelt Hotel. [6]

Milo Burcham—a dare-devil acrobatic flyer who had just returned to Los Angeles from a European exhibition tour—was among the many expected flyers. He held the world record for inverted flight. [7]

Foreign flyers and racers would compete with the best American pilots. Peggie Salaman stopped in from England before flying to Cleveland to enter the Ruth Chatterton Sportsman Pilots race.

Michel Detroyat from France brought two of his fastest Caudron-Renault planes for the Thompson and Grieve Trophy and one for the Shell events. [8] Flyers would use new planes and give aerial demonstrations the viewing public had never seen before.

Chapter Two

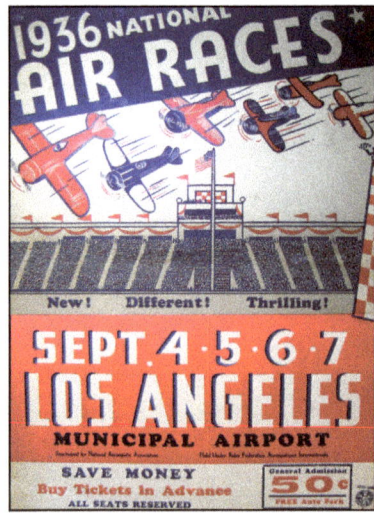 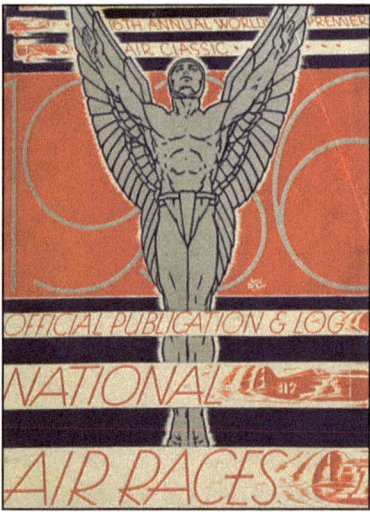

figure 02.02. The official poster and program for the Sixteenth National Air Races, Municipal Airport at Mines Field, Los Angeles, 1936. BHS Collection.

Large prizes drew the best flyers in the world:

1. The Vincent Bendix Trophy. Transcontinental speed dash from New York to Los Angeles. All types of airplanes. Men and women. Total purse: $15,000 ($332,146 in 2023 with inflation).
2. Charles E. Thompson Trophy Race. World's high-speed land plane classic. A distance of 150 miles in fifteen laps over a ten-mile course. Men only. Total purse: $20,000.
3. Louis W. Grieve Race. Planes with not more than 550 cubic inch displacement. Men only. Total purse: $10,000.
4. Three separate Shell Cup races for ships with 375 and 550 cubic inch motors. Men only. Total purse: $12,000.
5. Two separate Ruth Chatterton Trophy for sportsmen pilots races, sponsored by Ruth Chatterton. Men and Women. One from Cleveland to Los Angeles and one from Dallas to Los Angeles. Total purse: $1,000 for each race.
6. The Earhart Trophy, sponsored by Amelia Earhart. Women only. Limited to eight contestants chosen by a committee. A five-lap, twenty-five-mile-long race for ships with 800 cubic-inch motors and a maximum speed of 175 miles per hour. Total purse: $1,500. [9]

Pilots assembled at Floyd Bennet Field, in New York, forty-eight hours before the Vincent Bendix dash began, which would end at Mines Filed on the first day of the race. [10] Thirty flyers left Dallas, headed for Los Angeles, while sixteen Navy planes and twenty-seven Army pilots rehearsed stunts, formation flying, aerial attacks, and defense maneuvers for one of the most remarkable military displays ever seen at a civilian show.

Fourteen pursuit planes from the Third Wing, Boeing P-26A type, planned to arrive from Barksdale Field in Louisiana. Fifteen pilots qualified for the Thompson Trophy Race by proving their ships could fly 225 miles an hour or better.

The social elite mingled with leading military flyers, officers, and other dignitaries at a lavish Army and Navy Ball in the downtown Biltmore Hotel. Hollywood screen actors issued an invitation, printed on an elaborate scroll, encouraging the entire world to attend. W.C. Fields, Gary Cooper, Marlene Dietrich, Bing Crosby, George Burns, Gracie Allen, Claudette Colbert, Fred McMurray, Carole Lombard, Cary Grant, and others signed the scroll. Ten aviation officials from South and Central America scheduled a five-day visit to witness the events. [11-13]

The City Council adopted "a resolution requesting all departments, bureaus, commissions, and divisions of the city government to cooperate in every way to make the National Air Races a memorable and successful event." [14]

On 29 August, the race began in Cleveland when more than 100 male and female sportsmen pilots took off for Los Angeles in an efficiency and navigation competition, the Ruth Chatterton Trophy. [15] Noted women pilots included last year's winner Grace Prescott, Peggy Salaman from England, Canton-born Katherine Sui Fung Sun, Marjory Jane Gage, and twenty-year-old Cecil Hamilton.

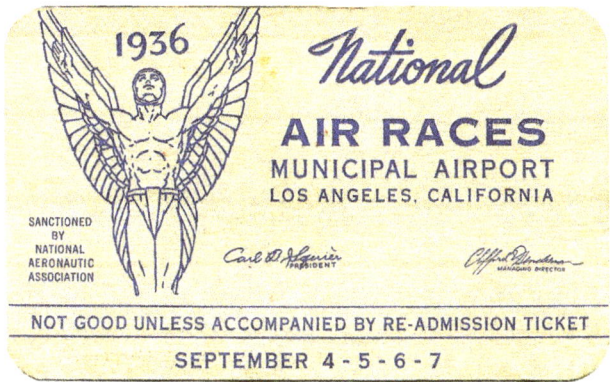

Figure 02.03. The 1936 National Air Race ticket. Made from duralumin—a metal used in racing planes—were sent to 1,000 members of the Early Birdmen Club of America, veterans who had flown together thirty years ago and planned to re-unite at the Writers Club banquet. [16] BHS Collection.

Other women included the Flying Secretary Evelyn Hudson of Glendale, the Flying Hostess Marjorie Page, A.C. Anderson from Phoenix, Adrienne and Edith Clark, Edna Gardner from New Orleans, and Genevieve Moore Savage from Coronado Island. The race's sponsor, Ruth Chatterton, flew as co-pilot with her pilot Bob Blair and led the group as the pathfinder. [17]

> The Aerial Nurse Corps of America could not have chosen a grander entrance for their inaugural post— this was the largest and most spectacular aerial event the city of Los Angeles had ever witnessed.

For the first time, women outnumbered the men in a speed dash for the Bendix Trophy: Amelia Earhart, Laura Ingalls from Long Island, Louise Thaden from Arkansas, and Marie Bowman from Burbank vs three men.

Although 1936 still had financial remnants of the Great Depression, this was the golden age of flight, and when the planes came out, people came out too. The new and exciting idea of flight enamored them.

The Junior Chamber of Commerce's inaugural parade encompassed thirty miles starting at City Hall and proceeding through Hollywood, Beverly Hills, Hawthorne, Inglewood, and the airport. Captain Eddie Rickenbacker, an American war ace, served as parade marshal. Thirty floats represented towns from San Diego to Santa Barbara.

The U.S. Army Air Corps, the U.S. Naval Air Force, and the U.S. Marine Corps staged combat flight maneuvers downtown. [18] After the demonstration, the aerial squadrons circled the parade line to the Municipal Airport at Mines Field. Seven bands followed the parade under the direction of J.T. Boudreau. KFAC described the march to its radio listeners as it passed their studios at 10:45. KFWB and KECA set up broadcasting areas at Mines Field. [19] Today, it's inconceivable to imagine a parade with thirty floats of celebrity pilots traveling from downtown to the Los Angeles Airport while low-flying military planes maneuver overhead.

The race officials declared the opening day as American Youth Day and gave 25,000 children free tickets to attend the races. At Mines Field, the bands sounded taps as a triple salvo of aerial bombs called for the lowering of colors at the start of day one. Ruth Chatterton, stage, film, television actress, novelist, and aviator, opened the show. [20-21]

Schimmoler must have felt the height of pride this day. She'd been thinking, planning, and learning the methods to begin this organization for seven years. Imagine her mixed emotions of delight and apprehension.

The attending dignitaries and thrilling events made this race unique, but the winning results created its historic nature. Some past races had allowed women to compete with men. But after Florence Klingensmith fatally crashed her Gee Bee Y during the 1933 Frank Phillips Trophy Race in Chicago, Bendix banned women from his race and required them to compete in separate women-only races.

Klingensmith had entered the race first. As she reached the grandstands, fabric loosened from the fuselage and fouled the engine. Instead of parachuting she veered off to avoid hitting the grandstands. The plane nose-dived at 350 feet. She tried to bail out, but it was too late; they found her parachute tangled in the fuselage. She died rather than kill the spectators.

> When male pilots died, officials would claim them victims of an accident. When female pilots died, they labeled them as incompetent.

Despite knowing she crashed from equipment failure, race officials and newspapers used her death against all female pilots. And they ignored her bravery. Her crash was the reason women were excluded from the 1934 Bendix Race. Earhart protested the decision by refusing to fly the actress Mary Pickford to Cleveland to open that year's races. Eventually, people realized that women's times and speeds were equal to men's. After pressure from female pilots, Bendix allowed women into the 1935 race. [22]

Louise Thaden's radio died almost immediately upon leaving New York; her co-pilot, Blanch Noyes, could not check ground speed or position. They would need to navigate the entire continent by dead-reckoning (estimates based on a previously known position). They'd borrowed a stock Beech C17R Staggerwing biplane, which had the back seat removed to install an extra 56-gallon gas tank and an extra 12-gallon oil tank in the luggage compartment. They were competing against twin-engine planes specifically designed for racing.

They stopped for fuel once in Wichita. They doubted they could finish before the 6:00 p.m. deadline because of the headwinds and turbulent storms. But they pushed on. During their descent, the glare of the Los Angeles sun, combined with a smoky haze from recent forest fires, blinded their forward view. They had to look backward over the tail to determine their position. When they landed at 5:10, they realized they had flown over the finish line in the wrong direction. Usually, they would stop in front of the grandstands, but they figured others had landed long before them; spectators would not care. They decided to proceed to the farthest area of the field, as unobtrusively as possible, toward a group of parked planes. As they taxied, a group of men followed them shouting and waving their arms.

"I wonder what we have done wrong now," Thaden asked Noyes. When they parked the plane, the men told them they'd won the race. "I won't believe it until the contest committee tells me," Thaden said. They'd flown the route in 14 hours, 54 minutes, and 46 seconds. Race officials had set aside $2,500 for the first woman to finish, never thinking a woman could win. And according to Thaden, Vincent Bendix looked a bit disappointed that two women had won. But they had. They took the $7,000 first-place prize plus the $2,500 as the first women to finish. Later Thaden learned the plane she'd piloted had 1,200 hours of flight time—practically a grandfather.[23]

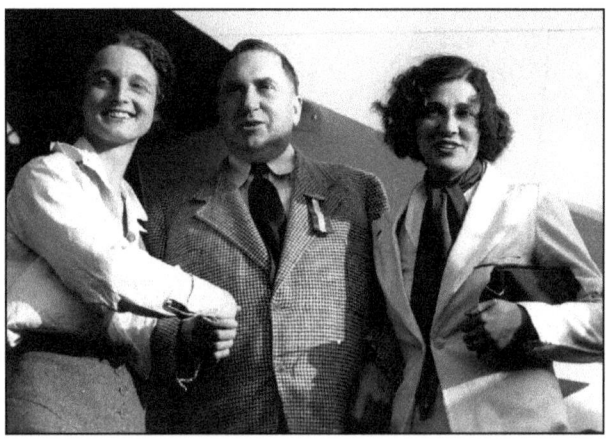

Figure 02.04. Vincent Bendix greets Louise Thaden, left, and Blanche Noyes after the race in Los Angeles, 4 September 1936. Bendix Corporation.

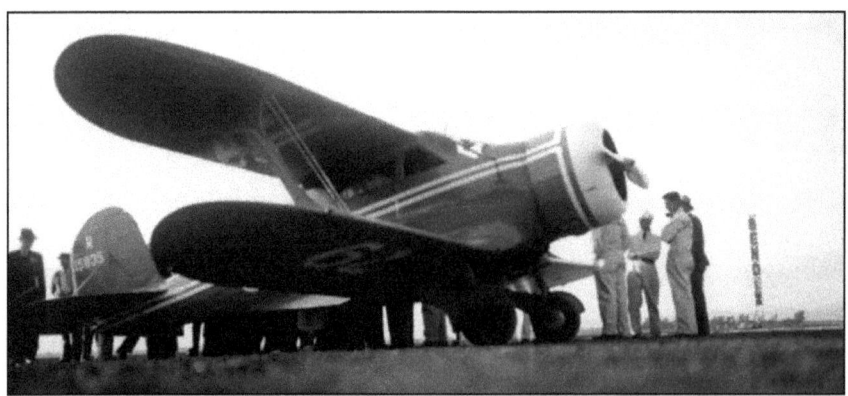

Figure 02.05. Their Beechcraft C17R-NC15385 at the end of the race in Los Angeles. Bendix Corporation photo.

Laura Ingalls crossed the finish line 45 minutes later in her Lockheed Orion and won second place. Amelia Earhart and Helen Richey finished fifth. Officials had to rethink the idea that women could not compete with men. [24]

Several Bendix racers crashed en route. Joe Jacobson parachuted to safety when his plane exploded over Kansas. He boarded a TWA and arrived in Los Angeles in time to compete in other races. Roscoe Turner crashed his plane over New Mexico. Benny and Maxine Howard's propeller accident resulted in a life-threatening crash that totaled their plane. Benny lost a leg. [25-26]

A pilot crashed to avoid a film camera truck that rolled onto the runway. Rudy Kling was landing immediately behind the crashed pilot when a car and a group of spectators headed onto the runway toward them. Kling tried to avoid them and hit the guide wire. He demolished his plane and the car. Neither pilot nor the driver was seriously injured. [27]

During the Shell Trophy race, veteran Oshkosh flyer S. J. Whitman gunned his homemade plane around the center tower. His motor died, and he plunged toward the ground. He maneuvered a dead-stick landing at 100 miles per hour but struck the antenna of an Army Northrop plane parked at the east end of the field.

They rushed him to the field hospital and treated him for severe facial lacerations—undoubtedly assisted by the waiting nurses. The ANCOA provided personnel for two field hospitals at the event. In four days, they delivered first aid to 220 persons. [28-29]

Most injuries were minor, but the ANCOA had trained to stabilize pilots with serious injuries. Some of the non-pilot injuries reported at field hospitals were: aged man requests oil for his glass eye, a man falls off a horse while patrolling the airport boundary, a dog-bite on a man's lip, and a woman's hand crushed in a car door. [30]

In the "Acrobatic Trio with Smoke," Hollywood stunt pilots Paul Mantz, Frank Clarke, and Easton Noble thrilled the crowd with loops, spins, rolls, power dives, and falling maneuvers. Other stunts included inverted flying, various tricks, and skywriting. While riding a motorcycle, Don Stevens jumped aboard a glider being pulled by an automobile. Faye Lucille Cox performed her famous delayed parachute jump from 10,000 feet. [31]

The "Star Spangled Banner" and aerial bombs opened the second day. A "March of Air Progress" parade of American planes filled the sky. Sixty service ships appeared on the eastern horizon. Seventeen attack groups burst into the air with flames spurting from their tailpipes. Betty Browning won the Earhart Speed Trophy at 157 miles per hour. [32]

Chapter Two

Despite the fog that threatened the final-day activities, the Labor Day crowd of 70,000 watched as French flyer, Lieutenant Michel Detroyat, broke the world speed record at 301 miles per hour and won the Thompson Trophy race. A massive fireworks display rocked the field midday. [33]

The Navy Grummans and eighteen new Northrop fighters staged a mock aerial dogfight. The Army squadron displayed a wing-to-wing snake dance designed to confuse attacking planes and antiaircraft. A Marine Corps detachment of eighteen Vought Corsairs initiated a power dive at a small yellow marker in the center of the field and blasted it with smoke bombs. [34]

The final day ended with a Mass Parachute Jumping Contest dedicated to the civic production of "Everyman"—the classic tale of the power of beliefs and the fear of death. The Texas Fire Chief Band played the finale.

At the close, pilots started a new fad: collecting autographs of fellow pilots and friends on their leather helmets. [35]

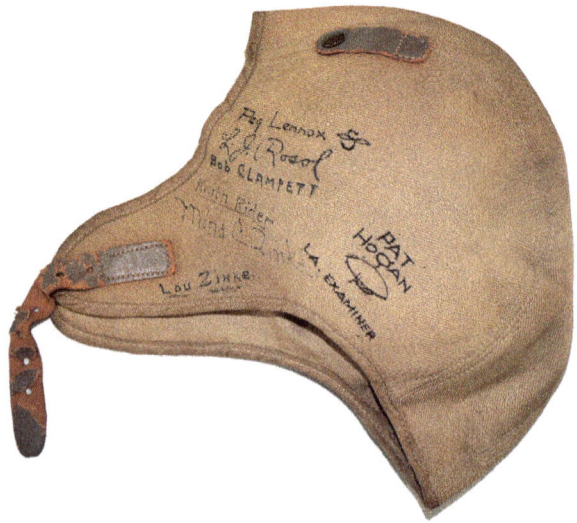

Figure 02.06. Schimmoler's leather race day helmet, with various autographs she collected, 1936. Author photographed at BHS.

Schimmoler had recruited thirty-three nurses for company A by the end of 1936. Twelve group members visited Schimmoler's movie-star friend, Victor McLaglen, on the set of his movie *Wee Willie Winkie* with the ultra famous child star Shirley Temple. McLaglen's business relationship with Schimmoler isn't known, but a Ninety-Nines newsletter briefly mentioned his association with the start of the Los Angeles ANCOA; research could not confirm the exact association.

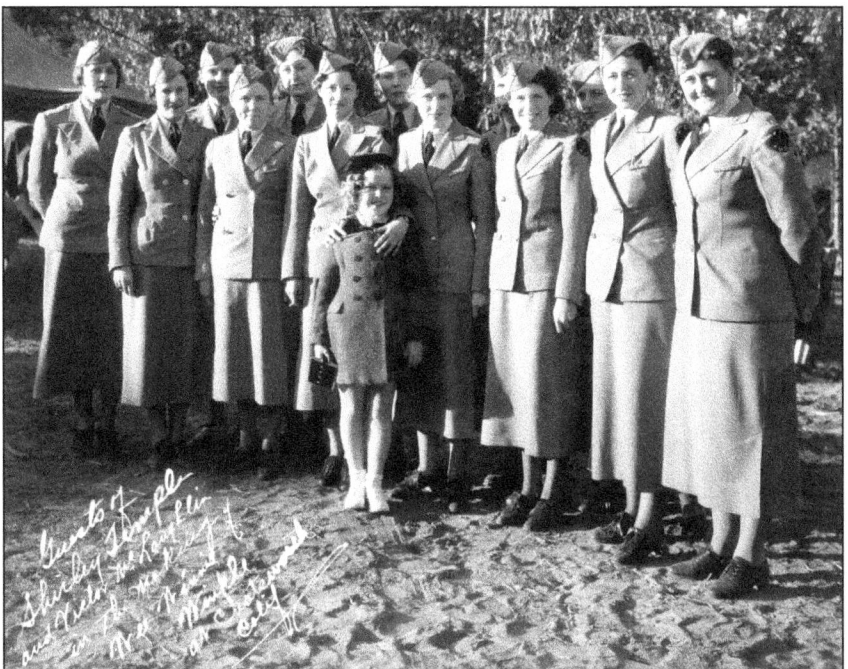

Figure 02.07. Twelve ANCOA nurses, Schimmoler, and Shirley Temple, 1936. The writing on the photo says, "Guests of Shirley Temple and Victor McLaglen in the making of *Wee Willie Winkie* at Chatsworth, California." BHS Collection.

The nurses and Schimmoler wear the Lafayette Esquadrille Blue uniform and garrison-style cap.[36] These caps have the embroidered words McLaglen and Medical (the complete wording is unreadable). They have added a circular arm patch, which became the official patch.

Several nurses have an additional crown-style patch set above the arm patch with an unreadable title. The unusual crown patch and McLaglen cap embroidery are not seen again in photographs, so this early McLaglen association must have changed. The name badges are the same style worn at the National Air Races. They still have no cap pins. Schimmoler continues to wear the oak leaf, but the group's style is moving forward. The official ANCOA uniform is taking shape.

The year 1937 proved busy for Schimmoler and the first ANCOA Company. The number of participants increased to 78. She split the geographic area and added two more Los Angeles County companies to the 1st Division: Company B in Pasadena and C in Santa Monica. By August 1937, they wore a pin on the forward section of the left curtain of the garrison cap.

Chapter Two

One of the nurses created a first aid field kit with supplies that contained an oxygen tank, bandages, scissors, tape, sutures, various medications, and wound-cleaning items.

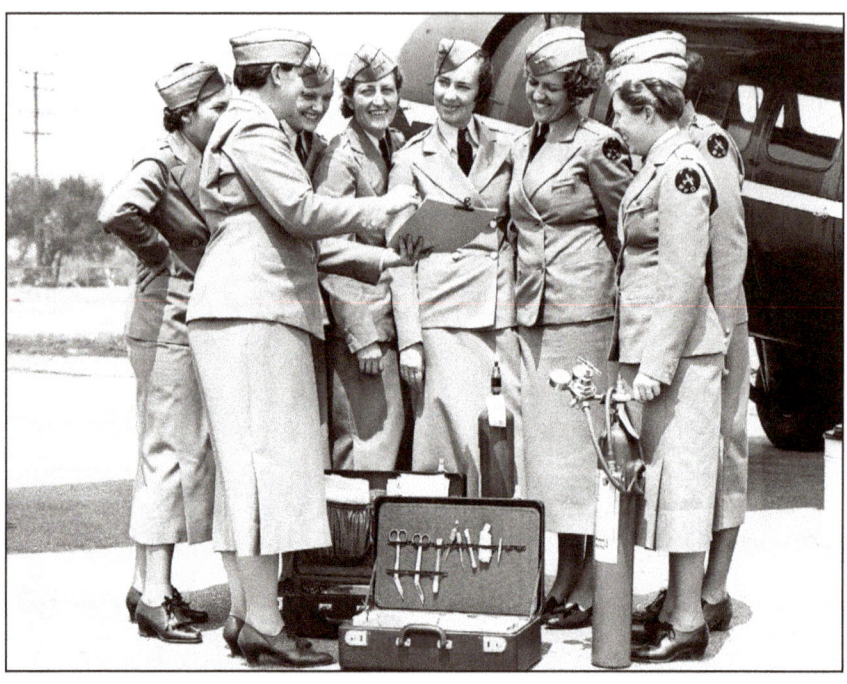

Figure 02.08. Lauretta Schimmoler and ANCOA nurses at United Airport in Burbank, California, display the first aid field kit, 2 August 1937. Left to right, Lauretta Schimmoler, Velma Cook, Jeanne Frederickson, Edith Corns, Shirley Weidman, Oro Brook, Gladys Daniels, and Frances Kurtz. Author's Collection.

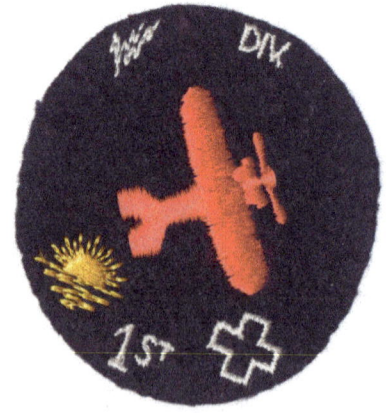

Figure 02.09. Schimmoler's ANCOA arm patch, 1936. An airplane of red cotton-silk embroidered thread facing at two o'clock; a yellow setting sun on an ocean horizon; the number 1st, for the division; and a Greek cross representing service. Above the airplane are lightning bolts to symbolize air communication and the word DIV for division.[37] Author photographed at BHS.

For the ANCOA National Headquarters, Schimmoler chose a three-room house opposite the Union Air Terminal at 2620 North Hollywood Way, Burbank. She leased it from co-owners Paul Mantz and her friend Amelia Earhart.[38] Mantz was a famous Hollywood stunt pilot, President of United Air Service, and the only three-time Bendix Race winner. Earhart, the most celebrated female pilot of all time and the first woman to fly solo across the Atlantic, mysteriously disappeared while attempting to circumnavigate the globe in June 1937.[39]

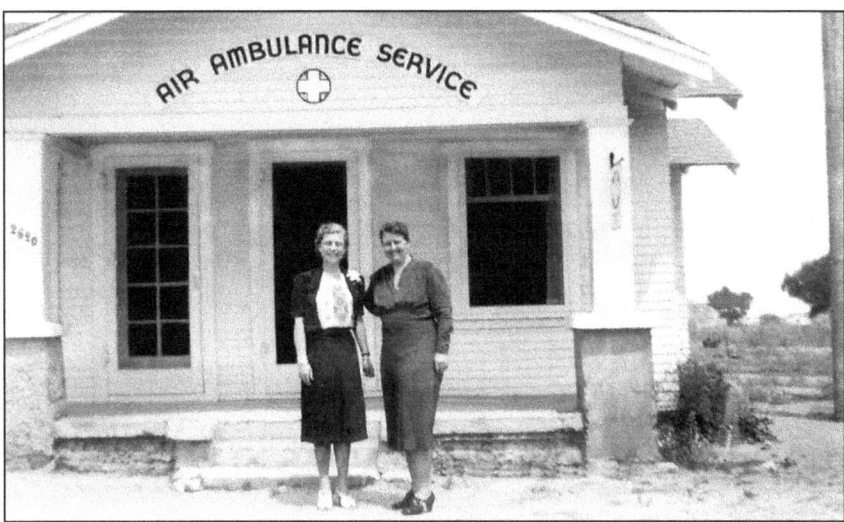

Figure 02.10. Lauretta Schimmoler, right, at the National Headquarters with Wanda Fill, RN. BHS Collection.

Figure 02.11. Lauretta Schimmoler working in the yard at the National Headquarters. MMM Collection.

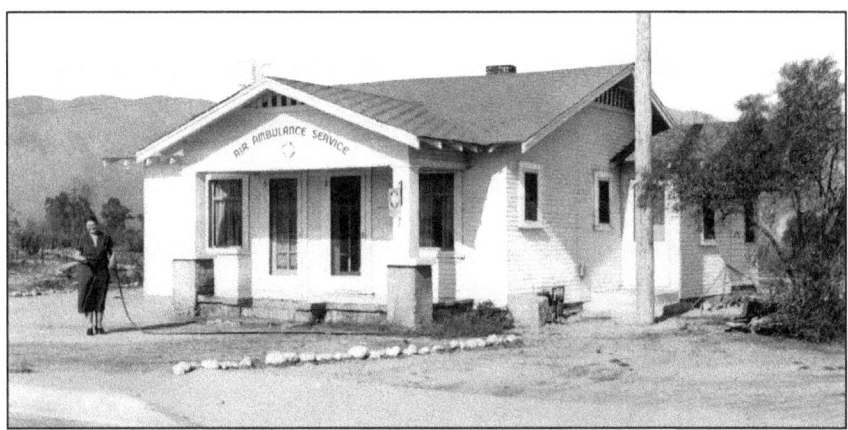

Chapter Two

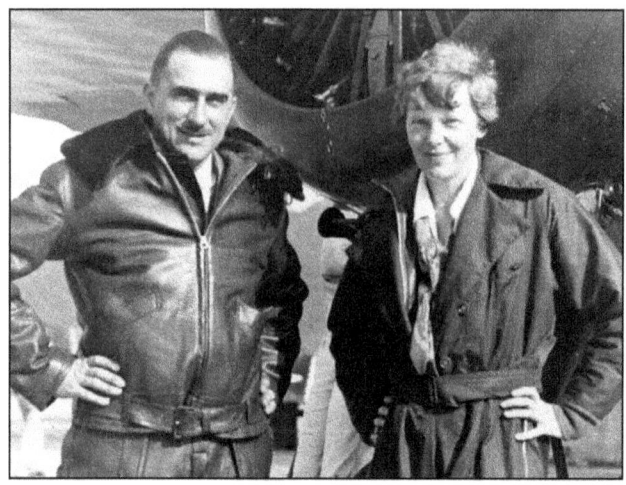

Figure 02.12. Famous aviators Paul Mantz and Emelia Earhart, c. 1936. Co-owners of the ANCOA's National Headquarters building in Burbank. Courtesy of San Diego Aerospace Museum.

Mantz must have thought the idea of an air ambulance sounded promising. On 17 May 1937, he called a meeting at Union Air Terminal to discuss forming the Southern California Aviation Medical Advisory Board. An elite group attended: Mantz; Schimmoler; Earhart; Dr. G.C. Gowan, Department of Commerce inspector; Dr. Isaac Jones, Department of Commerce; Dr. Harlan Shoemaker, intern instructor at General Hospital; Dr. Vincent Askey, secretary of Los Angeles County Medical Association; Dr. Nichol Smith, chief surgeon of Hollywood Hospital; and three other doctors. The board met to plan for emergency air transportation of the sick and injured. [40]

Mantz was Earhart's technical advisor and often her co-pilot. She'd slated him to sit as co-pilot on her first attempt to circumnavigate the globe in March 1937. That flight, however, was canceled. His illustrious career ended in tragedy when he died performing a movie stunt in Arizona in 1965.

Public knowledge of the ANCOA began in 1937. During one trip to Ohio that year, Schimmoler told a reporter:

> Aerial ambulances will soon be a common sight throughout the United States, I believe. Already in California, my staff is called on for one to six trips each week to speed ailing persons to distant cities for medical and surgical treatment, so it is not only in the event of a war that these nurses will come in handy. [41]

Nurses who did not qualify to become an Aerial Nurse, or perhaps did not want to fly, could join as ground crew. Titles included Nurse-Medical Nurse-Radio, First Aid, and General Detail (Dietitians, kitchen, and messengers). They divided the departments into sections: [42]

        Medical   Section 1. Aerial Nurse
                              Section 2. First Aid Unit
                              Section 3. General Provisions
        Radio   Section 4. Communications
        General Detail Section 5. General Provisions [43]

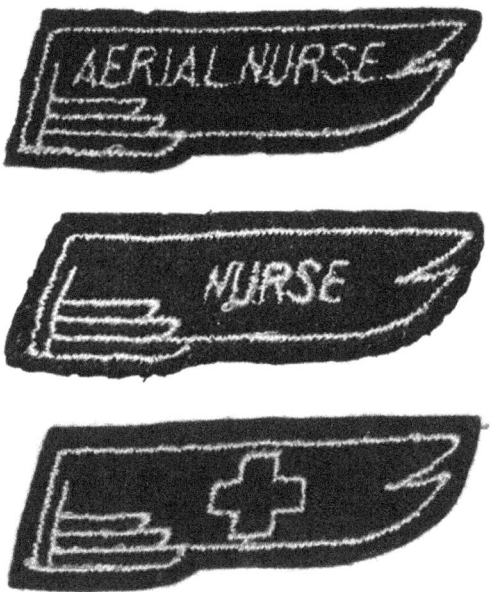

Figure 02.13. ANCOA pocket patches. The Aerial Nurse pocket patch, the Ground Nurse pocket patch, and the First-Aid pocket patch. Later, when the Aviation Emergency Corps began, those members would use the first aid pocket patch. Author photographed.

In early 1938 they developed pocket patches for each group: nurses wore a patch that said nurse, aerial nurse, or a patch with the white Greek Cross for those who worked in first aid. Both the nurses and lay personnel wore the first aid patch. The patch style was inconsistent among nurses—some photos show nurses wearing the first aid pocket patch even though they were well-known as aerial nurses. No patch with General Duty could be located in Schimmoler's archives or photographs.

Chapter Two

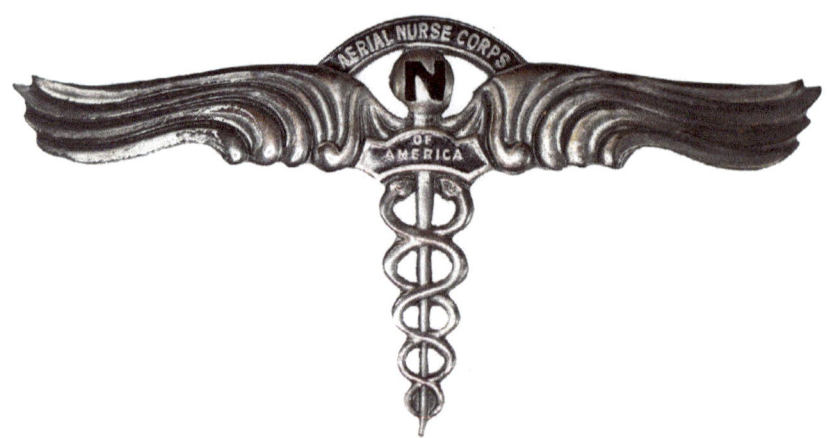

Figure 02.14. Lauretta Schimmoler's ANCOA cap pin. Silver-plated brass with black enamel, 2 ½ inches wide and 1 ½ inches tall, with a drop-in swivel catch. They could wear an identical pin, about 1 inch wide, as a tie tack or dress pin; it was either silver-plated or gold-filled. Author photographed.

The elongated wings designate the departments. AERIAL NURSE CORPS is set on a rainbow above a Hermes wand (the Caduceus). Apollo, the Greek God of medicine and healing, gave Hermes the wand as he was a messenger for the gods. An N for nurse is set on the wand's handle. A small banner with OF AMERICA sits between the wings.

Per the *Regulations Manual*, Commissioned Officers wore rank insignia bars on the left shoulder loop of the coat made from silver or gold metal. The bars are visible in many photographs but are small and difficult to see. Schimmoler didn't wear them; her pin archive did not contain officer rank insignia bars.

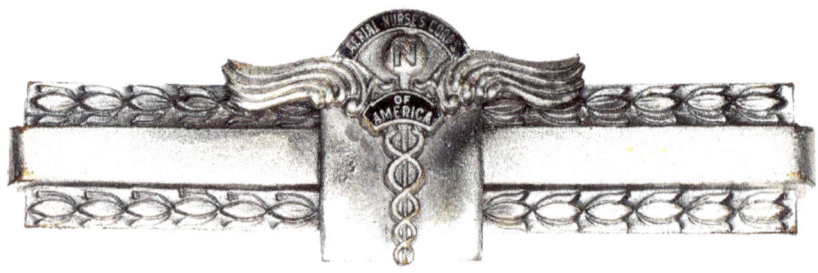

Figure 02.15. Lauretta Schimmoler's scarf pin, 1939. In her archive, this insignia is labeled as a scarf pin. The manual lists parachute scarves as part of the official uniform. The scarf, however, isn't seen in any photographs; perhaps they wore a scarf at special events. Author photographed.

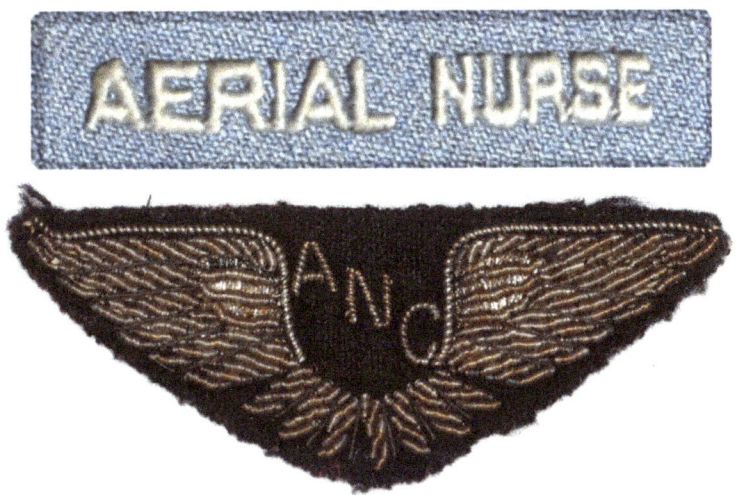

Figure 02.16. They wore a blue embroidered Aerial Nurse badge in their first year, before they created the pocket patch. Schimmoler wore the same embroidered badge but with the word Pilot.

Figure 02.17. Schimmoler's Commander Patch, 1937. Schimmoler created a unique patch for commanders. Oddly, she used only the ANC letters on the commander patch instead of the complete ANCOA. While ANC did fit better inside the wing design, it created scrutiny because the Army Nurse Corps also used ANC on early pins. Author photographed.

Schimmoler returned to the site of the 1937 National Air Races in Cleveland when she flew back home for a stay in Ohio.[44] She visited Bucyrus to attend a party her sister held in her honor.[45] At this point, she'd become a Bucyrus celebrity—the hometown girl had made her mark.

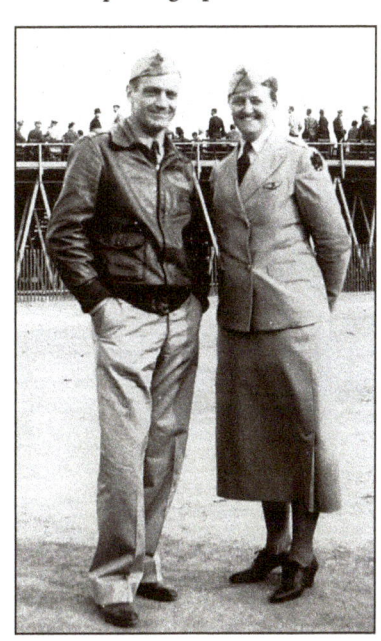

Figure 02.18. Schimmoler with Bill Leisy, an Overseas National Airline's pilot, at the National Air Races in Cleveland September 1937. Schimmoler is wearing the ANCOA commander patch. MMM.

Only Schimmoler would have worn the new ANC Commander Patch in 1937; she did not begin to appoint other nurses as commanders until 1938.

Chapter Two

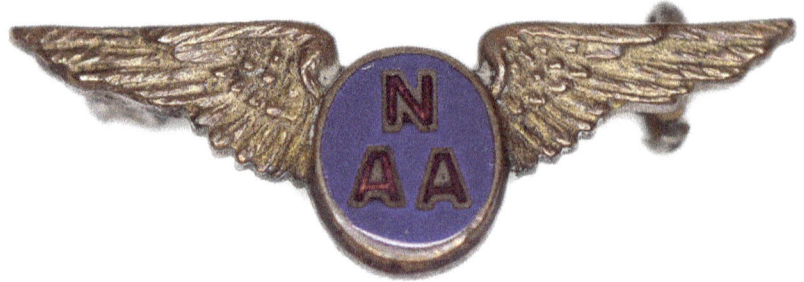

Figure 02.19. Schimmoler's 1931 National Aeronautics Association pin. Most ANCOA nurses used this NAA pin as their tie tack on the summer/indoor uniform. Author photographed.

Although Schimmoler's archive contained an ANCOA tie tac, it does not appear in any archived photographs. Instead, most members donned the NAA pin when they used a tie tac.

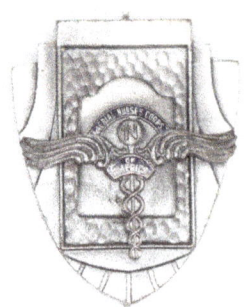

Figure 02.20. Schimmoler's ANCOA tie tac. Author photographed.

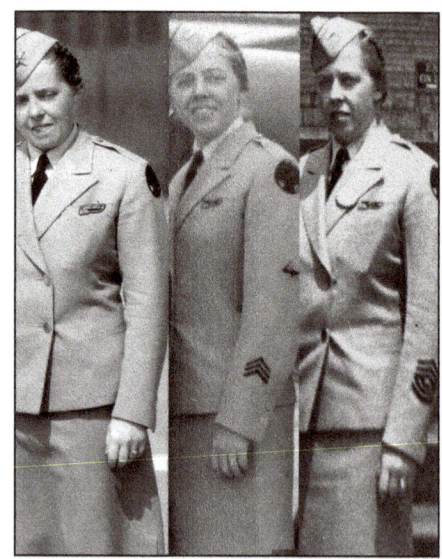

Figure 02.21. Marie O'Brien, of Dayton Company 5-C, wearing various chevrons.

Some members used chevrons on the formal jacket sleeve, but wore them inconsistently; few chevrons are visible in photos. The middle photo chevrons represent a Sargent title; at the right is O'Brien as a Sergeant Major.

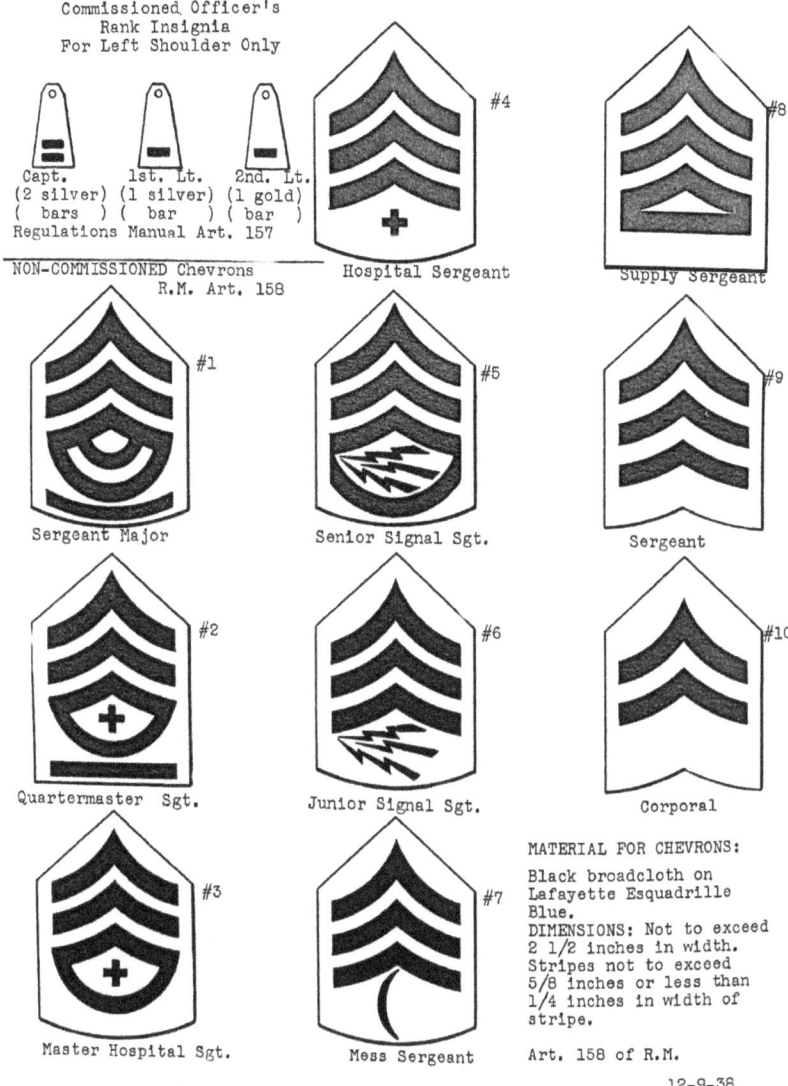

Figure 02.22. The Chevron and Rank Insignia chart, 1938. Leora Stroup Papers, AMEDD. The *Regulations Manual* showed an array of chevrons for non-commissioned members and the rank insignia bars for Commissioned Officers, but they only used a few of the titles listed under the chevrons. Schimmoler might have created them for the Corps to use during a national emergency if they needed additional hospital, messenger, or mess personnel.

Chapter Two

Schimmoler established a Board of Governors *pro tem*. The members assumed the duties and positions of Division Commanders until Schimmoler made official policies and appointments in the various Corps areas. The following nurses from Company A-1 comprised the Board of Governors *pro tem*:

- 1st Division: Ora Brook, RN
- 2nd Division: Lavinia Hodgkins, RN
- 3rd Division: Shirley Weidman, RN
- 4th Division: Marie Wallace, RN
- 5th Division: Margaret Derenia, RN
- 6th Division: Lucille Hurst, RN
- 7th Division: Phyllis Brewer, RN
- 8th Division: Elizabeth Tintorri, RN
- 9th Division: Frances Yeoman, RN [46]

The *Los Angeles Times* printed articles about the Corps which helped with the recruitment. Schimmoler set the following qualifications for application into the Corps:

- Agree to volunteer for three years
- American Citizen
- Age 21-35
- Height 5'2" to 5'8" with a weight corresponding to age and height
- Pass a physical examination for air duty fitness
- Member of her state's nursing association
- Member of the American Nurses Association
- Member of the First Reserve of the ARC (American Red Cross) [47]

Most of the requirements were understandable, but why would she insist ANCOA nurses be First Reserve members of the American Red Cross?

Early in the twentieth century, the ARC maintained a unique relationship with the military from previous war experience. The Army Nurse Corps (ANC) began in 1901, but mainly functioned during wartimes; if the U.S. was not engaged in a war, the ANC employed few nurses. If a war started, many eligible nurses would be needed quickly. The Red Cross maintained a list of First Reserve Nurses who qualified and were willing to join the Army Nurse Corps immediately when called. The requirements for First Reserve included being unmarried, under forty, in good health, and a graduate of an approved nursing school. [48]

Schimmoler had initially envisioned the ANCOA only as an aerial nurse ambulance—a trained medical transport group. At some point, she included a second goal of readiness: to prepare to assist during national emergencies and help the military with evacuation during wartime.

This goal stated the ANCOA would provide technically trained, physically qualified personnel to fulfill the requirements of the U.S. Army Medical Department and Navy Nurse Corps in national emergencies, under military supervision, for aerial nurse duty in air transports at airports and air bases of the Army, Navy, and Marine Corps in time of national and civic emergencies. [49]

By requiring them to be Red Cross First Reserve, she knew they were qualified to fulfill the second goal—even though she had yet to obtain positive acknowledgment from the Red Cross. In fact, she had received quite the opposite.

In 1933 Schimmoler had sent a letter to Clara Noyes, the Director of the ARC Nursing Service, and asked, "If I were to interest nurses and train them for air duty, would I be rendering my country a service?" Noyes replied, "There would seem no point attempting to organize a special group of nurses for this (Emergency Flight Corps) purpose." Obviously, that didn't deter Schimmoler from developing the ANCOA, but she didn't contact any ARC official again for several years. [50-51]

> ...they had become quite suspicious of her actions. What did she really want? What were her motives?

Schimmoler didn't realize the ARC had already been closely interested in the ANCOA. And they had become quite suspicious of her actions. What did she really want? What were her motives? By 1937 Schimmoler's fame had traveled to Maynard Carter, Chief of the Nursing Division, at the League of the Red Cross Societies in Paris. Carter wrote to Ida F. Butler, the Director of Nursing of the ARC, apparently curious about the ANCOA. Butler replied to Carter:

> My Dear Mrs. Carter, It is pleasant to receive a letter from you. I am particularly interested in its contents about the Aerial Nurse Corps of America because it has not yet been officially recognized by the American Nurses Association (ANA). In fact, I am quite sure that the President and Founder, Lauretta M. Schimmoler, is not a nurse.
>
> I have already written Mrs. Alma H. Scott, Director of the American Nurses Association at her New York headquarters, not only on the question of the ARC recognizing the ANCOA, but also whether the ANA would take any cognizance of the ANCOA organization. [52]

Chapter Two

The American Red Cross, the American Nurses Association, and the Army Nurse Corps exchanged information about the ANCOA and Schimmoler. Should they take legal action or ignore her? Schimmoler was blissfully unaware of these exchanges; their remarks were not kind.

The ARC did not appreciate she had implied a connection between the ANCOA and the Red Cross when none existed—Schimmoler hadn't even discussed the requirement that ANCOA nurses should be First Reserve Nurses with anyone at the ARC. They thought that omission was wrong. Moreover, the ARC alone had been designated, by law, as an auxiliary air to the Army's medical department in times of emergency. They didn't need or want the assistance of the ANCOA.

The Army Nurse Corps was also skeptical—the ANCOA occasionally used the same ANC initials as the Army Nurse Corps. Schimmoler also used the term Corps areas in describing the ANCOA territories. The Army used Corps areas for the division of the states. [53]

The American Nurses Association, particularly the California State Nurses Association, argued Schimmoler wasn't a nurse. Butler was privy to letters from the Secretary of the ANA to the CSNA, which did not hide any feelings:

> She is not a nurse. She is a great promoter with the ability to attract because of her personality, but she is not a woman of either culture or education. It is a very great surprise to me that nurses with high standards of education and enrolled in the Red Cross Nursing Service would be willing to organize with a leader who is not one of their professional group. [54]

Butler wrote again to Carter and told her about the letters she had read:

> After consultation with Mrs. Scott, I decided to discuss with our Legal Advisor, Mr. Hughes, whether I would in any way be entangling the Red Cross if I were to write to the promoter of this organization, Lauretta Schimmoler, to express my surprise that she would not have communicated with the Director of the Red Cross Nursing Service before making, through her literature, the requirement that she had made enrollment in the Red Cross Nursing Service one of the requirements for membership in the Corps, and also the requirement that the applicant shall have had the Red Cross First Aid and Life Saving Course.
>
> I will make the letter, of course, as friendly as possible and ask for further information as we are interested. [55]

Mr. Hughes advised Butler not to communicate directly with Schimmoler as a letter "might be misconstrued and might be used for publicity in a way of which we would not approve." [56]

Butler told Carter she had also talked to Major Julia Flikke, Superintendent of the Army Nurse Corps. As Butler understood it, Flikke had been advised by her commanding officer to completely ignore the ANCOA rather than raise any confusion about Schimmoler's use of Army terms.

> "...unaffiliated auxiliaries offer more romance than war has ever seen before."

Butler had also written to Admiral Cary Grayson, Chairman of the ARC. He took a proactive stance; he did not want the Red Cross to be left out of a potential Aerial Nurse Corps creation. Grayson asked Butler to draft a letter for his signature to the Surgeon General, Major General Charles R. Reynolds. He made it clear the Red Cross was ready to organize their Aerial Nurse Corps if the Surgeon General thought it to be a good plan. [57] Reynold did not believe they would need it expectantly:

> We recognize the airplane will be used as a transportation agency in time of war, and it may be that especially in the secondary evacuation in the rear area or the theater of operations, and in home territory, there may be a need for specially trained nurses. However, this need will not exist, in my opinion, in the combat zone, or at least the employment of women nurses for front line evacuation will not be required. [58]

Reynold raised concerns. He asked Grayson to discuss the matter further, "... to forestall activities on the part of any unaffiliated auxiliaries in the field which offers more romance than war has ever seen before." [59] The military had even influenced fashion—the tailored uniform-style became de riguer.

In the fall of 1937, Schimmoler learned Brigadier General Henry "Hap" Arnold had visited California. Arnold was a General in the Air Force and a pioneer airman—the Wright Brothers had taught him to fly—and he contributed to the early development of flight. [60] Schimmoler wrote him a letter. Hap replied on 14 October 1937:

> Just a note to express my regret that I didn't get a chance to see you while out on the coast and talk over the Aerial Nurse Corps of America program. I hope, however, that on my next trip out I will have more time and will be able

> to discuss the subject with you in detail. I believe there is a place in the scheme of things for such an organization, but just what that place is I will be unable to definitely decide until I know more of the details. [61]

Schimmoler must have felt elated. Finally, someone had paid attention to her idea. But her joy did not last. She wrote back to Hap on 3 November. By this time, Hap had learned of the ANCOA from the medical division chief, Colonel Grow. Grow had contacted Major Flikke and drafted a letter for Hap to sign. [62] Schimmoler received his reply:

> I do believe, however, that inasmuch as the American Red Cross has been designated by law (Army regulation 850-75) that this organization is in effect in time of emergency an auxiliary air to the medical department of the Army, it would be advisable that you should work in conjunction with that organization... Not only should your members be individually a part of the Red Cross, but your entire organization must be incorporated in or acting closely with, and under supervision of, the American Red Cross. He included a copy of the Army regulation with his letter. [63]

She replied to Hap that the Aerial Nurse Corps did maintain copies of Army regulation 850-75; she had discussed her project with the Red Cross but "the personnel in the office were not air-minded and could not see the need for nurses to be educated." She hoped he would show them where her service could be of value. [64]

Schimmoler's fame made the military rounds. Statements from the Surgeon General's office and the Assistant Chief of the Medical Section highlight their stagnant ideas. Even those in the Air Corps lacked enthusiasm:

> Nurses are not required to be, nor is it deemed necessary that they be assigned to the Air Corps for the rendition of nursing service in the air, inasmuch as enlisted men in the Medical Department are taught first aid.
>
> If commercial aviation companies require nurses, which at present I can't visualize, it is a matter which has nothing to do with the Medical Department of the Army.
>
> The present mobilization plan does not contemplate for the extensive use of aeroplane ambulances. For this reason it is believed that a special corps of nurses with qualifications for such assignment will not be required. [65]

Since Schimmoler had no success with the General Hap route and was unaware that Grow had previously discussed the ANCOA with Flikke, she decided to write directly to the Army Nurse Corps. On 23 April 1938, she sent a letter that included a four-page summary of the objectives and accomplishments of the ANCOA. She ended the letter by saying:

> With the hope that this statement of aerial nurse work and our objectives will be of interest to you and convince you that the work warrants good will. Your suggestions and cooperation are invited to assist the patriotic young women of this organization to better equip themselves to assist in furthering the interests of commercial aviation in times of peace, and providing for them a definite place in the scheme of national defense in the event of a major national emergency. Your suggestions on this last phase of our work are particularly desirable.[66]

On 28 April, Flikke wrote back her tepid reply:

> It is, of course, an undisputed fact that aerial travel is of very vital importance and will become increasingly more so in the future. From your letter and other information that has come to me unofficially during the past few months, it would seem that you have a very well-planned organization. If your motive is to care for commercial aerial transportation, your success is no doubt assured.
>
> In the Army, however, we have a well-organized corps of nurses, and flying is not unknown to them. I venture to say that the majority of them have experienced the thrill of traveling by air, and when necessary to transport a patient from one section of the country to a hospital some distance away, a doctor and a nurse board a plane and accompany the patient.
>
> To us, a nurse in a transport plane is like any other nurse that has a special assignment, such as being a surgical nurse, anesthetist, laboratory technician, etc.
>
> In times of peace, very few calls are made for such assignments. If we should become involved in a conflict, any trained nurse to whom air travel is not distasteful could be so assigned so that at the present time at least there seems to be no factual justification for a group of nurses being segregated and called aerial nurses. Nor does it seem

Chapter Two

> advisable to have two organizations with such similar nomenclature that confusion may result therefrom.
>
> As you know, the reserve nurses have always been supplied by the American Red Cross—a practice which we hope will continue. Perfect harmony and cooperation exist between the Army, Navy, and Red Cross, and efficient service has always been rendered. [67]

Flikke sent Butler a copy of the letter she had sent to Schimmoler and information about the ANCOA. Butler replied:

> After reading it, I am very skeptical about the soundness of the organization and I believe that you and I are following the safe course in not committing ourselves. Your letter in reply to Miss Schimmoler's was very fine. [68]

> **This wasn't the first time someone told her, "No!"**

The lack of enthusiasm within the military and the Red Cross did not dissuade Schimmoler. This rebuff wasn't the first time someone told her, "No!" She would not stop; she continued to develop the ANCOA despite setbacks from the military and professional nursing organizations. She didn't hesitate to expand her lofty goals:

1. An establishment of Divisions of the organization in at least one major city in each state.
2. To maintain field hospitals and emergency rooms at all sanctioned air races, and at all air meets and air shows.
3. To improve and increase air ambulance service over the country, including making available to the medical profession proper and adequate air nursing facilities, with special attention to protections for patient, pilot, and other passengers.
4. To establish definite requirements for personnel who fly in air ambulances, especially for the physical and the technical qualifications.
5. After adequate testing and proving of the organization's principles of operation, to present the Aerial Nurse Corps of America to the American Red Cross, for their assignments in national emergencies.
6. Recognition by both the Army Nurse Corps and the Army Air Corps.

Figure 02.23. The *Regulations Manual*, 1940. Leora Stroup Papers, AMEDD. Schimmoler wrote and copyrighted with the Library of Congress a sixty-three-page *Regulations Manual*. Each new cadet received a copy of the book, which detailed the rules and regulations in three chapters: the Departments, the Uniform, and Administration.

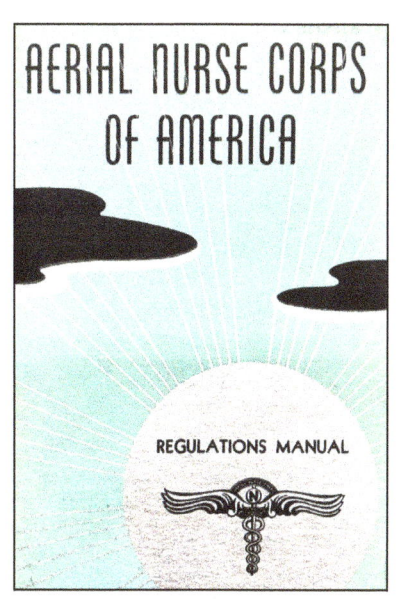

Schimmoler began the monthly newsletter, *Flashes*. Members from the ANCOA companies sent a page of articles to the editor each month. She and her assistant compiled them, wrote announcements from GHQ, mimeographed them on their Speed-O-Print machine, and mailed it to all members. *Flashes* allowed members to communicate among the companies about activities, successes, rank promotions, recruitment encouragements, aerial nurse history, and flight education opportunities.

Figure 02.24. *Flashes* Editor Aileen Crain, left, and the Assistant Editor, Sue Ottig.

Crain edited almost all issues. Shirley Weidman edited the first four and Edith Corn edited a few issues after Weidman's. Colorized clipping, MMM.

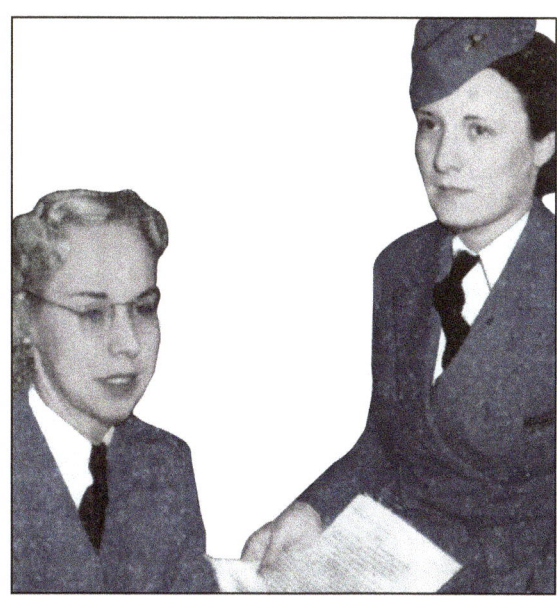

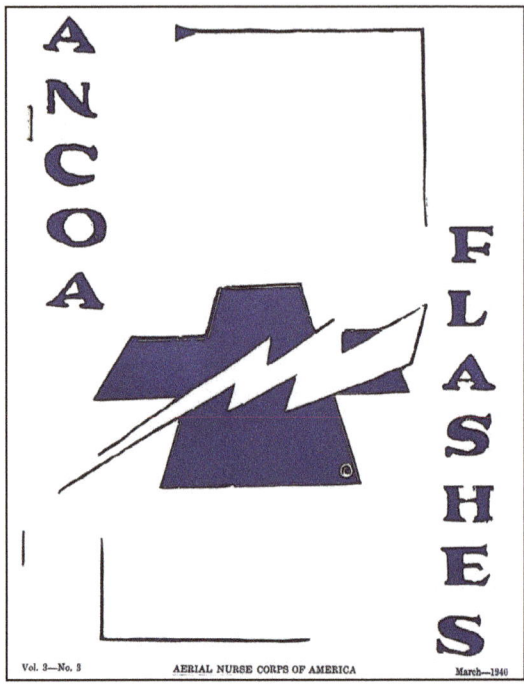

Figure 02.25. *Flashes* Newsletter, March 1940. Leora Stroup Papers, AMEDD.

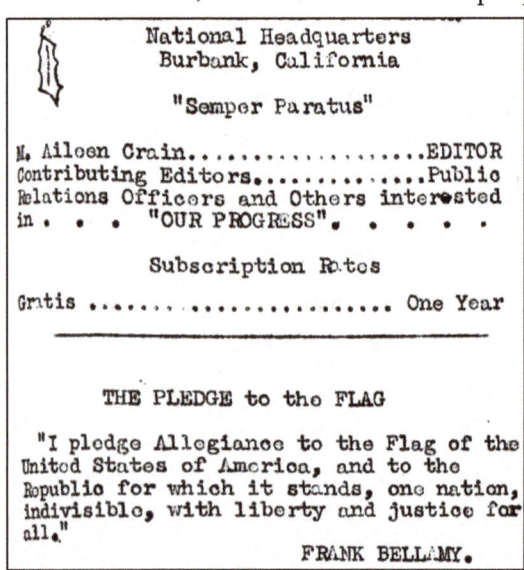

Figure 02.26. The *Flashes* Masthead, December 1938. BHS. Editor Crain included the ANCOA motto "Semper Paratus" (always prepared) and the Pledge to the Flag—the original version, written before 1954, which did not include the phrase "under God." 69

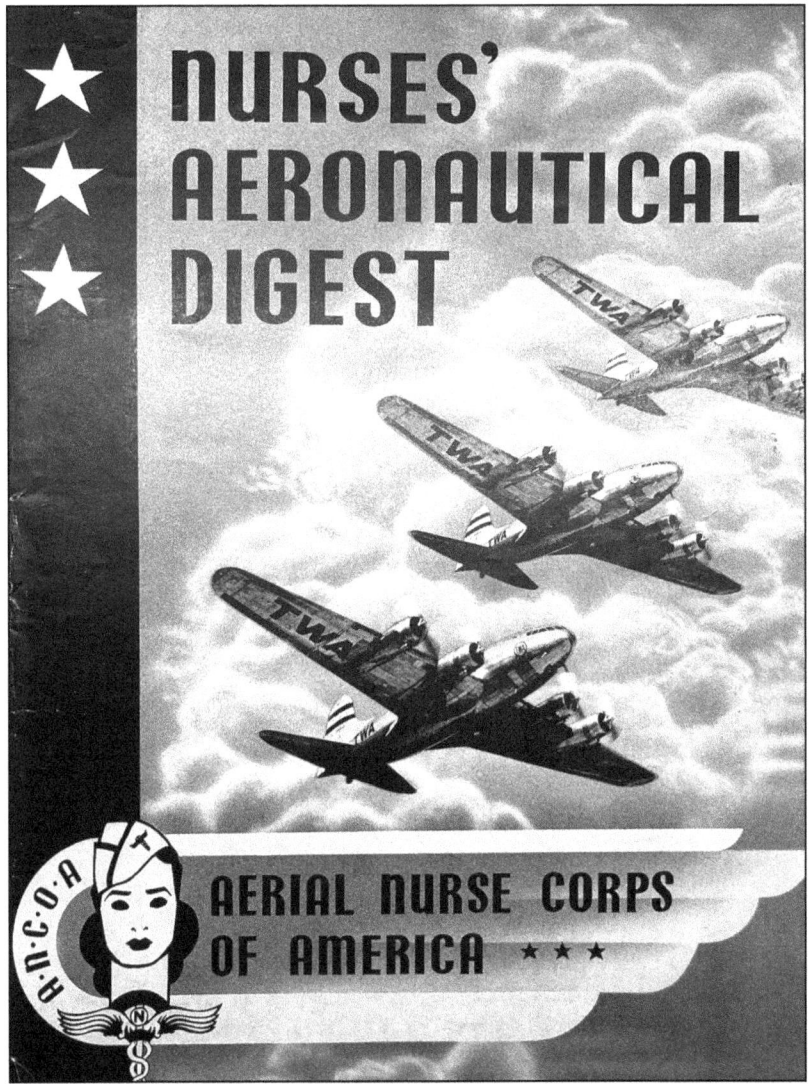

Figure 02.27. The *Nurses' Aeronautical Digest*, October 1940. AMEDD.

In 1940 the ANCOA produced a glossy publication, *Nurses' Aeronautical Digest*—the first and only volume. The professional magazine featured TWA Stratoliners on the cover. The contents contained educational articles: "Physiotherapy, Color Blind Pilots, Progress, Activities at the National Headquarters," and comments from company officers. They dedicated the first volume to the California State Nurses Association as they attempted to become more professionally aligned with the nursing organizations. They continued to publish *Flashes* every month.

Chapter Two

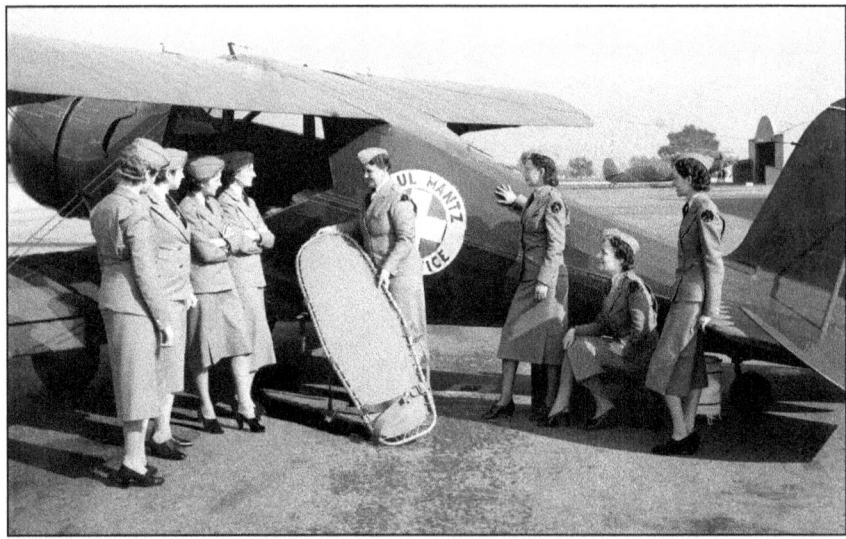

Figure 02.28. Aerial Nurses, left, Schimmoler, and members of the First Aid Department. Schimmoler holds the stretcher she designed, 1938. MMM.

The group discussed the best method of admitting a stretcher into a four-place airplane—called four-place because it held four people. Not all planes were suited for patient transport; the door and configuration of this cabin made it difficult to house a stretcher.

To determine if the plane was fit for transport, they would measure its height at the widest part of its door, compare it with the height of their shoulders, and compare the trailing edge of the wing with the height of their knees.

The group calculated that a nurse would need to lift shoulder high and step knee high while holding up the stretcher to get the patient into this plane. Schimmoler, therefore, did not recommend this four-passenger Beech airplane as an air ambulance.

As was the custom of the time, hard-working nurses wore skirts and heels. Wearing pants wasn't yet a socially acceptable norm for women. During WWII, pants became ubiquitous as women became employed in factories.

The ANCOA began staffing non-air show events—gas model airplane contests, boat shows, or any event where injuries might occur. The word aerial in their name didn't imply they would only work around events with airplanes; it meant they were prepared to transfer those injured as quickly as possible. They would transport by air ambulance, if necessary, and ground ambulance if the location was close.

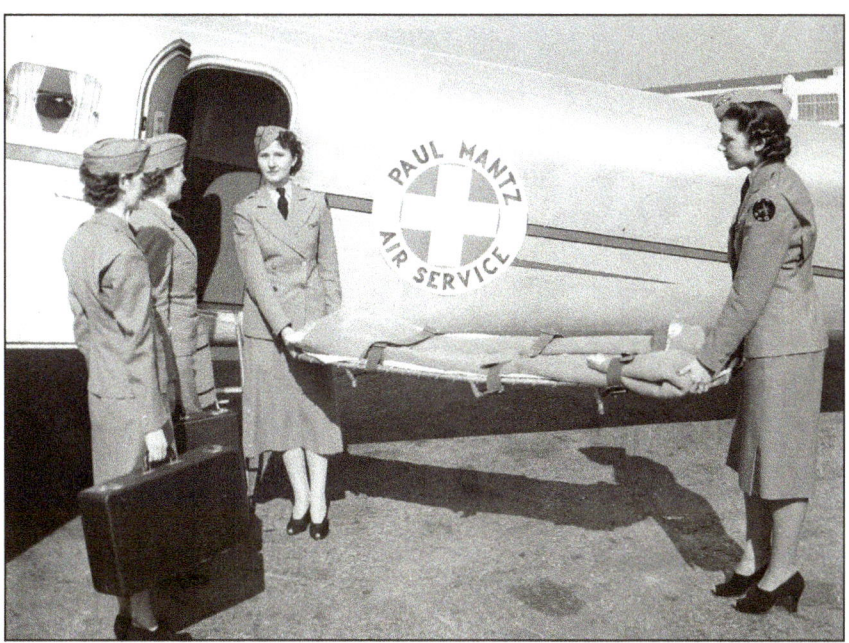

Figure 02.29. ANCOA members load the Schimmoler-designed stretcher into a plane, 1938. Cecelia Getsfred, original ANCOA member #8, looks at the camera; other members are unidentified. MMM Collection.

Unlike the other plane, this Paul Mantz airplane met the door height and trailing edge of the wing criteria; the group deemed this plane suitable for patient transport; the nurses were always ready for emergencies with their handy first aid field kits.

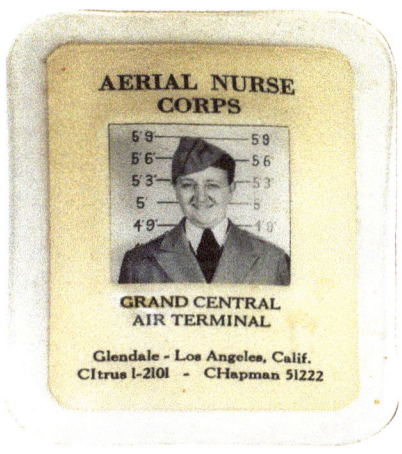

Figure 02.30 Schimmoler's ID card for Grand Central Air Terminal. BHS.

Chapter Two

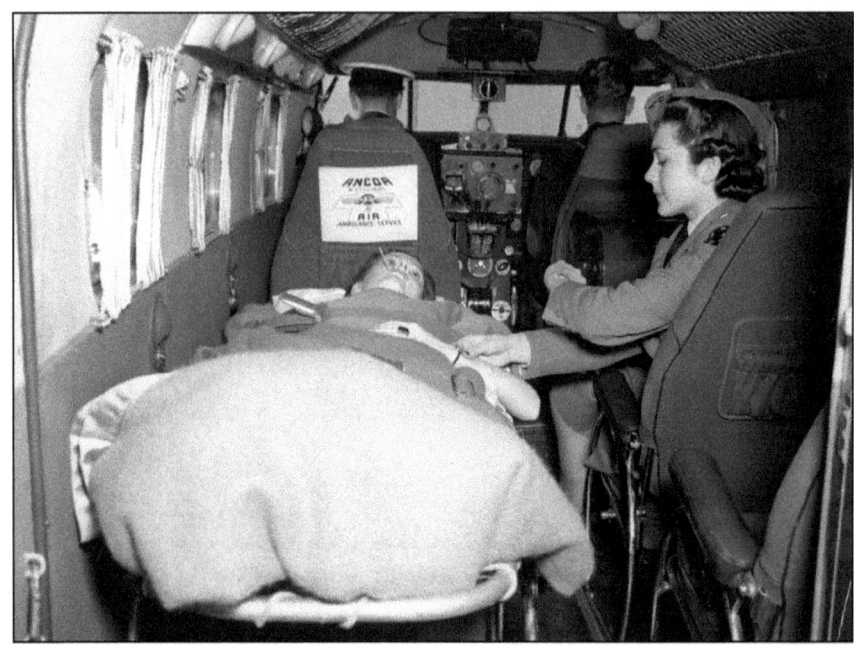

Figure 02.31. Jeanne Lipis, RN, of Company A, First Division, transports a patient aboard a Lockheed Electra. MMM Collection.

Myrtle Martin, RN, recounted a typical landing experience in the life of an ANCOA nurse transporting a patient. A monoplane bearing the ANCOA logo on the fuselage approached Burbank Airport. The nurse picked up the microphone and reassured the patient they would land soon:

> Myrtle Martin calling Burbank Tower. 'Burbank Tower answering Myrtle Martin. Go ahead.' Arriving Union Air Terminal, Burbank, approximately 7:38. Please clear me to ANCOA headquarters—patient resting, pulse 82, temperature 98.8. Will call again over Glendale. That is all.

A short time later, the plane settled down on the airport runway and taxied toward a hangar at the end of the field, where an ambulance waited to complete the trip to a hospital in Los Angeles. Martin turned the case over to the nurse detailed to ground duty and made her way to headquarters to file a report of the trip.[70]

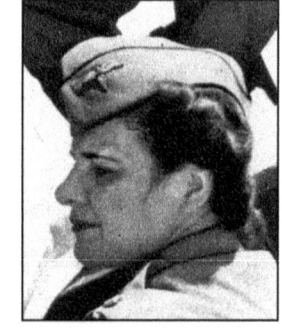

Figure 02.32. ANCOA air-transport nurse Myrtle Martin, RN. MMM Collection.

In August 1938, O.J. Whitney, Inc., at Floyd Bennet Airport in New York, contracted with Schimmoler to become their west coast air ambulance representative. Whitney owned two planes designed for air ambulance service, one that held two stretchers. The ANCOA would arrange transport, assist with the transfer into the aircraft, and accompany the patient in the air if needed. Schimmoler's idea for nurses to accompany private patients across the county had begun. *Flashes* mentioned Captain Lucille Hurst, RN, was in the middle of an "Aerial Tour…as her patient prefers to fly and does not go on any tours without her Aerial Nurse."[71]

The ANCOA became fully organized by 1938. Schimmoler had created divisional areas even before the various groups formed. She divided the ANCOA into three wings. She located the National Headquarters in Burbank, California, with two additional Regional Headquarters in Newark, New Jersey, and Cleveland, Ohio. The regional wings were divided into nine divisions. Divisions were divided into companies by cities as groups formed.

Aerial Nurse Corps of America		
Wings, Divisions, Companies		
National Headquarters: Union Air Terminal		
Burbank, California		
1st Wing Headquarters: Union Air Burbank, CA	2nd Wing Headquarters: Newark Newark, NJ	3rd Wing Headquarters: Municipal Cleveland, OH
1st Division Headquarters: Burbank, CA **Companies** A-Los Angeles, CA B-Pasadena/ Glendale, CA C-Santa Monica, CA/ Phoenix, AZ D-San Diego/ La Jolla, CA E-Bakersfield, CA F-San Francisco, CA K-Seattle/ Tacoma, WA L-Boise, ID	6th Division Headquarters: Atlanta, GA **Companies** A-West Palm Beach, FL B-Fort Lauderdale, FL 7th Division Headquarters: Balto., MD **Companies** A-Washington, D.C. B-Johnstown, NY 8th Division Headquarters: Newark, NJ **Companies** A-New York, NY 9th Division Headquarters: Boston, MA No Company formed	2nd Division Headquarters: San Antonio, TX **Companies** A-Denver, CO 3rd Division Headquarters: Omaha, NB **Companies** A-Ingleside, NE 4th Division Headquarters: Chicago, IL **Companies** A-Chicago, IL B-Milwaukee, WI C-Decatur, IL 5th Division Headquarters: Cleveland, OH **Companies** A-Detroit, MI B-Cleveland, OH C-Dayton, OH D-Dayton, OH E-Toledo, OH F-Lancaster, OH G-Cincinnati, OH

Chapter Two

The 5th Division, Company A, began in Detroit on 5 May 1938, after Leora Stroup, RN, officially joined. Stroup was already a nursing leader, a pilot, and a member of the 99s. Schimmoler and Stroup met in Cleveland at the 1933 National Air Races and discussed the idea for the ANCOA.

The following month, on 24 June 1938, Merle McGriff, RN, joined and organized Company C in Dayton, Ohio. By the end of 1938, McGriff had recruited thirty-eight nurses. Stroup's Company A had a slower start—she only recruited fifteen by the end of that year—but both companies soon became equal in size and together made the 5th Division the second largest.

The *Company Commander's Handbook* stated a company should consist of thirty registered nurses, eighteen first aid workers, and six radio operators: the captain, an adjutant who served as the secretary, a quartermaster who doubled as treasurer, a public relations officer, an athletic instructor, a mess officer, a photographer, a recruiting officer, and a color guard.

Not all companies could meet this large requirement; the roster lists some companies as having only a few members. Schimmoler would later change this requirement so more members in outlying areas could join.

Each company consisted of the Medical Department, a Communications Department, and a General Detail Unit. The Medical Department of thirty registered nurses and their eighteen assistants performed first aid work. The Communications Department had four licensed radio operators and two assistants. A General Detail Unit included two dietitians, two messengers, and twenty-four kitchen workers—this was the ideal company complement. They only required a General Detail Unit during national emergencies.[72]

The ANCOA included active and associate members. Registered nurses, pilots, licensed radio operators, and physicians were active members. Associate memberships were unregistered graduate nurses, nursing students, and persons who had distinguished themselves in allied medical, aeronautic, and social sciences. Schimmoler granted honorary memberships to donors and others who assisted the organization in valuable ways.[73]

In the summer of 1938, at least twenty national newspapers ran a curious advertisement from Schimmoler—it contained no explanation about the group or contact information except her name. All used the exact phrase:

> More and more we are coming to need nurses who are available instantly to go by air with patients who need special medical service.– Maj. Lauretta M. Schimmoler, president and the founder, Aerial Nurse Corps of America.

ANCOA

Perhaps Schimmoler hoped this ad would pique nurses' interest in joining. Whatever the reason for the ad, their numbers began to increase in 1938.

End of Year	Number of Members	Numbers added
1936	33	33
1937	78	45
1938	175	97
1939	233	58
1940	387	154
1941	545	158
1942	610	65

The yearly membership totals were abstracted from the official ANCOA roster Schimmoler kept. But the roster number is incomplete—photos and correspondents contain additional names not listed on Schimmoler's roster; the actual numbers are higher.

Schimmoler introduced various aeronautic associations to the ANCOA; the associations welcomed the ANCOA into their organizations. The National Aerographic Academy presented Schimmoler with the Aero Educational Research Organization plaque and a certificate of membership for her idea to create the ANCOA and promote women's aviation.[74]

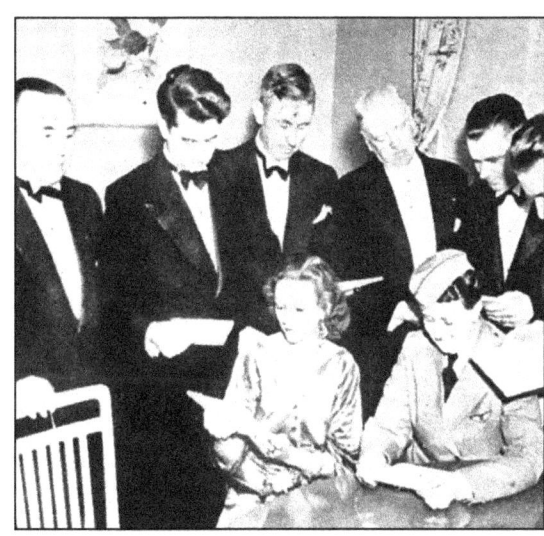

Figure 02.33. Dr. John Carruthers, left, presented Schimmoler with an Aerographic Educational Research Organization Plaque and Certificate of Membership, May 1937. BHS Collection.

The founder of the National Aerographic Academy, Dr. John Carruthers, presented awards to Schimmoler and others. Schimmoler is seated at right.

Chapter Two

The National Aeronautics Association (NAA)—called the Aero Club of America before 1922—verified national and international flying records set at the National Air Races in the 1920s and 1930s. Schimmoler joined the NAA in 1931. In July 1938, the NAA recognized the ANCOA as its official nursing organization.[75] ANCOA members were encouraged to join to help maintain their membership quota, although Schimmoler didn't state the desired number.[76]

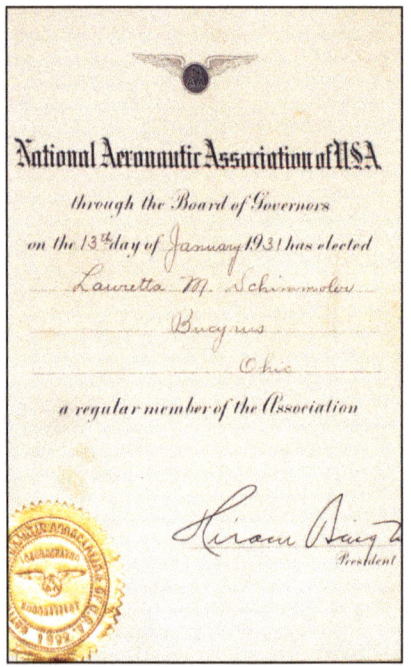

Figure 02.34 Schimmoler's NAA certificate. BHS Collection.

Figure 02.35. A *Flashes* advertisement to join the NAA.

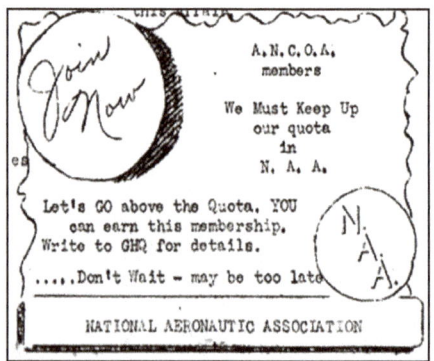

Schimmoler had developed a relationship with United Air Lines. Not only was one of their flight surgeons on the Aviation Advisory Council, but she reported in February's 1938 *Flashes*, "By mutual arrangement between United Airline Lines and the ANCOA, recently completed applications for future stewardess position will now be received at our office in Burbank." She would train them using the ANCOA program.[77]

Before WWII, all airline stewardesses were RNs, so this association made sense. Airline stewardess was a prestigious job for a nurse and the market was competitive. Perhaps some nurses heard the airlines hired ANCOA members and joined for a line on their resume. Stroup complained the airlines had appropriated many ANCOA nurses.[78]

Schimmoler filed the required paperwork with the Secretary of the State of California, and on 8 February 1938, the ANCOA became incorporated. They'd chosen a President, Vice-President, Secretary, Treasurer, Aviation

Advisory Council and the Nursing Advisory Committee by then. The Board of Governors had changed from the original *pro tem* and included officers from various companies. The final board included no original *pro tem* members.

Staff
OF
Aerial Nurse Corps of America
INCORPORATED

NATIONAL OFFICERS

President, Founder and Director of Aviation Activities
LAURETTA M. SCHIMMOLER
National Headquarters - - - - - Burbank, California

Vice-President and Chief-of-Staff (in charge of Nursing Dept.)
RUTH G. MITCHELL, R. N.
390 Central Avenue - - - - - Oakland, California

Secretary
MERLE McGRIFF, R. N.
1040 Fidelity Med. Bldg. - - - - - Dayton, Ohio

Treasurer
LEORA B. STROUP, R. N.
246 E. Alexandrine - - - - - Detroit, Michigan

Board of Governors
RUTH G. MITCHELL, R. N. (Chairman)   MERLE McGRIFF, R. N., 5th Div.
MARGARET HELTON, R. N., 1st Div.   LEORA B. STROUP, R. N., 6th Div.
LILLIAN JENSEN, R. N., 2nd. Div.   ROSE MARIE STERBERG, R. N., 7th Div.
MYRTLE MARTIN, R. N., 3rd Div.   ANTOINETTE HAEZART, R. N., 8th Div.
ELLEN McNEILL, R. N., 4th Div.   AMANDA STEWART, R. N., 9th Div.

Aviation Advisory Council
ARTHUR S. DUDLEY (Chairman)
Sacramento - - - - - - California
Member Executive Committee, National Aeronautic Association
COLONEL JOHN H. JOUETT
Pres. Aeronautical Chamber of Commerce - - Washington, D. C.
JAMES WEBB
Member Executive Committee, N. A. A. - - - Brooklyn, N. Y.
COLONEL A. D. TUTTLE, M. C.
Flight Surgeon, United Air Lines - - - Chicago, Ill.
One additional appointment not complete at time of going to press.

Nursing Associations, Advisory and/or Study Committees
California—RUTH G. MITCHELL, R. N. (Chairman)
Michigan—LOUISE KNAPP, R. N. (Chairman)
Ohio—MERLE McGRIFF, R. N.

ORGANIZED GROUPS
1st Div.: Co. A-1—Los Angeles; Co. D-1—San Diego; Co. F-1—San Francisco; Co. K-1—Seattle.
4th Div.: Co. A-4th Chicago; Co. B-4th Milwaukee; Co. C-4, Decatur, Ill.
5th Div.: Co. A-5th Detroit; Co. B-5th Cleveland; Co. C-5th Dayton.
8th Div.: Co. A-8th New York.

"The Army has its nurses—the Navy has its nurses. I am glad to see the Air is going to have its nurses—and such women as can be of assistance in aviation," says a Civil Aeronautics representative.

Figure 02.36. Incorporation staff list from the ANCOA booklet, 1938.

In 1938 the ANCOA joined the Los Angeles Sheriff's Aero Squadron. Los Angeles County had created the Sheriff's Airplane Detail in 1929—designed to investigate thefts and crimes connected with the air industry. They re-named it the Sheriff's Aero Squadron and re-designated it for rescue and disaster service in 1933.[79]

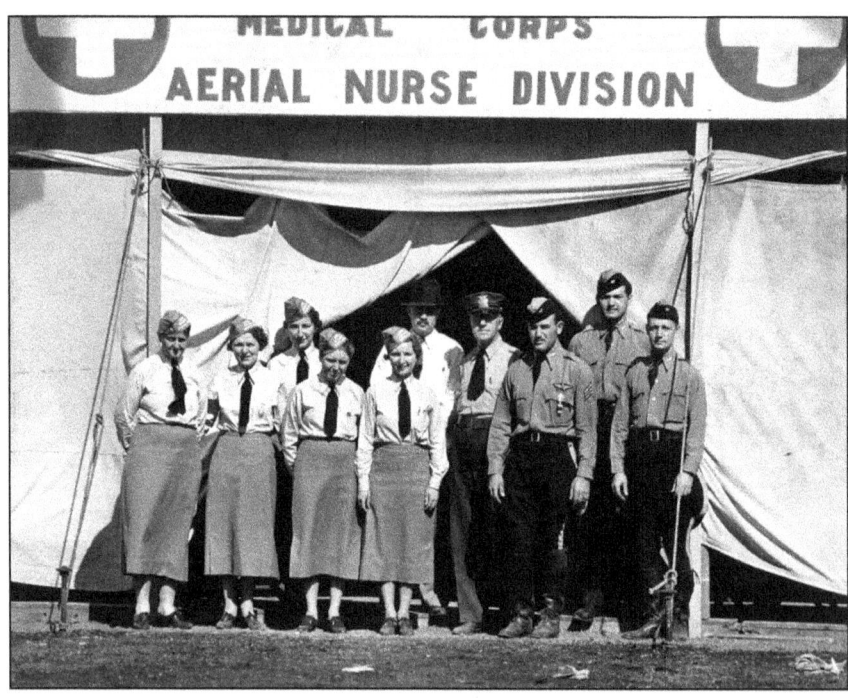

Figure 02.37. ANCOA nurses with the Los Angeles Sheriff's Aero Squadron. Schimmoler is far left. Captain Claude Morgan is at the center in the light-colored Sheriff's uniform and hat. BHS Collection.

Deputy Sheriff, Captain Claude Morgan, was a wartime flyer and a Major in the U.S. Aviation Reserve Corps.[80] The all-volunteer, deputized reserve officers of the Sheriff's Aero Squadron searched for lost individuals in the mountains and deserts, aided in capturing fugitives, and assisted in major disasters. The volunteer owner-pilot crew maintained their planes at no cost to the county—all those who flew were veterans from private charters or aerial pioneers. Membership was by invitation only. Captain Morgan invited the ANCOA to become an auxiliary emergency unit of the Aero Squadron. They were the perfect complement and practiced maneuvers with the Squadron at an annual event.[81]

The National Advisory Committee for Air Progress formed in September 1939, with 150 people from various air transport groups and corporations.

ANCOA

The ANCOA, listed under Schimmoler's name, was the only women's service organization included among the dignitaries. The Air Progress committee planned to formulate the American Aviation's aims and achievements and compile an extensive manual of proceedings for each participating city. [82]

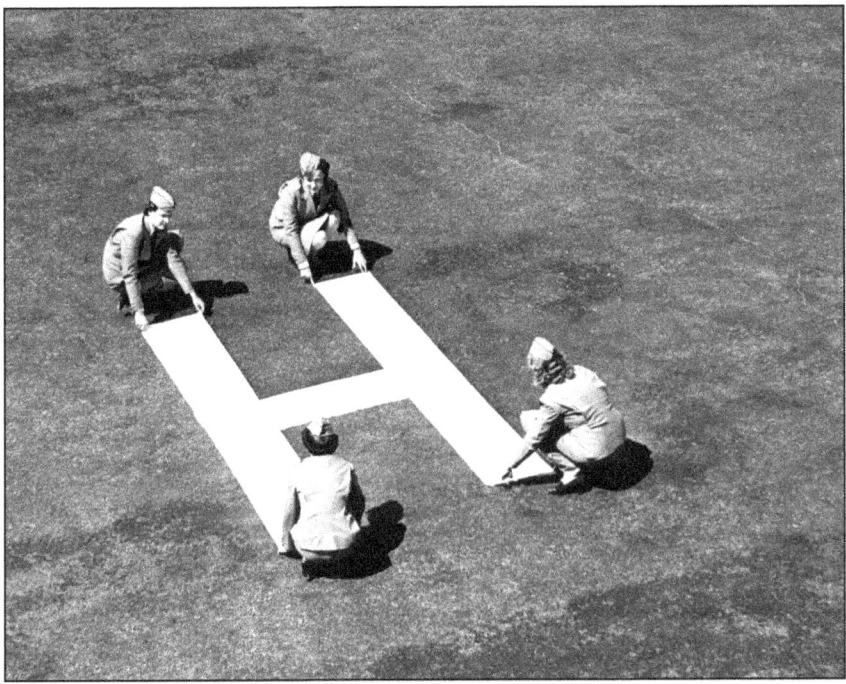

Figure 02.38. ANCOA nurses practicing the aerial message bombs. They displayed the letter H here to signal HELP—doctors and nurses needed urgently. Leora Stroup Papers, AMEDD.

The Los Angeles group tested a device they called aerial message bombs. When dropped from a plane, a tiny charge burst the package open, and a capsule with a compartment containing letters floated down. A small parachute attached to the capsule helped slow its descent.

Those awaiting rescue could arrange letters to form messages. The bomb contained six letters cut from muslin strips, ten feet by twenty feet. Each letter signified a code: H indicated help, doctors and nurses needed urgently; F meant send food; A was first aid kits only; T for need water; and O, everything OK. The pilot would dip a wing to signal he understood.

Schimmoler conceived of and designed the message bombs, including the code. After she created the model pack, she presented it to Captain Morgan.

The Civil Aeronautics Authority granted them permission to stage a test drop at 400 feet to determine how low pilots needed to fly to read the letters.

The Aero Squadron taught the ANCOA dietitians a technique to pack the food containers they planned to drop. The rescuers thought it could be helpful for train wrecks in isolated areas, earthquakes, or floods. [83]

While they did sponsor balls and dinners, the ANCOA was not a social group: strict rules applied for attendance, behavior on the job, and proper attire. They constantly sought out work and training to improve themselves and the new aerial nurse specialty they were building.

Schimmoler and the other commanders made it their business to know about air meets of all sizes. They asked permission from those in charge to set up their first aid stations and field hospitals. Schimmoler followed her creed of "Act first, then talk." She said the best advertisement was showing them, in action, in newspaper articles and magazines. "Action speaks better than words." [84]

> The lay person waits for something to turn up; the ambitious one goes out and turns it up.
>
> *Lauretta M. Schimmoler*

During the 1930s and early 1940s, ANCOA photos and articles appeared in *Popular Science, Aviation Flying, Popular Mechanics, American Modeler, The Trained Nurse and Hospital Review, National Aeronautics, American Aviation, the American Journal of Nursing* and other publications. In 1939 *National Aeronautics* reported, "Scarcely a first-rate aviation event has been arranged without the assistance of the local Aerial Nurse Corps." [85]

To increase their knowledge, they toured aircraft manufacturing plants, studied Morse Code, and Third-Class Radio requirements. They completed Red Cross Courses and local military men taught them marching drills.

They attended the Aviation American Legion's parachute demonstrations and the Women's Aviation Aeronautical Association. They sought out all aviation activities to broaden their knowledge.

They believed they should maintain good physical condition. For sports, they roller skated; they laid out tennis courts to learn and participate in the game. They organized a pistol team, owned three pistols for team use, and practiced at a local firing range.

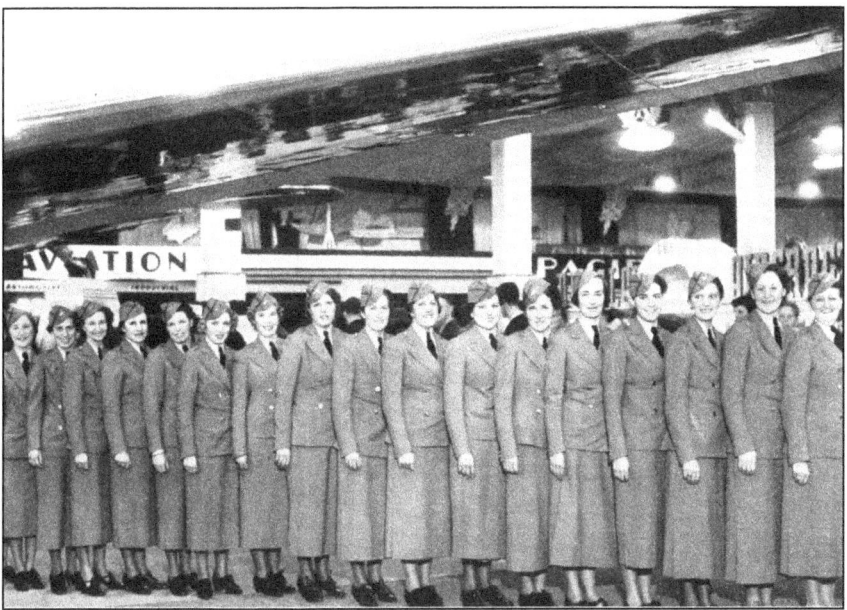

Figure 02.39. The Division 1 members standing under the wing of a huge airliner at Union Air Terminal, June 1938. Leora Stroup Papers, AMEDD.

Musical members created a band called the Kitchen Cabinet Orchestra, which performed at various outings. They undertook a theoretical study and survey of airports; they planned to obtain drawings and detailed information concerning all major airports and landing fields.[86] They embodied the very definition of industrious.

Schimmoler broadened the scope of air ambulance service. She prepared sketches, recommendations and proposals, which she submitted to the Surgeon General. No reply. Was it because she wasn't a nurse? She decided to find out. She traveled to Washington to meet with department heads and receive a direct answer.

She attended the 1940 Air Congresses in Washington, D.C., Sacramento, Denver, and New Orleans. At each meeting, she presented her paper, "Air Ambulance Service," where she appealed for specific structural changes in civilian aircraft to improve the assembly of stretchers, always stressing the safety and adequate care of the patient. She said about the conferences:

> At each, I was accorded courteous commendation by those interested, but always there appeared a doubtful reaction… I was suggesting something that appeared quite radical and untried.[87]

At the Air Congress in Washington, she met with the Air Force, Congress, and the Chief of the Army Nursing. The Chief of Army Nursing told her:

> You have a wonderful idea, but you are ten years ahead of us. If only you were a nurse, we could find a place for you.

She left Washington disheartened, but, as usual, she was not discouraged. She knew in due time they would recognize the worth of her idea. [88]

Schimmoler met with many U.S. aircraft operators to recommend methods to improve the safety and comfort of transported patients and acquaint them with the Aerial Nurse Corps. Based on her input, one manufacture changed a new model's entrance and compartment walls to facilitate improved stretcher loading.

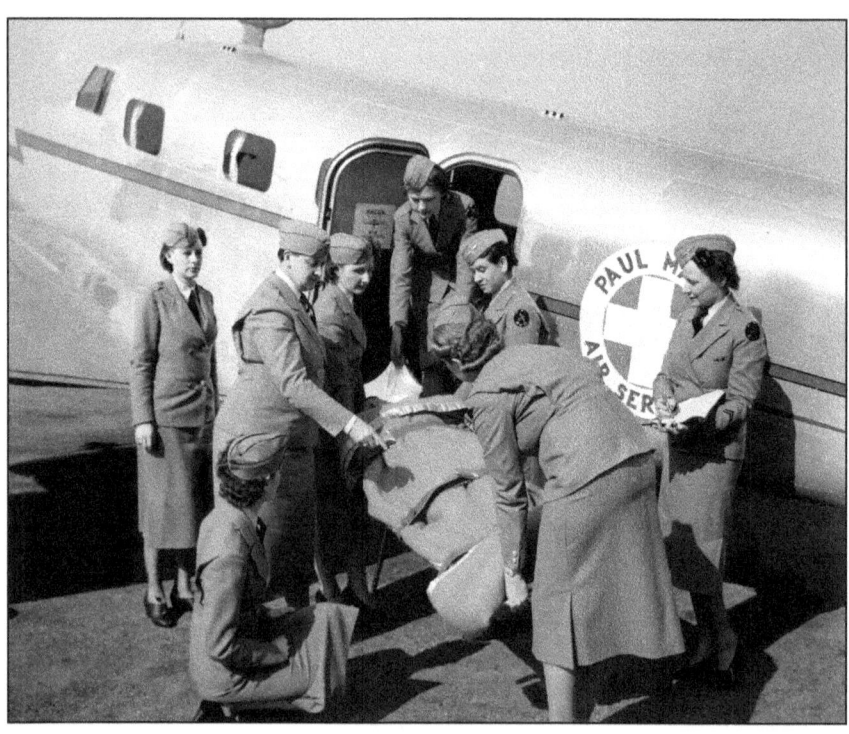

Figure 02.40. Company A-1 loading a patient into a Paul Mertz plane at Union Air Terminal, 1938. An ANCOA sign hangs on the loading door. Schimmoler is pointing at the stretcher she designed. BHS Collection.

Schimmoler designed her stretchers to fit inside smaller aircraft and to improve patients' comfort. Due to the planes' resting tilt, the angled landing gear made loading and unloading patients more difficult. When manufacturers created tricycle landing gear, those planes were more valuable for air ambulances because the patient remained level: when they stopped to refuel or during a weather layover, the patient could rest more comfortably flat than at an incline.

She frequently reminded the nurses of the importance of their pioneering endeavor, as she did in this *Flashes* article:

> Nurses, do you know there are NO regulations governing airplanes used as air ambulances and that today, any civilian owner of an airplane is allowed to carry an injured person anywhere without question, regardless of the condition of the airplane, consideration of horse-power, interior dimensions, or qualifications of the pilot. Should any nurse be allowed to ride in an airplane with a patient?
>
> Nurses, you owe it to your profession to institute a rule not to allow any mechanic or pilot to take an injured person alone in an airplane. You, one of you, should be riding in that airplane, and you should know the Civil Air Regulations and know that you are fit for this duty.
>
> We sincerely hope those who read this will think of this air service as something serious, and far from the so-called glamorous that seemingly surrounds aviation. Help us to safeguard that which is beautiful. Life.
>
> Who will be the first to approve of this necessary training and recommend the Aerial Nurse Corps of America be a distinct and separate nursing department serving aviation? Will it be Ohio, the scene of the founding, or will it be California, the proving grounds? [89]

Between 1936–1939, the ANCOA treated over 1,000 individual cases at twenty-eight major air events, including the National Air Races of 1936, 1937, 1938, and 1939. They received no payments for their first aid services.

They cared for contestants, spectators, and employees. The nurses and first aid group assisted with flying food and medical supplies to the victims of three floods through their membership in the Red Cross. [90-91]

Although they enjoyed their participation in the group—they frequently stated their joy in belonging to it—their writings in *Flashes* portrayed a sense of dedication and value they attached to their part in developing this new aerial specialty.

Chapter Two

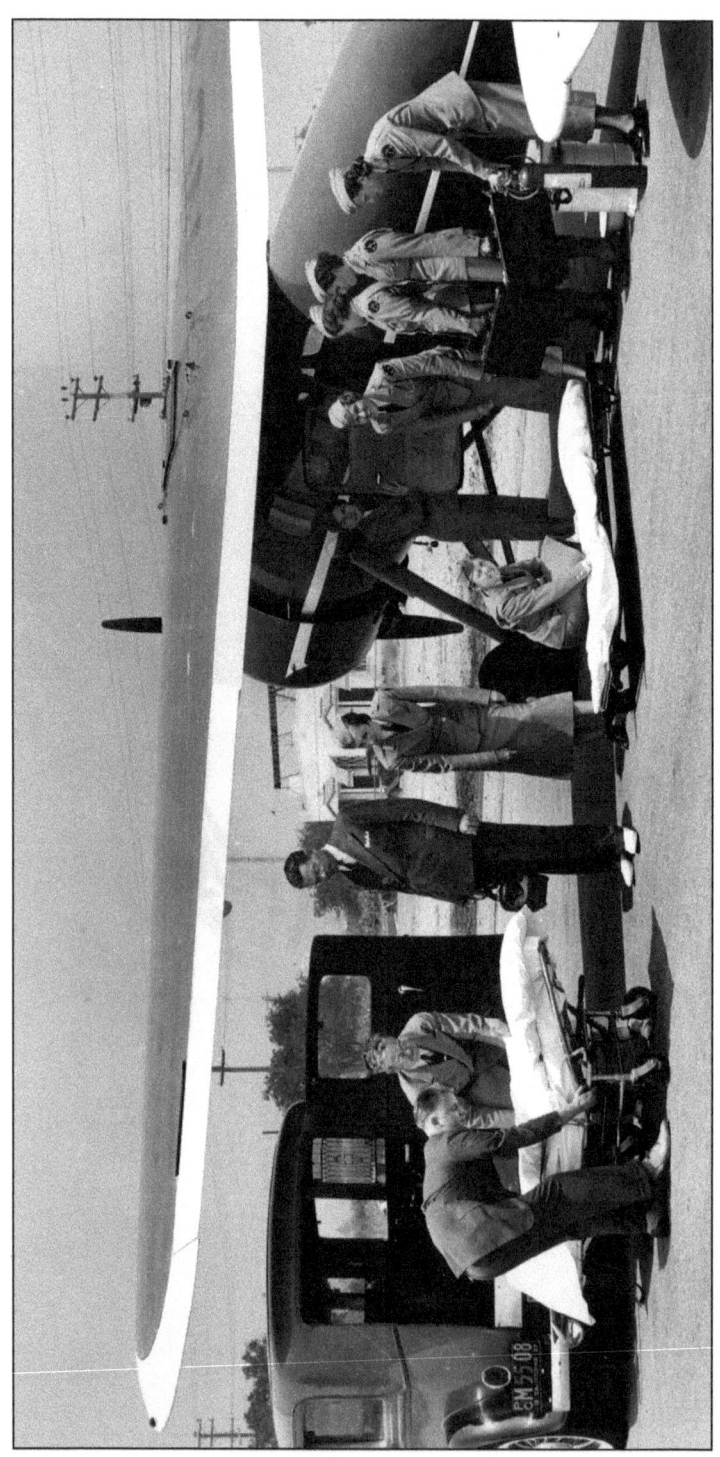

Figure 02.41. Practicing to transfer patients from a ground ambulance to an air ambulance. The white building in the background is the Spitz Flight Recorder building, 1937. Leora Stroup Papers, AMEDD.

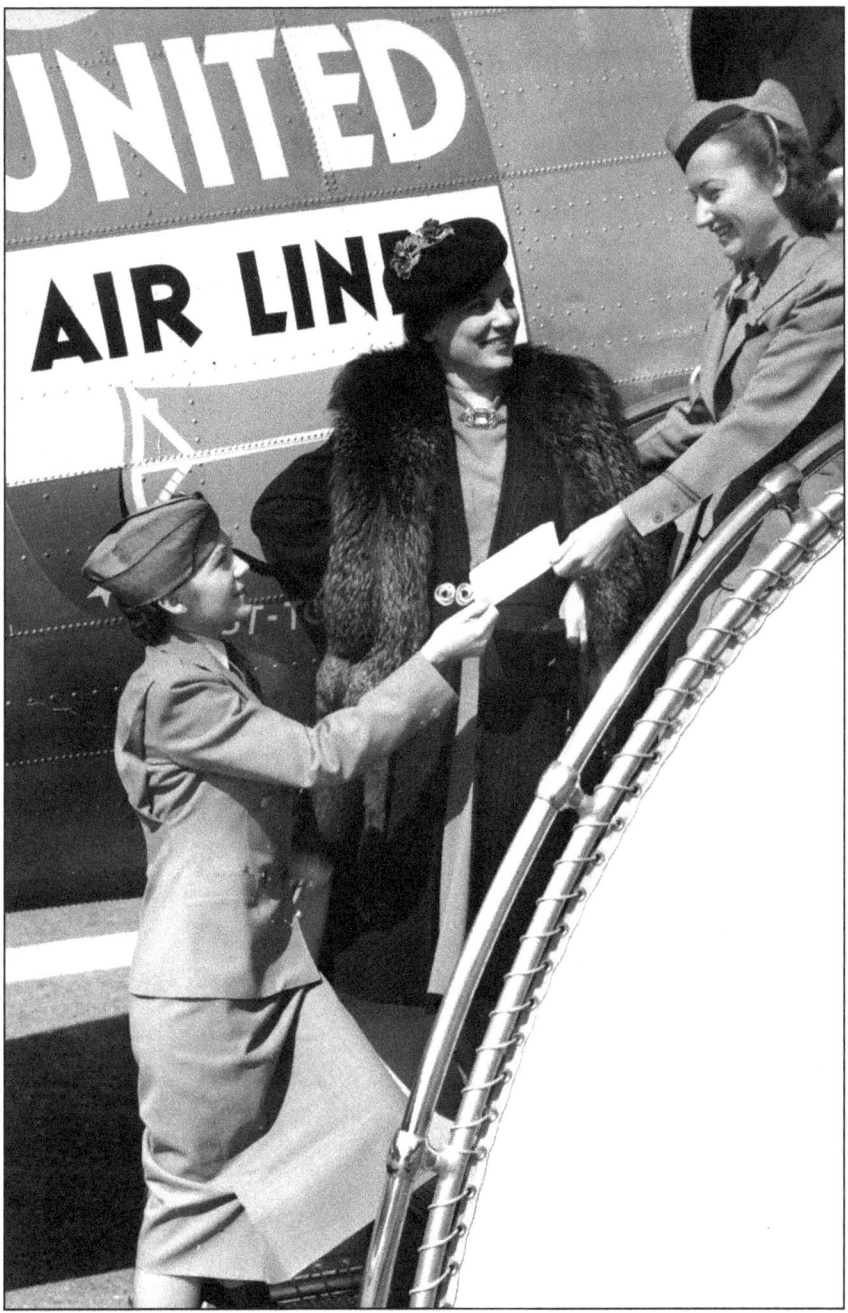

Figure 02.42. Captain Lucille Hurst, RN, escorted a business owner over 15,000 miles on a regular airline, as her patient would only travel if her Aerial Nurse accompanied her, 1941. Leora Stroup Papers, AMEDD.

Chapter Two

By 1941 the nurses had flown more than 25,000 miles while on duty; one nurse, Capitan Lucille Hurst, accompanied a patient over 15,000 miles on a regular airline, ready for any nursing needs, as she attended to urgent business.[92] No list is available of all the air shows the ANCOA staffed or the patients they escorted, but they discussed a few in *Flashes*:

- The Gas Model Airplane Association of Southern California Semi-Annual Contests
- The Airshows in Linda Vista, California
- Lansing, Michigan, Air Shows
- Amateur Aerial Maneuvers in Vandalia, Ohio
- Springfield, Ohio, Municipal Airport Airshow
- The Society of Automotive Engineers, Aviation division meeting
- Hurst flew to Mexico to accompany a patient in a private yacht
- National Aircraft and Boat Shows, Southern California
- Dayton, Ohio, Air Shows
- Detroit, Michigan, Air Shows
- Lansing, Michigan, Air Shows
- National Model Meet, Detroit, Michigan
- American Legion Air Show, Bakersfield, California
- Pageant of Air Progress Air Show, Los Angeles, California
- Ushers for Dayton's Civic Ceremony honoring the Wright Brothers

> Perhaps by the time I grow up we will ride in airplanes like people ride trains and buses today. I shall never forget my first ride, thanks to you.

One unusual event they sponsored, in association with United Air Lines, was to accompany fifteen children, from the Los Angeles County Orphans Home, on a ride aboard the United Air Lines Mainliner. Three members, Elizabeth Tintorri, RN, Rose Marie Sternberg, RN, and Schimmoler, accompanied the children. When they returned to earth they said, "We wanted to stay up forever!"[93] After the flight, Schimmoler received letters from the children expressing gratitude:

> The ride I had in the Mainliner was the biggest thrill I have ever had. Some interesting things we saw were Catalina Island, Hollywood Bowl, the mountains, and many other things. That was the first time I have ever been in an airplane and, I think it was a very good idea. Perhaps by the time I grow up we will ride in airplanes like people do in trains and buses today. I shall never forget my first ride, thanks to you.—Ellen Owen

ANCOA

Schimmoler prepared the *Aviation First Aid Duty Manual*. After completing their training, she required every nurse and First Aid Attendant to pass an exam based on the manual. She took pride in the booklet and she registered its copyright in 1939. The detailed manual listed a step-by-step Emergency Medical Setup for air events, including all the necessary items:

- Preliminaries
- Types of Events
- Class 2 Air Events
- Class 1 Air Events
- Qualifying Dashes
- Establishment of first aid stations
- Plates
- Civil Air Regulations
- Personnel
- Operations
- Miscellaneous Do's and Don't

She thought it prudent to teach essential knowledge for peace and war, so she included classes in chemical warfare. The military trained only a few officers in chemical warfare during that time; the ANCOA nurses received this training most military didn't know.[94] She developed a home course, *Chemical Irritants*.

As always, Schimmoler wanted more. She arranged for the Williams & Wilkins Publishing Company to provide her with an exclusive edition of Vedder's book, *The Medical Aspects of Chemical Irritants*. When Schimmoler wanted something she never hesitated to ask.[95]

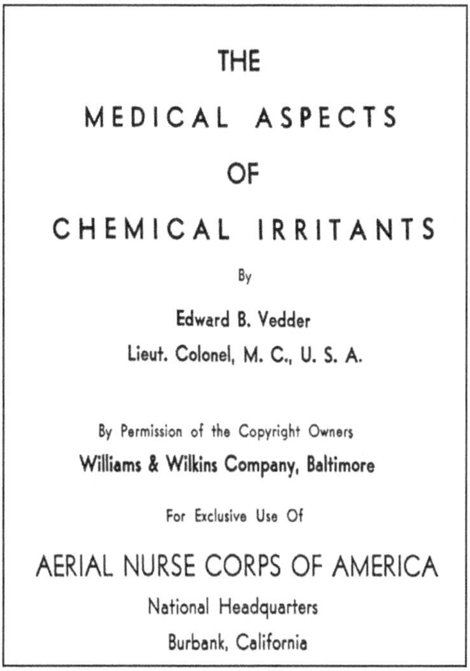

Figure 02.43. The title page of *Medical Aspects of Chemical Irritants,* Williams & Wilkins Company publishers, prepared for the exclusive use of the ANCOA nurses. Leora Stroup Papers, AMEDD.

THE

MEDICAL ASPECTS

OF

CHEMICAL IRRITANTS

By

Edward B. Vedder
Lieut. Colonel, M. C., U. S. A.

By Permission of the Copyright Owners
Williams & Wilkins Company, Baltimore

For Exclusive Use Of

AERIAL NURSE CORPS OF AMERICA

National Headquarters
Burbank, California

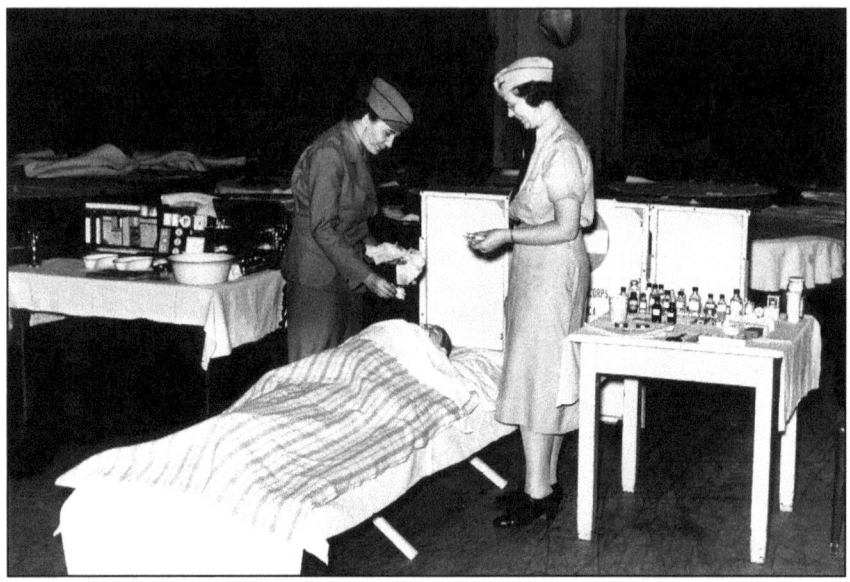

Figure 02.44. The Dayton, Ohio, ANCOA nurses during a chemical warfare class, 1940. MMM Collection.

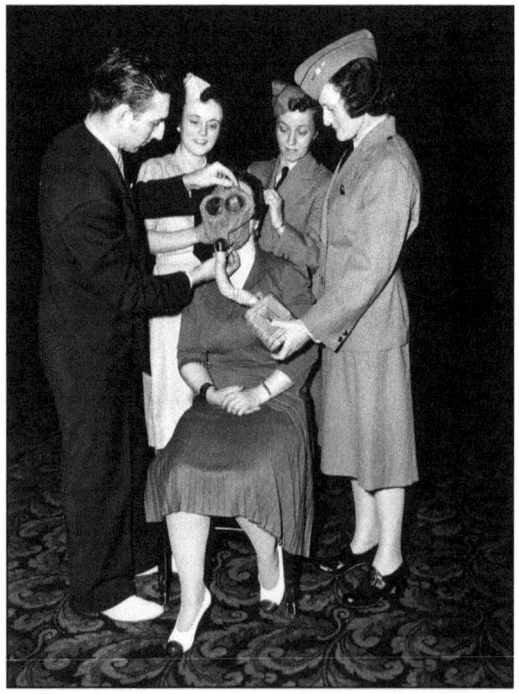

Figure 02.45. Gas mask demonstration during chemical warfare class, 1940.

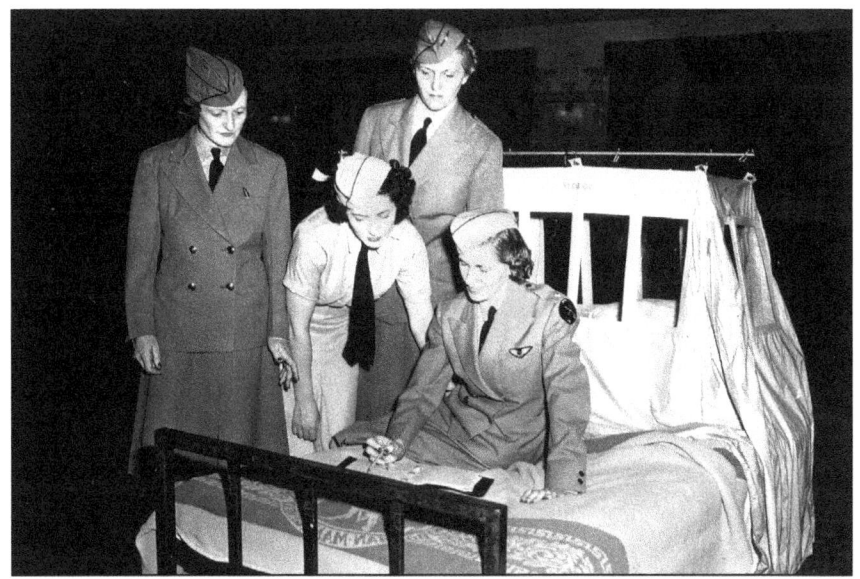

Figure 02.46. ANCOA discussing aerial first aid, Merle McGriff, Dorothy Kyle, Ruth Maurer and Irene Anderson, 1940. MMM Collection.

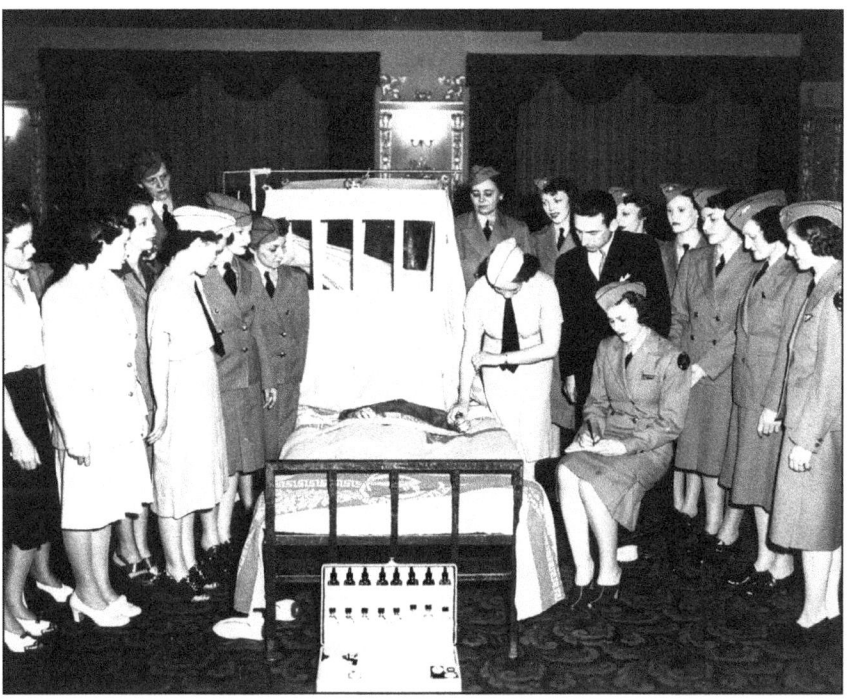

Figure 02.47. The care of the patient recovering under an oxygen tent, 1940.

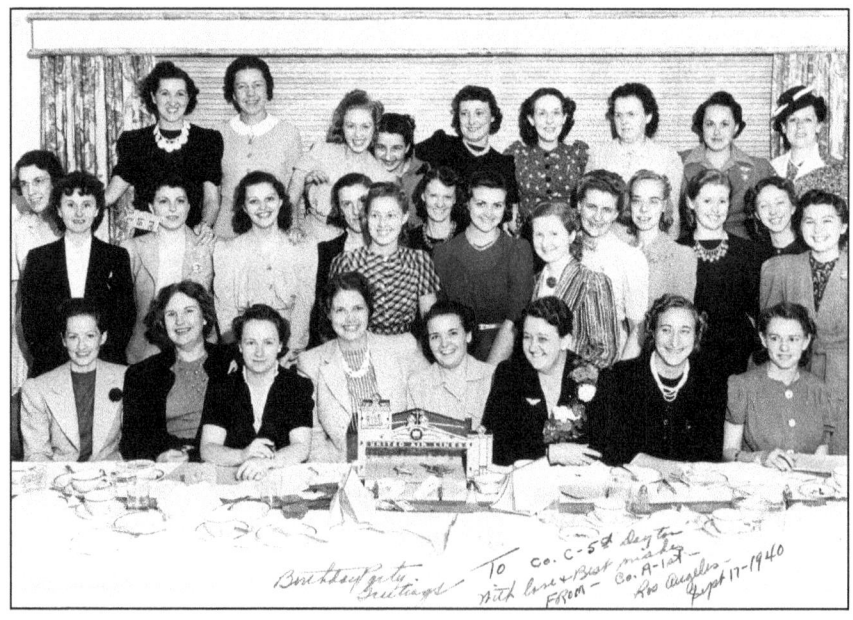

Figure 02.48. Company A-1 in California organized a birthday party for Ohio Company C-5, and sent a photo with "greetings and best wishes," 17 September 1940. MMM Collection.

The birthday celebrants: Top row, left to right: Rose Mare Sternberg, RN; Lorraine Wilson, first aid; Martha Pfister RN, Sylvia Wexler; Sue Atteng, First Aide, Finger Printer; Clara Jane Light RN, Helen Doke, First Aide; Artie Hart Blair, First Aide; Pauline Busch. Center row, left to right: Jeanne Lipis, RN; Agens Danonran, RN; Lillian Jensen RN; Ailen Crain Carrigan, RN; Doris Nystrum; Olga Kiesel RN, Dorothy Regan, RN; Dorothy Andrews, First Aide; Edith Parkor RN; Loretta Windsor, RN; Toni Hoezark, RN; Esther Eklund RN, Seated, left to right: Lida Dolan Radis; Sophie Jevne, RN; Joy Johnson, First Aide, Athletic and Drill Officer; Edith Stark RN, Captain Myrtle Martin, RN, Commander 1-C; Lauretta Schimmoler; Mary De Korte, RN; Florence Walden.

While the military, the American Red Cross, and the professional nursing organizations were leery of Schimmoler and her motives, the nurses who knew her and worked closely with her were not. They loved and trusted her and frequently expressed appreciation for her efforts and actions toward advancing women's independence in their repressive society.

The ANCOA sought to embrace the emerging societal paradigm for women, which they demonstrated in their actions and words. Rose Marie Sternberg, a Company A-1 Aerial Nurse, wrote in a 1939 *Flashes* newsletter:

Isn't there rather a whole new spirit among women today? Aren't women more curious about life? Aren't women less willing to be put off with the rather sentimentalized picture of life that men tried to give them in the past? The answer to this is that our horizons are wider these days. [96]

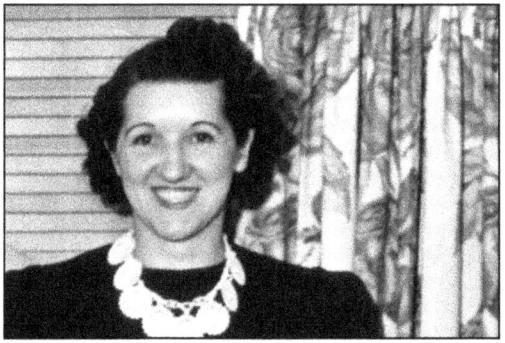

Figure 02.49. Rose Marie Sternberg, 1940.

Another aerial nurse, Ruby Bolch, related what membership in the ANCOA meant to her:

> I only wish I could find words to express this feeling more vividly of what it means to me to belong to the Aerial Nurse Corps of America. It's value to aviation and our country. I wish I could make others see the progress that ANCOA has made and is making, which I feel will be recorded in nursing history in the years to come.

Bolch wrote a poem expressing gratitude to Schimmoler for creating the Corps:

> To Our Colonel
> Years behind have been hard for you
>   to climb.
> But being sincere, selfless, and cheerful,
>   you shine.
> We look into our mirror and see our
>   small reflection
> And compare it to your example of
>   real perfection.
> Colonel, your inspiration cannot be
>   surpassed
> You've given us courage to go forward
>   at last.
>   Ruby Bolch RN, Recruiting Officer, Co.A-1 [97]

Schimmoler told a reporter she'd spent $20,000 of her savings to enlist recruits.[98] With inflation that's $442,861 in 2023.[99] The amount sounds large; it could be a misprint; Schimmoler didn't appear to have abundant funds. Nevertheless, she spent a large sum to start the group.

She collected fees from the enlistees: an initiation of five dollars and monthly dues of fifty cents. The local company sent half of the dues to National Headquarters and retained the other. While nurses didn't receive payment for their work in the field tents and first aid tables, they did receive compensation when they attended a patient on board a flight—at the same rate as the customary working pay in their area.

Like other para-military organizations, they maintained strict rules and were not hesitant to use them. The newsletter frequently listed members who Schimmoler discharged. In one *Flashes* article, they printed a warning:

> If YOU do not comply with the Regulations, no one is to blame, and don't send letters of apology, for GHQ will not file them…we are too busy with the ACTIVITIES of our ACTIVE members.
>
> No organization can accomplish anything with such a large membership unless all work…in the Aerial Nurse Corps, all have a chance. Our initiative will give you this…no one will put it in your hand unless you show the interest expected of you.
>
> DON'T BE SURPRISED IF YOU GET DISCHARGED. We have a definite reason for this.[100]

Those who could not function physically or technically in the aerial nurse role were not allowed in the air. The application to join stated it in the section on the ANCOA's aims:

1. To awaken and promote a wide and intelligent interest in Aviation and Aviation Medicine.
2. To increase the safety factors by reducing the hazards of the untrained and physically disqualified nurses for air ambulance duty. This is a serious matter. There is a vast difference between riding as a passenger and being on duty with a sick patient.
3. To enlist only those physically and technically qualified.
4. To provide, especially to the hospitals, those nurses who are qualified for Air Ambulance duty.
5. To provide educational training for this highly specialized form of duty.
6. To provide our nation with an Air Unit—second to none.

ENLISTMENT AGREEMENT
AERIAL NURSE CORPS
OF AMERICA
(INCORPORATED)
National Headquarters
2620 Hollywood Way—Burbank, Calif.

№ 21

I HEREBY AGREE to pay the sum of Five Dollars ($5.00) as an enlistment fee in the Aerial Nurse Corps of America, with the understanding that in the event national subsidy is obtained and/or received by the Aerial Nurse Corps of America, the above amount of initiation fee will be refunded to me provided I am an active member in good standing, and providing terms of national subsidy permit such refund.

I HEREBY PLEDGE myself to support and defend the Constitution of the United States of America, and agree to abide by and conform to the Rules and Regulations now in force and which may hereafter be adopted by the General Staff of the Aerial Nurse Corps of America.

Date July 24-1940 Leora B. Stroup
Signature of Applicant

RECEIPT FOR ENLISTMENT FEE

I hereby acknowledge receipt of $5.00 enlistment fee from above applicant.

This Space for use of G. H. Q.
Application received
( ) ACCEPTED ( ) REJECTED
Approved
Chief of Staff

Leora B. Stroup
~~Company~~ ~~Commander~~ Quartermaster general
Company A— Division 5th

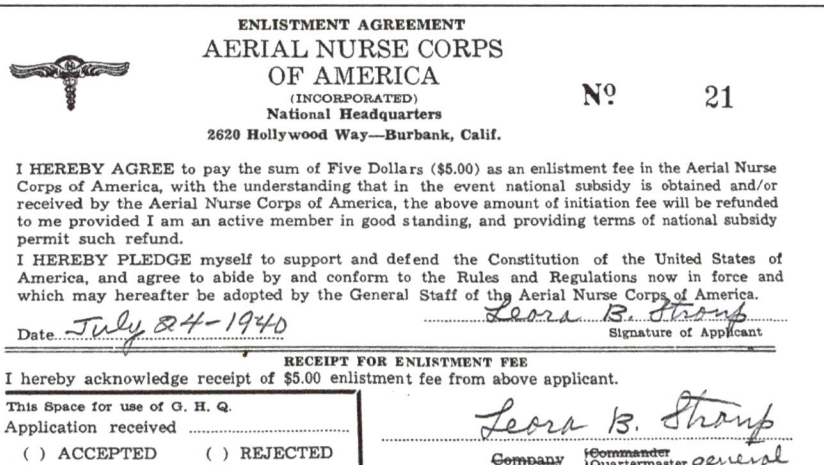

Figure 02.50. The ANCOA enlistment agreement and fee, 1937. AMEDD.

ANCOA cadets studied to receive a Radio Telephone Operator License (third class) from the Federal Communications Commission. Applicants needed to pass a test called Element One and Element Two. [101]

The United States of America
NUMBER P 19 4866
FEDERAL COMMUNICATIONS COMMISSION
RADIO TELEPHONE OPERATOR LICENSE
THIRD
(Class)

This certifies that LEORA BELLE STROUP possesses the requisite qualifications for and is a licensed radio operator authorized to operate any licensed radio station of the class specified by the regulations of the Federal Communications Commission governing the issuance of radio operators' licenses.

This license is granted under the authority of the Communications Act of 1934 and the terms and conditions thereof and of all legislative acts, executive orders, and treaties to which the United States is signatory, and all rules and regulations of the Federal Communications Commission, which are binding upon radio operators, are made a part hereof as though specifically set out in full herein.

Neither this license nor the rights granted hereunder shall be assigned or otherwise transferred to any other person.

This license was issued at Detroit, Michigan on June 2, 1939, and will expire at three o'clock A.M., Eastern Standard Time June 1 1942.

Special Endorsement:
The holder hereof has been issued verification card form 758-f. June 2, 1939.

Emery H. Lee
Examining Officer kmc
By Direction of the
Federal Communications Commission.

Leora B. Stroup (Licensee) Emery H. Lee (Examining Officer) (Secretary)

(THIS LICENSE IS NOT VALID UNTIL SIGNED ABOVE BY BOTH THE LICENSEE AND THE EXAMINING OFFICER, AND THE OATH OF SECRECY EXECUTED ON THE REVERSE HEREOF.)

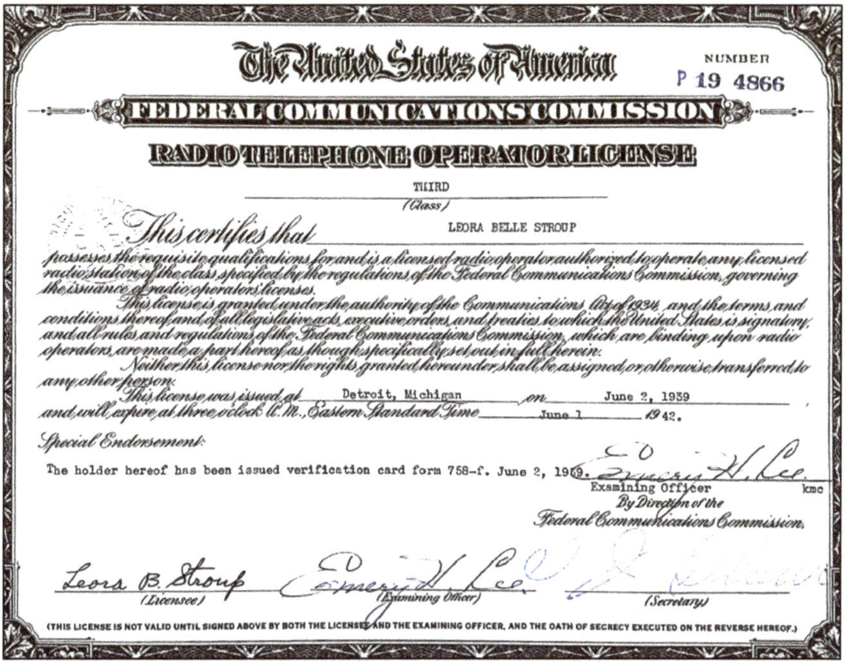

Figure 02.51. Stroup's Radio Third Class License, 1939. AMEDD.

Chapter Two

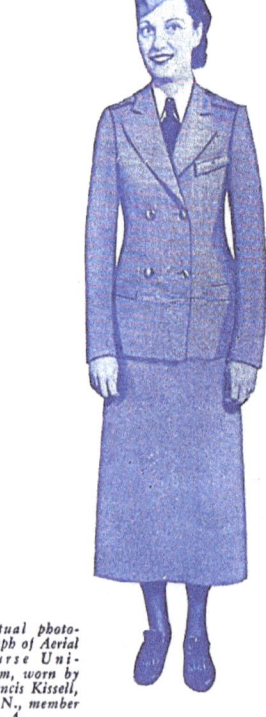

AERIAL NURSE CORPS of AMERICA *Regulation* **UNIFORM**	French Blue Serge Coat.............$20.00
	French Blue Serge Skirt........... 10.00
	Overseas Cap 1.75
	Blue Broadcloth Shirt................. 1.25
	Black Officers' Tie...................... .75
	Division Emblem........................ 1.00 (shoulder)
	Department Emblem.................. .65 (pocket)
	Cap Emblem .... 1.75 (2½" pin)
	A small Pin 1¼", to be worn on the dress, is also available 1.00
	White broadcloth shirts may be purchased by individuals to be worn on special occasions.

Actual photograph of Aerial Nurse Uniform, worn by Francis Kissell, R. N., member Co. A.

Furnished by

JOSEPH PANITZ & CO.
MANUFACTURERS OF
Uniform Clothing and Trimmings
426 SOUTH SPRING STREET
LOS ANGELES, CALIF.
TUcker 2205

Figure 02.52. A *Flashes* advertisement for the formal blue uniform with the coat and a skirt, 1937. Leora Stroup Papers, AMEDD. This early uniform ad showed the embroidered writing on the overseas cap and name tag, but sold a cap pin, a dress pin, and the emblems. The rules required hems to measure 12 inches from the floor or 14 inches in Cuban heels.

In 1938, *Flashes* happily reported K.M. Myers Company of Los Angeles, had manufactured a light tan summer/indoor uniform dress—designed by Schimmoler, of course, and worn with a tie. The dress must have been a welcome addition as the members could wear a lightweight garment at summer meets instead of the hot formal coat.

While Schimmoler kept the 1st Division busy with air meets in the Los Angeles area, the 5th Division grew to rival the 1st Division in size and intent. Two committed leaders made this possible: Leora Stroup, RN, of Company A, Michigan, and Merle McGriff, RN, of Company C, Ohio. Schimmoler quickly promoted them to commanders. Initially, they joined their companies at field hospitals in Ohio. Later when both companies grew, they staffed events separately. Both nurses were pilots. Schimmoler continued this custom of promoting nurse-pilots to commander positions, although not all commanders were nurse-pilots.

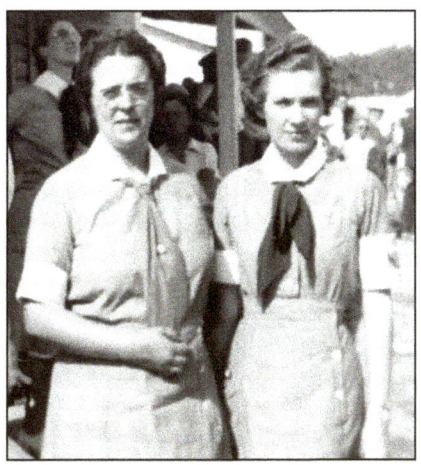

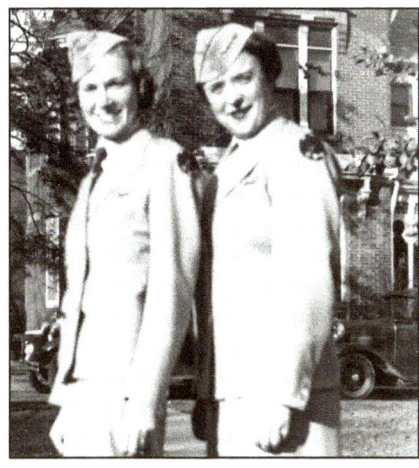

Figure 02.53. Leora Stroup, left, and Merle McGriff, Cleveland Air Race, 1938, before owning the official ANCOA uniforms.

Figure 02.54. Merle McGriff, left, and Leora Stroup, later in 1938, now both wearing the official ANCOA uniforms. MMM Collection.

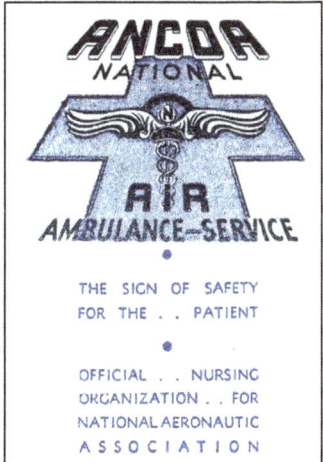

Schimmoler copyrighted her Air Ambulance Emblem with the Library of Congress, which would last for twenty-eight years by the law of the time.

Date: January 15, 1938
Entry: Cl.G2 No. 28301
Emblem: Caduceus on a cross of four equidistant arms.

Figure 02.55. ANCOA National Air Ambulance-Service Emblem, 1938.

Chapter Two

Schimmoler furthered her public outcry for officials to understand what she hoped to accomplish—what she knew she needed to do. Her articles in newspapers and flight publications continued. She appealed to professional flying audiences with her "Safety Procedures," piece in *National Aeronautics Magazine's* trade journal. She explained that simply flying sick patients to their destination with so-called "mercy flights" was not enough; this new charter service, the dedicated Air Ambulance, required new considerations.

She appealed to pilots—something she could do. She wasn't a nurse, but she was a pilot, and just as nurses might circle the wagon with nurses, pilots did the same for pilots. She understood commercial pilots were most concerned about making money as they transformed their four-seater or six-seater planes into comfortable conveyances for the sick. But she cautioned them they were unaware of critical details:

> Safety procedures for the comfort of the patient, doctor, or nurse are far from the operator's thought. As a consequence, the patient is not calm. The mental reaction of an urgent flight, 'We much get the patient to a certain destination within a given time,' is not paramount. Unfortunately, if the doctor or nurse is not entirely familiar with the many technicalities, the pilot must consider they are little or no help at all in the preparation of the airplane for correct ambulance use.
>
> The pilot, of course, is not expected to be expertly schooled in medical procedures, nor should the pilot be expected to assume the responsibility of the patient. Pilots and operators invite trouble if they accept an ambulance flight without professional assistance.
>
> The Aerial Nurse Corps of America is preparing to establish an Air Ambulance registry…all airplanes suitable for ambulance work will be listed…nurses are being trained for this type of duty and will be available to suit each case. [102]

Despite her detractors, she knew her idea was valuable. And although other groups may have considered this, some had even begun to entertain the idea of training aerial nurses, no one else in the U.S. had proceeded with Schimmoler's characteristic gusto. No one else had moved forward on the idea. No one already had a cadre of trained nurses ready and anxious to fly. While other famous women were making their aeronautical mark with distance and speed, Schimmoler's was more altruistic. Yes, she ensured her name was always attached to the idea, but it seemed less of a hedonistic venture than breaking a speed record.

While Schimmoler lived in a world of possibilities, the military maintained their short-sightedness: they could see no reason to train nurses for aerial duties. Lieutenant Colonel Platt, Assistant Chief of the Medical Section, advised the Superintendent of the Army Nurse Corps:

> The Army is not building any hospital airships or airplane ambulances. When necessary to transport ill or injured Army personnel, transport or bombing-type airplanes are used. Nurses are not assigned on these planes." [103]

How dare Schimmoler implicate!

The American Red Cross's oversight didn't abate either. By early 1939, Mary Beard had replaced Ida Butler as the Director of Nursing. Beard became concerned the ANCOA was even more determined. She thought that the nurses respected Schimmoler too much; they almost deified her—the great founder of the organization! Advertisements continued to run, with their subtle references, implying the Red Cross approved of the ANCOA. Beard didn't like that Schimmoler had an advertisement using "RED CROSS NURSES" in large print followed by "are interested in..." in small print. How dare Schimmoler implicate!

Schimmoler mainly used the words "Red Cross" for a headline attention-getter and in her list of ANCOA qualifications. This author couldn't find an abundance of advertisements misusing the "Red Cross" words in posts, magazine articles, historical newspapers, or clippings from Schimmoler's, Stroup's, or McGriff's archives. Schimmoler occasionally mentioned the Red Cross, but after searching historical newspapers that included ANCOA membership details, she couldn't locate many with disconcerting words. Beard might have overreacted.

Beard again contacted Mr. Hughes, the ARC legal advisor:

> Rather recently, we have heard of efforts to organize in New York where an enrolled Red Cross nurse is helping to promote it. Miss Schimmoler is trying to get a large group within her Aerial Nurse Corps of America to enroll in the Red Cross first reserve. This, of course, is a laudable idea, but not when it promotes a nurse reserve outside the Red Cross and which is growing so fast. You remember we consulted both the Army and Navy to know whether they wanted the Red Cross to go in for this sort of a reserve for them, and they said no. Would you be willing to talk with me about it again? [104]

Chapter Two

A memo from Beard to Hughes the following month indicated that Beard had communicated with Schimmoler. Beard told Hughes that Schimmoler had unfortunately manipulated her into a conundrum:

> If we reply to this letter approving what these nurses are doing, she will undoubtedly give publicity to this approval. If we do not approve it, she will publish this disapproval, and I do not like either position. I shall be very grateful for your help. [105]

Looking for usable trouble, Beard's assistant Virginia Dunbar, gathered the various publications and newspaper advertisements about the ANCOA:

> As I read all of the material from the Aerial Nurse Corps of America (newspaper clippings, letters, printed bulletins, etc.) I was impressed with the number of references made to the Red Cross.
>
> Some of the notices were very short so that a reference to the Red Cross stood out. I felt the statements were decidedly misleading as they certainly inferred a connection with the Red Cross (and the Army). [106]

Beard wrote to Schimmoler with praise of her prior promise to cooperate, to warn that her actions could confuse the public, and to advise her again the Red Cross would promptly supply trained aerial nurses if and when they needed them:

> You were kind enough also to give us your assurances of the desire of your group to cooperate fully with our society. There is, we believe, a practical method in which this cooperation may be made to be effective, namely by exercising constant care to have the public fully appreciate the special and the separate fields in which both of our organizations are engaged.
>
> As you know, we maintain a reserve of nurses who may be needed for duty with the United States Army and Navy. If and when there would be such a need by these branches of the Government for nurses, especially trained in aviation matters, the Red Cross will proceed to meet this need.
>
> It would be most unfortunate if those directly connected with nursing and the public, in general, did not clearly understand the services which both our organizations are fostering. [107]

Although the ANCOA nurses were not privy to the details, the scrutiny of their organization did not go unnoticed. Aerial Nurse, Major Stromme, offered her opinion in a *Flashes* commentary:

> In spite of criticism, the Red Cross came into being; in spite of criticism, the Army and Navy Nurses Corps were organized; in spite of criticism, Aerial Hostesses provide their value, and in spite of criticism, the Aerial Nurse Corps, in my opinion, will occupy its place alongside these other organizations whose chief aim is service to humanity.
>
> There are many nurses who show great skill in a hospital; there are some who exercise skill under adverse conditions, but few indeed will be able to exercise that skill in the air without training. The time will not be far distant when aerial ambulances and hospitals may be part of our scheme of living, and the pioneers in this development are the Aerial Nurse Corps of America. [108]

Other groups attempted to help the ANCOA establish credibility with the nursing hierarchies. The President of the National Aeronautics Association, Gill Robb Wilson, wrote to Mary Beard and asked the society to "take a constructive interest" in the ANCOA, as they were "valued affiliates of the National Aeronautic Association...anything you can do to assist them." [109]

To ease some of the mistrust that arose because she, not a nurse, was the President of a nursing organization, Schimmoler promoted Vice President Ruth Mitchell, RN, to Chief of Staff. Mitchell delivered a speech at the 1939 California State Nurses Association meeting in San Francisco. She explained the aim of the ANCOA and outlined a plan to establish a connection between them and state nurses' associations:

> This proposal has always been the plan of the Founder to have someone direct the nursing activities and thus meet all requirements of the nursing standards. This is wholly a nursing project and is designed to serve the daily needs of the public through aeronautical means.
>
> Advisory Counselors are to be chosen in each State and will thereby represent her respective State Nurses Association. They will act as advisors within the ranks of the Aerial Nurse Corps on professional requirements, as well as mediators within the association for the future demands to be made in aviation for the safety of the nurse, the patient, and the aircraft operator.

Mitchell recommended the California State Nurses Association establish an advisory council to investigate the ANCOA, accept it as a nursing project, and endorse its activities. The ultimate goal was recognition by the national headquarters of the American Nurses Association (ANA):

> The passing of the Nurse Practice Act gives the California State Nurses Association (CSNA) the right to determine who is qualified to care for the sick on land, in hospitals, homes, etc., and it is only logical for them also to determine who is qualified to care for the sick in the air and for all aviation activities.
>
> The establishment of this Advisory Council for the Aerial Nurse Corps will make this possible and through the council, the standards for future aeronautical nursing will thus be determined by a recognized nursing board. [110]

But Mary Beard did not give up her scrutiny of them. She discussed her concerns with the ANA about Schimmoler's inferred connection to the Red Cross and alerted them to problems the ANA might also experience:

> There is no connection, formal or informal, between the American National Red Cross and the Aerial Nurse Corps of America. This should be borne in mind, inasmuch as one may read in the pamphlet from which I have just been quoting such a statement as the following: The Aerial Nurse Corps should be called into service through the American Red Cross, the Army, the Navy, or any other civic or military group placed in charge at the time the emergency should arise.
>
> In at least two states, an approach has been made to the state nurses' association, and these state nurses' associations have considered the appointment of an advisory committee on the ANCOA. I am unable to say whether or not such advisory committees are now active or even that they were ever actually appointed.
>
> On more than one occasion during the past two years, there were conferences about aerial nursing between the representatives of the Army Nurse Corps, the Navy Nurse Corps, and the American Red Cross. Each time the Red Cross has been assured that neither the Army nor the Navy wishes any special action in regard to the services of nurses in the air. [111]

Despite Beard's dismissive attitude, the CSNA did appoint an ANCOA Advisory Committee, as Mitchell had suggested, and assigned Gladyce L. Badger, RN, to represent the CSNA. Schimmoler and Mitchell prepared their list of recommendations they hoped the CSNA would adopt and sent it to Badger:

> We recommend the approval and recognition of the Aerial Nurse Corps of America for the development of an aviation department for the nursing profession under the National Defense Program.
>
> Recommendation to the CSNA for their formal approval standards and for enrollment of the Aerial Nurse Corps of America, which includes memberships in the American Nurses Association and American Red Cross Nursing.
>
> Recommendation for the creation of an Aerial Nurse Corps roster within the Red Cross Nursing files for any and all forms of aviation duty for any national emergency under the direction of the American Red Cross. [112]

Badger flatly refused to sign the list of recommendations. [113] On 30 October 1940, she sent Beard copies of letters Schimmoler had sent and her replies:

> I think great confusion exists, and in my letter, I have tried to clarify my position as a member of the Advisory Committee of which I was appointed to by the CSNA. [114]

Schimmoler had said:

> Inasmuch as they have asked us to appoint a committee to confer with the Special Committee in the ANA, and inasmuch as we already have a functioning committee in the CSNA–ANCOA Advisory Committee, we believe it is only fitting and proper that this Committee represents ANCOA before the ANA Committee. [115]

Schimmoler had seemed to imply that Emily K. Eck, the chairman of a Special Committee appointed by the ANA, had asked her, Schimmoler, to appoint an ANCOA committee to confer with this Special Committee. Badger made it clear with her reply—she would not cooperate:

> It is evident there is confusion regarding the relationship of the CSNA Advisory Committee to the ANCOA and its individual members. First of all, I wish to make clear my

> relationship to the ANCOA by stating the following facts: I am a member of the California State Nurses Association, and as such, I was appointed by the State Association on the Advisory Committee to the ANCOA. I am not a member of the ANCOA.
>
> From your letter, it is my understanding the chairman of a Special Committee appointed by the ANA has written to you, asking you to appoint a committee to confer with this Special Committee. It would seem to me that such a committee is intended to be composed of ANCOA members. In view of the above, I am returning unsigned the recommendations you attached for my signature.

Badger talked to some younger nurses during the California State Nurses Convention. They said Schimmoler had suggested that when they send their Red Cross First Reserve enrollment application, they should indicate a preference for service in the Aerial Nurse Corps. She explained to the nurses the Red Cross would return their applications since the only Reserve provisions they offered were either in the Army or Navy.[116]

The CSNA Special Committee met to review the ANCOA information. Committee members consulted officials of the airline companies and superintendents of the Army and Navy Nurse Corps. Emily Eck, the committee chair, prepared an outline of content for what they agreed the training of aviation nurses should include.[117]

Beard's assistant forwarded a report to her on a meeting that indicated Schimmoler was willing to step down from her leadership position of the ANCOA and leave it in the hands of nurses as soon as she felt the organization could take care of itself. Schimmoler was not likely to disappear from the scene, however, as Dunbar explained:

> The nurses in the group are concerned to find the proper way for Miss Schimmoler to continue to give what they consider has been her great contribution, especially in the field of the construction of aeroplanes for transporting sick people safely.
>
> A great deal was made of the fact that the ideal place for Miss Schimmoler would be on the national advisory committee to the Red Cross on the use of airplanes in disasters.[118]

By now, Beard seemed to have developed at least some degree of respect for Schimmoler, which was evident in her letter to the CSNA:

Schimmoler…is one of those promoters who frequently establish something which is needed and which turns out in the end to be much better than one would have expected it to be in the beginning.

Not one of our nursing organizations, no leading school of nursing, nor any other professional group has tried to promote an organization of nurses who understand conditions surrounding patients traveling by air. Nor has the Army, the Navy, or the Red Cross done this.[119]

> ### Had Beard had begun to soften?

But the Special Committee of the ANA concluded they could not support the ANCOA under its current organization. They gave their reasons for denying support and listed their requirements—if it would ever go forward:

I. That formal recognition of the ANCOA in its efforts to develop aviation instruction and training for the nursing profession be withheld for the following reasons:

(a) The ANCOA organization itself is non-professional in that its President is a layperson—she is not a nurse.
(b) The training which the ANCOA nurses are receiving at the present time, in the opinion of the committee, does not prepare them adequately for the nursing service they would be expected to render in a disaster.

II. That in view of the above recommendations, the ANA advise that the State Advisory Committees to the ANCOA, which have been appointed, be dissolved.

III. That if the ANCOA should reorganize and select as its President, a qualified professional nurse, the ANA would consider ways and means of developing a close affiliation with the ANCOA organization.

IV. That a short course of instruction designed to prepare graduate nurses for nursing service in the air, be made available to qualified nurses.

V. That the National League of Nursing Education be asked to develop an outline for such a course.

Chapter Two

VI. That the outline be sent to the American Red Cross for a trial in several of the Red Cross Chapters to determine its professional effectiveness.

VII. That recommendation IV be referred to the Nursing Council on National Defense.

VIII. That the American Red Cross be requested to organize a Reserve of nurses qualified to constitute an organized group for any and all forms of nursing duties in aviation in the event of civic or national emergencies. [120]

The Special Committee submitted its report to Julia C. Stimson, President of the ANA, 16 May 1941. [121]

Schimmoler promoted Leora Stroup—a fellow Ninety-Niner, long-time friend, and Company Commander of the Detroit Company—as the new ANCOA president. Schimmoler sent her a congratulatory telegram. [122]

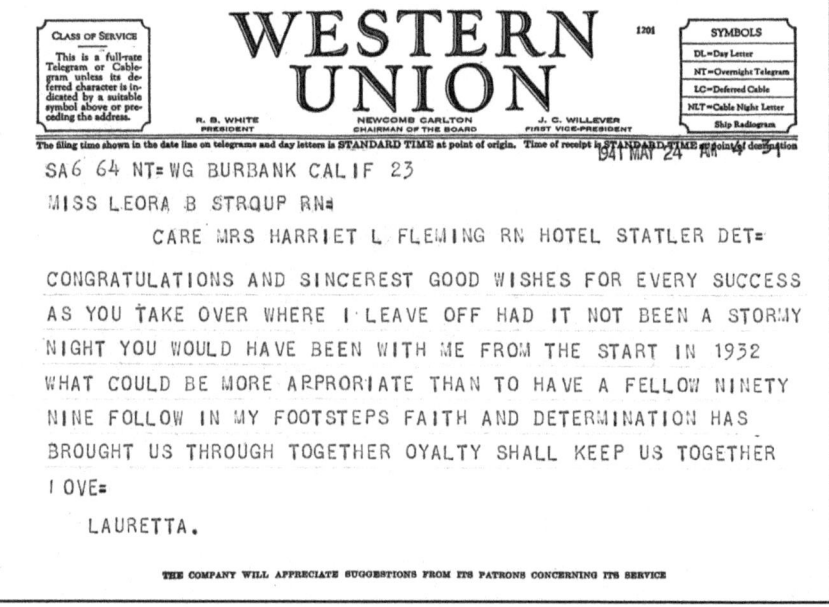

Figure 02.56. Schimmoler's telegram to Stroup, 24 May 1941. AMEDD. She copied it to Harriet Fleming of the CSNA—not a moment's delay for the leaders to know her intent. The 1932 reference concerns when Schimmoler traveled to Cleveland for the opening of Vi-Air-Ways, hung the 99s emblem on the office balcony, and coined the name Emergency Flight Corps. Stroup had planned to attend the opening, but a storm hampered her ability to fly.

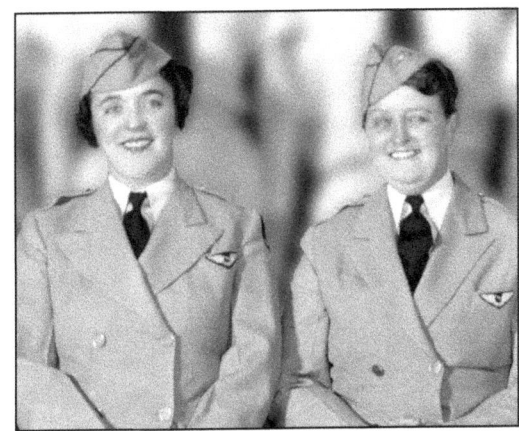

Figure 02.57. Leora Stroup and Lauretta Schimmoler, c. 1939. MMM Collection.

Stroup had been promoted to Quartermaster in 1940 and to the Director of Nurses in February 1941. Now in May 1941, she became President—the entire ANCOA was hers to command. She created a plan to reorganize and comply with the requirements of the Special Committee:

1. The organization to be an all-nurse group
2. An emphasis on greater coordination with all local and all national defense organizations
3. More State Nursing Association Committees as Advisories
4. A simple form of Constitution and By-Laws be adopted to fit the present emergency needs
5. An effort for increased membership
6. Lowered membership fees
7. Simplification of clerical procedures for leaders of local groups
8. A monthly educational publication on aviation nursing, research, and current events to all members
9. Consideration of the courses of study by local Leagues of Nursing Education with a view toward help and approval
10. A conference of the nurse-leaders of the Great Lakes area this month
11. Submitting the new set-up of the organization to the ANA Special Committee to get their help, guidance, and support
12. Formal approval by the Board of Directors of the American Nurses Association [123]

Stroup also began formulating her improved educational plan and detailed new entrance requirements for the nurses. She had created a solid proposal that should have been acceptable to professional nursing organizations and the Red Cross. It's unclear if her designs went forward even for a day; no documentation states they had implemented the changes. While it appeared they had settled the future of ANCOA, its unfortunate demise remained on the horizon.

Chapter Two

The National Aviation Emergency Corps (AEC)

Schimmoler had created an auxiliary group on 13 March 1941, which she named the National Aviation Emergency Corps—usually shortened to the Aviation Emergency Corps (AEC). The AEC allowed her to organize the clerks, radio operators, and first aid workers of the Corps who were not nurses. This complied with the new requirement that only nurses comprise the ANCOA. The Aviation Emergency Corps focused on home defense with preparations for emergency services at airports and aircraft plants.

Douglas Blintliff, the Corps public relations director, said that 75 to 225 of the Aviation Emergency Corps were in training to staff the Southland's airfields and plants. The two hundred women in service at Lockheed Air Terminal (formally Union Air Terminal) would also cover the Lockheed and Vega plants. The Municipal Airport detachment would service Douglas and North American. [124]

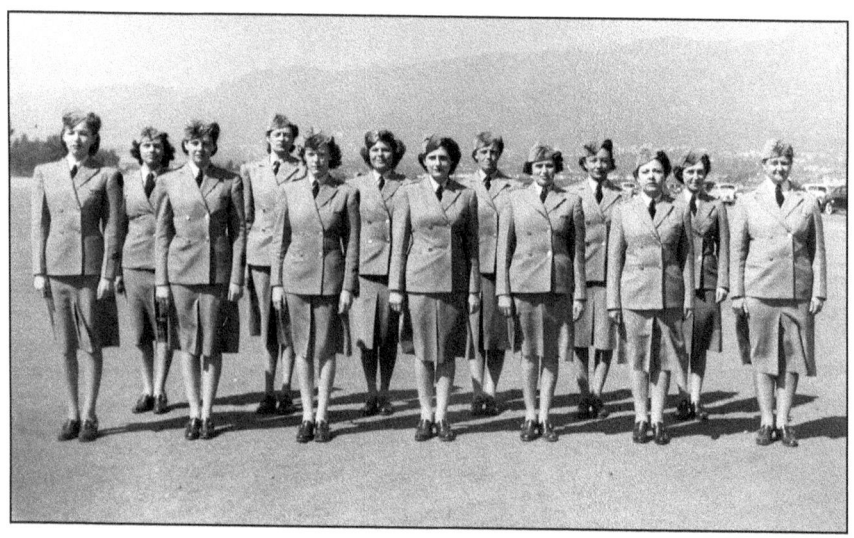

Figure 02.58. The Aviation Emergency Corps, West Los Angeles Platoon, California, Lauretta Schimmoler at right, 1941. MMM Collection.

Stepping down from her leadership role must have been difficult for Schimmoler. She alone developed the idea for the ANCOA. She had implemented her research and made something where nothing had been, and now the nurses had taken away her role. But she was a practical person in many respects; she knew to keep her treasured idea alive, she had to make the changes the nurses insisted on.

All was not lost—she could still command the AEC. She put her momentum behind them. Before, they had been a side group to her; now, she would spend her time developing this ANCOA auxiliary while Stroup reorganized the nurses.

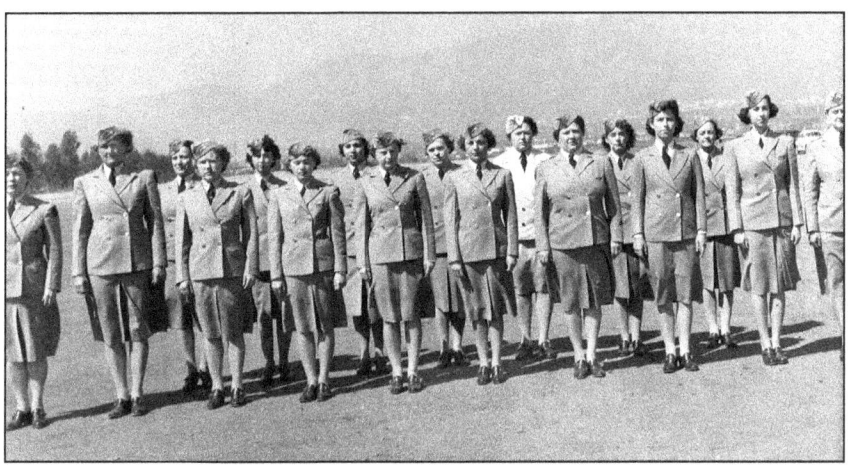

Figure 02.59. The Aviation Emergency Corps, Glendale Platoon, California. Lauretta Schimmoler at right, 1941. MMM.

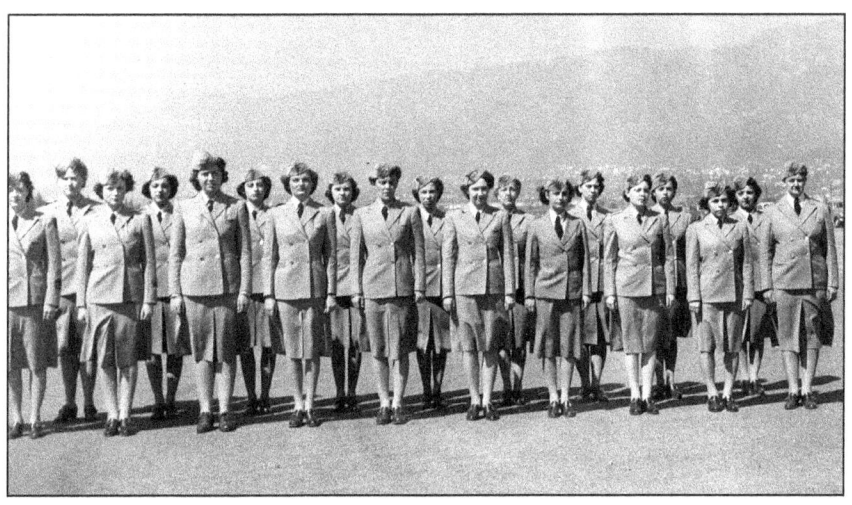

Figure 02.60. The Aviation Emergency Corps, Los Angeles Platoon, California, Lauretta Schimmoler at right, 1941. MMM.

The AEC wore the same uniform and arm patch as the ANCOA nurses. Schimmoler created a distinctive cap pin for the group but utilized the original first aid pocket patch.

Chapter Two

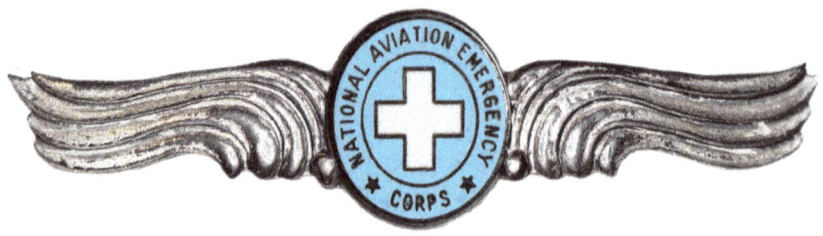

Figure 02.61. The National Aviation Emergency Corps cap pin, 1941. The new cap pin retained the elongated wings from the nurse's pin. An embossed Greek cross was set in the center—the international symbol of first aid. NATIONAL AVIATION EMERGENCY CORPS and two stars surround the cross. Author photographed.

Schimmoler joined the group and donned the new AEC pin on her cap; she retained her ANC commander patch. Several newspapers announced the start of the National Aviation Emergency Corps as an essential group for home defense. [125]

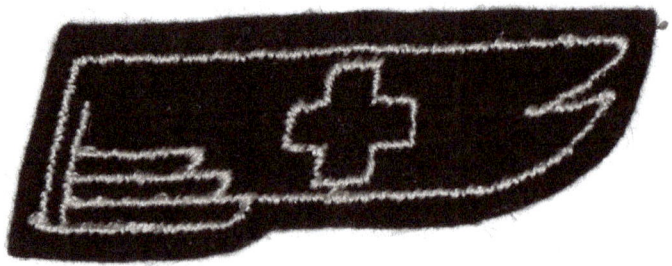

Figure 02.62. The Aviation Emergency Corps pocket patch, 1941. Author photographed at BHS.

The ANCOA and the AEC planned to expand their partnership with the Sheriff's Aero Squad. Schimmoler organized a "get-acquainted meeting" with the Squad at the Aviation Beach Club in Santa Monica—a South American supper dance. [126]

The Dayton Ohio Company formed an active Aviation Emergency Corps. Commander Merle McGriff, as energetic as ever, remained highly engaged in the success of the ANCOA.

On to the next phase, Schimmoler must have thought. How could she have known that a force more devastating to the ANCOA than the interference of the nursing organizations would soon dismantle her years of work.

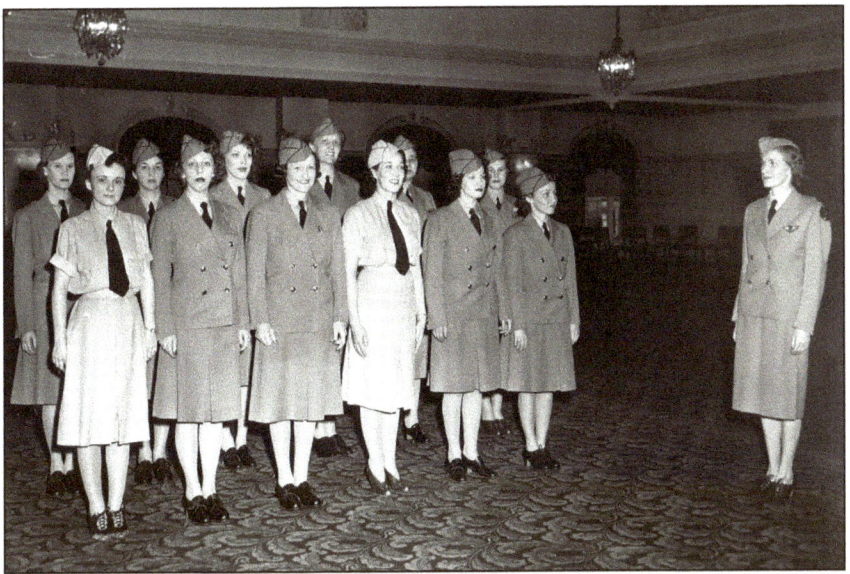

Figure 02.63. The Aviation Emergency Corps, Dayton, Ohio, Platoon, 1941. McGriff at right. Their cap pins identify them as AEC. MMM Collection.

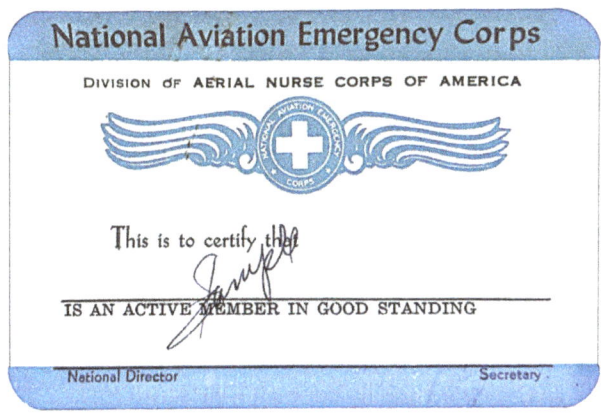

Figure 02.64. ID card for the National Aviation Emergency Corps. AMEDD.

Chapter Three
The WWII Effect

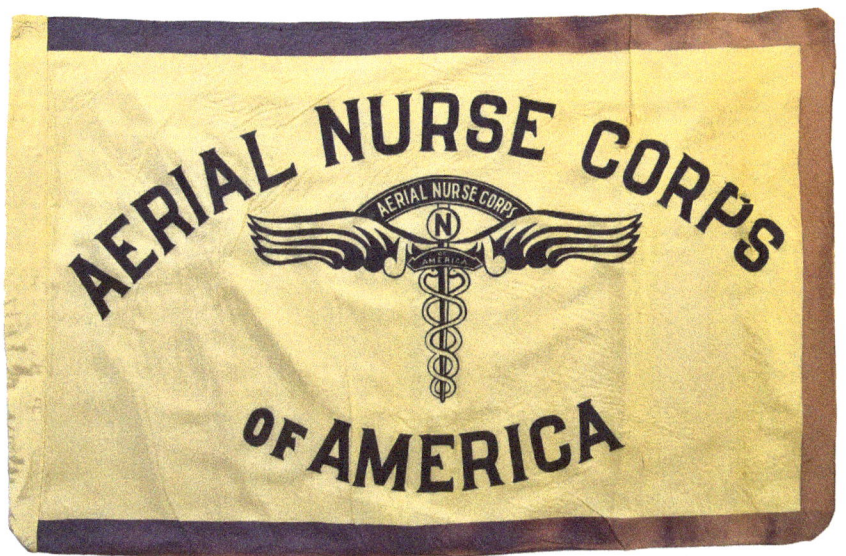

Figure 03.01. The official flag of the Aerial Nurse Corps of America, 2017. Courtesy of Ken LaRock, National Museum, USAF.

Schimmoler must have heard rumblings about a proposed start of the Civil Air Patrol (CAP), a civilian reserve organization for homeland defense. She wrote to the Director in October 1941 to inquire if ANCOA could affiliate with CAP. Reed Landis, Aide to the Director, replied they were setting up the Civil Air Patrol as a division of the Office of the Civilian Defense. CAP would be entirely voluntary for ground and flight personnel and open to men and women. They would offer national training. He said:

> Beyond a doubt, there will be a great need for service such as is rendered by groups similar to yours. However, this must essentially be a national organization to be thoroughly effective, and we hope members of your group will feel it possible to volunteer their services in the Civil Air Patrol. No organization will be affiliated with the Civil Air Patrol, but enlistment is open to individual applications.
>
> We would like to take this opportunity to commend to the Aerial Nurse Corps of America for the splendid preparatory

work they have done in emergency peacetime effort. Further details pertaining to the Civil Air Patrol will be available within the next few weeks through the Wing Command of the Civil Air Patrol, the State Departments of Aviation, and from the airport managers. [1]

The Civil Air Patrol opened its doors on 1 December 1941 [2] and it would permanently alter the direction of the ANCOA. Schimmoler had one week before everything changed for the group, before the world as she knew it, and as everyone else knew it, changed forever.

The following week, on 7 December, the Japanese bombed Pearl Harbor in Honolulu, Hawaii. The following day the Civil Aeronautics Authority grounded all aircraft except commercial airlines. [3] Private planes within 150 miles of the coastlines couldn't fly until further notice. [4] Schimmoler had struggled against the Red Cross, the nursing organizations, and the military, but she couldn't fight the effects of World War II.

With civilian planes down and no first-aid tents to staff or any patients to accompany, the ANCOA lost its basic function. Schimmoler left no words describing disappointments if she had any. Perhaps speaking such thoughts in light of the war felt trivial. Since the ANCOA had previously worked with the Sheriff's Aero Squadron, Schimmoler offered their services for ground support in whichever capacity they could fit.

By 11 January 1942, the Aero Squadron had assigned the Aviation Emergency Corps to fingerprint applicants for CAP volunteers. They worked Monday through Friday in four-hour shifts from 1:00 pm to 9:00 pm. Schimmoler reminded them after each shift:

> Clean the equipment and have it in readiness for the next day. You are reminded that promptness and neatness in your work will merit higher commendations. [5]

The government allowed pilots to keep flying if they joined CAP and parked their planes in a designated area with a 24-hour guard. Commander Bertrand Rhine of the California Wing sent an urgent call for pilots, radio operators, parachute riggers, and other help. He hoped owners of the 2,500 planes and the 3,000 licensed pilots would volunteer. Rhine directed volunteers to Grand Central Air Terminal, where "The Sheriff's Aero Squadron and the Aerial Nurse Corps of America are supervising." [6]

The National League of American Pen Women, a progressive press union for women writers and other artists, did their part and held several benefits to buy first-aid material for ANCOA's use with CAP. [7]

Although the director of CAP had made it clear in his previous letter to Schimmoler that CAP would not affiliate with any organization, their premier newsletter issue indicated otherwise:

> The Aerial Nurse Corps of America have volunteered as an auxiliary unit to the California Wing of the Civil Air Patrol. They are completely equipped through experience and supplies to serve in the field with the CAP even on an instant's notice.
>
> Members of the clerical division of the ANCOA have been serving at California Wing Headquarters since the office opening. Their assistance has been invaluable with organizational work of the California Wing. [8]

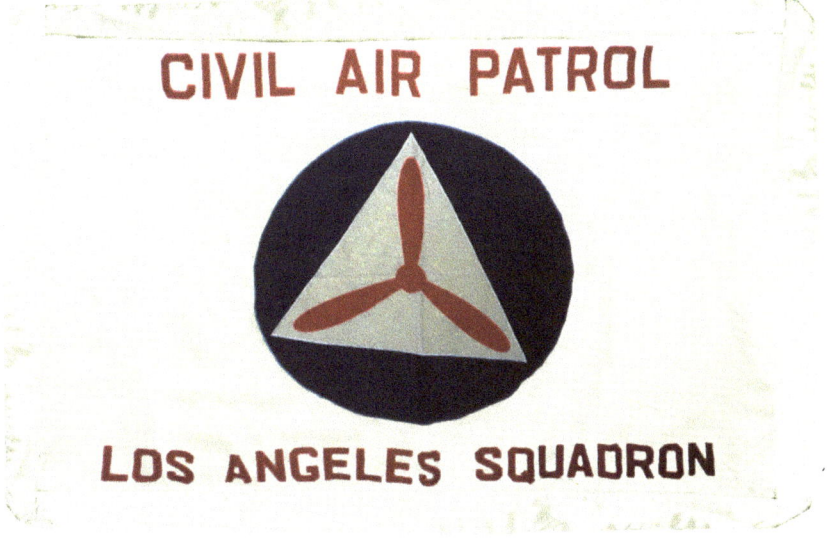

Figure 03.02. Los Angeles Civil Air Patrol flag, 1942. Author photographed.

A uniform shortage existed at the beginning of CAP; they rationed CAP uniforms. [9] Schimmoler requested to General Curry that ANCOA continue to use their own uniforms. He agreed, and she told Stroup, "Washington gave us their official sanction to wear them." They retained the Aerial Nurse pocket patch and ID badges but used the CAP shoulder patch and pin.

She further advised Stroup… "the CAP emblem is the same size, so they should stitch it on top of the ANCOA patch. If it's too bulky, they should remove it carefully because after the war, CAP will, no doubt, muster and fold up. ANCOA, of course, will go on." [10]

Chapter Three

Eventually, CAP became an auxiliary of the Air Force, awarded that status because of its history of military flying. The CAP Air Force members wore Air Force uniforms and used a mix of Air Force and CAP pins when on duty for the Civil Air Patrol.[11]

Shimmoler's CAP and Civil Defense patches and pins. Author photographed.

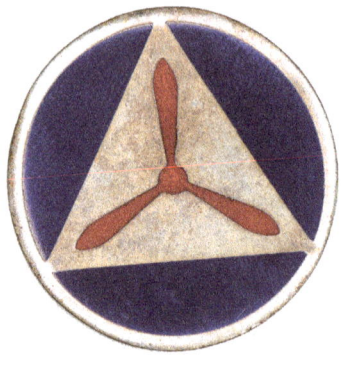

Figure 03.03. CAP pin, worn on the cap.

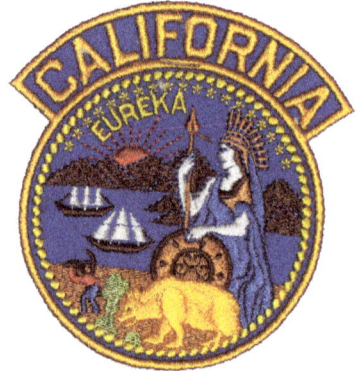

Figure 03.04. California CAP arm patch.

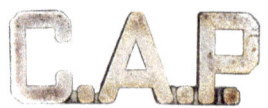

Figure 03.05. The Civil Air Patrol insignia lapel pin.

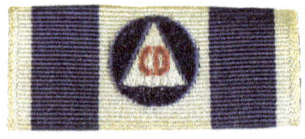

Figure 03.06. The Civil Defense ribbon, 1800 hours of service.

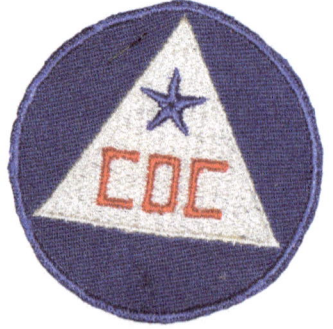

Figure 03.07. A Citizens Defense Corps patch with a star. The star above indicated the person was a staff member.

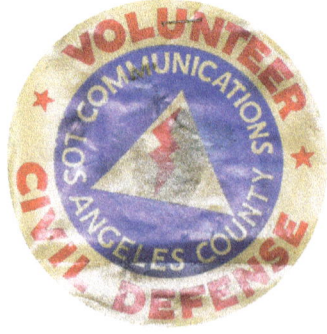

Figure 03.08. Communications Dept. Civil Defense sticker. The lightening bolt signified a Messenger Service Volunteer in Los Angeles County.

Schimmoler's three positions with the Civil Defense were as an Assistant Instructor, as Battalion Clerk with the Sheriff's Rifle Auxiliary, and as first aid instructor for the Sheriff's Department.

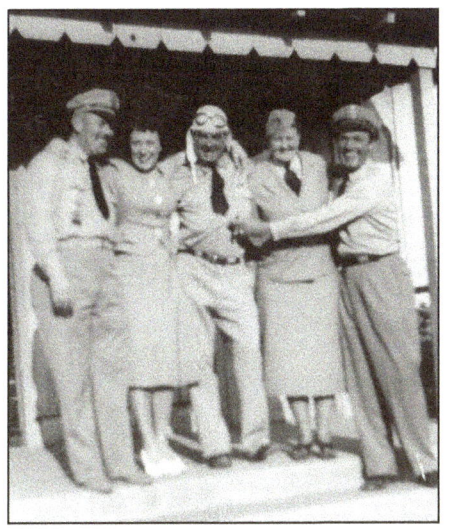 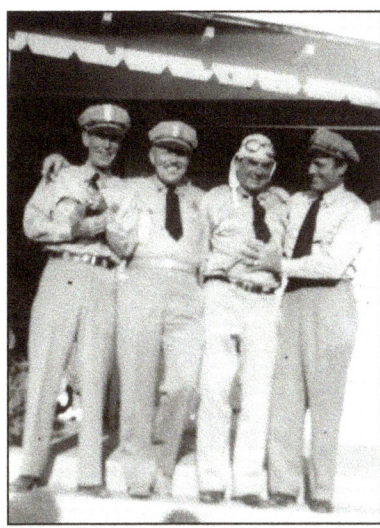

Figure 03.09. Schimmoler, fourth from left, with the Aero Detail Members. Figure 03.10. Sheriff's Aero Detail Members at the Sheriff's Rodeo, Santa Anita Race Track, 1942. Chief Kidder, Claude Morgan, Tex Rankin, and Dan King. BHS Collection.

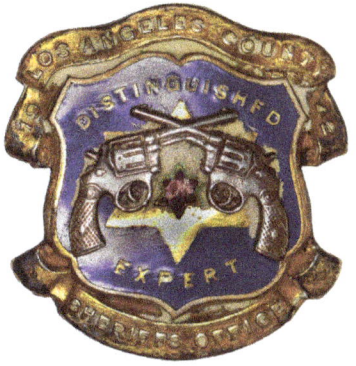 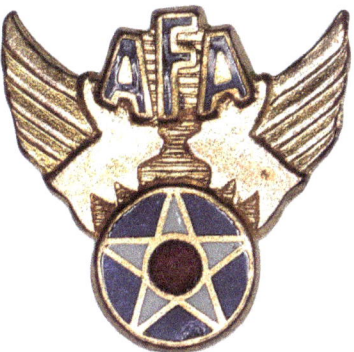

Figure 03.11. Schimmoler's Expert Rifle Medal with Distinction, awarded to Schimmoler by Lieutenant Griggers, the Chief of Aero Detail at the Los Angeles Sheriff's Department, 1942.

Figure 03.12. The Air Force Association of the Los Angeles Wing pin given to Schimmoler in 1942. Author photographed.

Chapter Three

Little is known of nurse Ruby Tallent—her uniform, ID, and patches are shown to demonstrate the actual colors of the uniform as most photographs from the era are in black and white. The reverse side of her ID states she had an affiliation with the Sheriff's Aero Squadron; she joined the ANCOA in April 1942 as member #594. Images courtesy of Centurion Auctions.

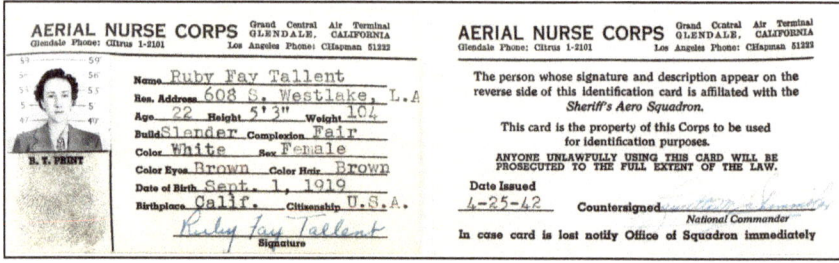

Figure 03.13. Identification Card, Ruby Fay Tallent, RN, 25 April 1942.

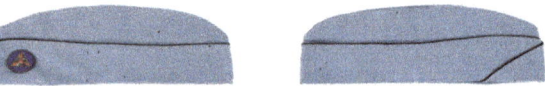

Figure 03.14. Tallent's ANCOA/CAP field cap with CAP pin, 1942.

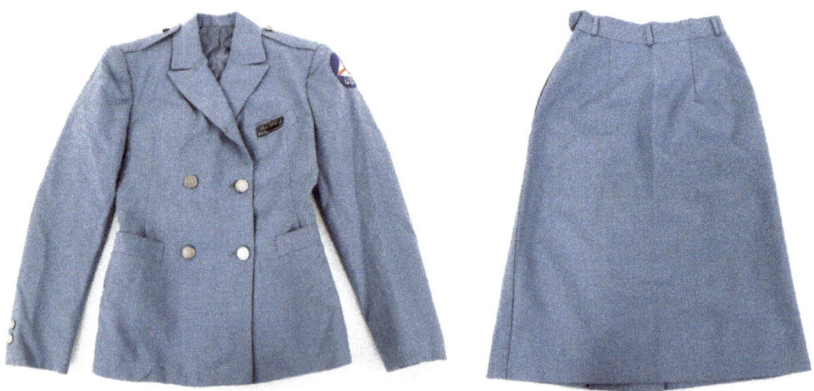

Figures 03.15. and 03.16. Blue ANCOA jacket and skirt Tallent wore with CAP, 1942. Note the combination of the CAP arm patch with the Aerial Nurse pocket patch.

Figure 03.17. An unknown patch from 1942. The W could have stood for Wing or Women's. Many CAP Wings had unique local patches. The patch was unattached to Tallent's uniform.

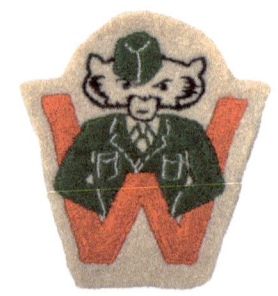

Merle McGriff McAfee, Dayton's Commander, taught a twenty-hour first aid course Washington required for all CAP members. CAP also required forty hours of infantry drills. [12]

The Dayton Company volunteered for the Civil Air Patrol. The *Journal Herald* printed the group's final story on their CAP emergency training day in October 1942:

> Army bombers roared overhead. Small training planes landed and took off in continuous streams on Municipal airport runways. Against this realistic backdrop, Dayton's Aerial Nurse Corps of America administered first aid to an accident victim and transferred her to an ambulance plane for transport to the hospital. While others of their profession answered the call to colors with the Army, Navy, or the Marine Nursing Corps, these blue-uniformed nurses are putting their shoulders to the Victory wheel at home.
>
> The ranks of the nursing profession, already seriously depleted by the demands of the armed forces, are not strained by enlistments of ANCOA members. These girls continue their daily work and swing into action with CAP after office and hospital hours. For the last two months, this group has gone through the paces with CAP under the direction of Squadron Commander Roy McGuire. [13]

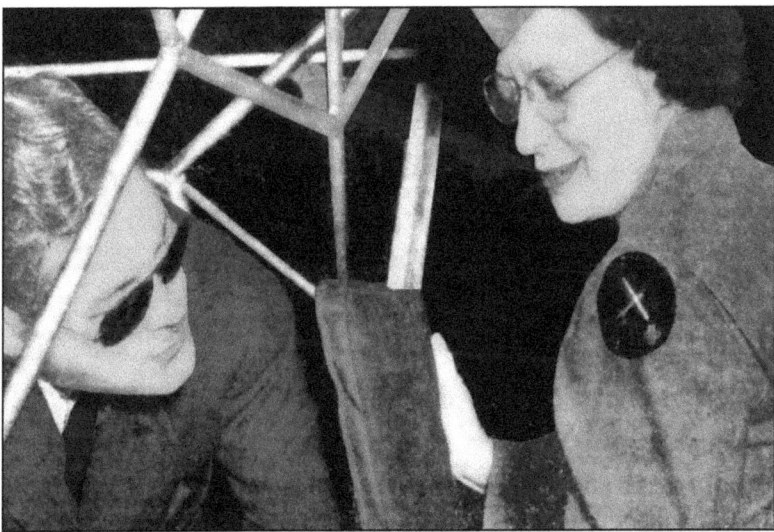

Figure 03.18. Suzanne Finke and Public Relations Employee W. J. Mitchel of the Aeronca Corporation discuss placement of the patient stretcher, 1942.

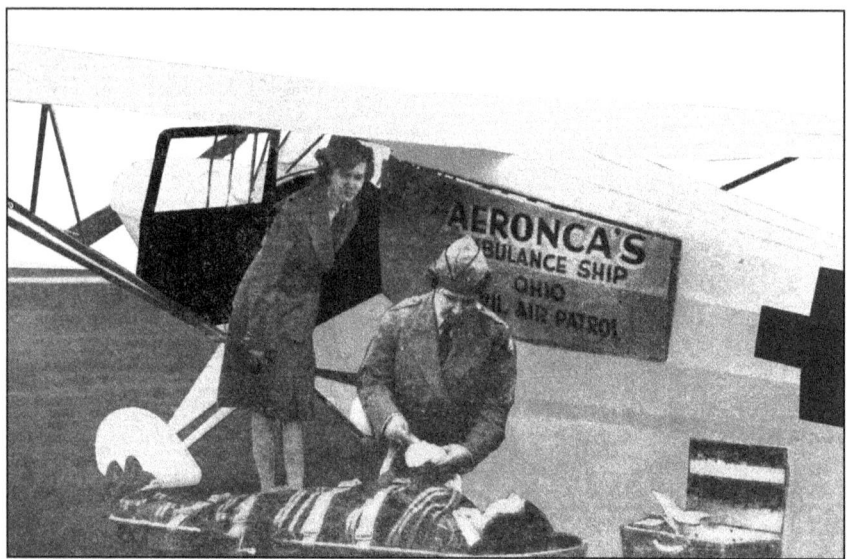

Figure 03.19. During the training day, Mae Moore applies a bandage, as Lucille Geary observes, 1942. Colorized clipping, MMM Collection.

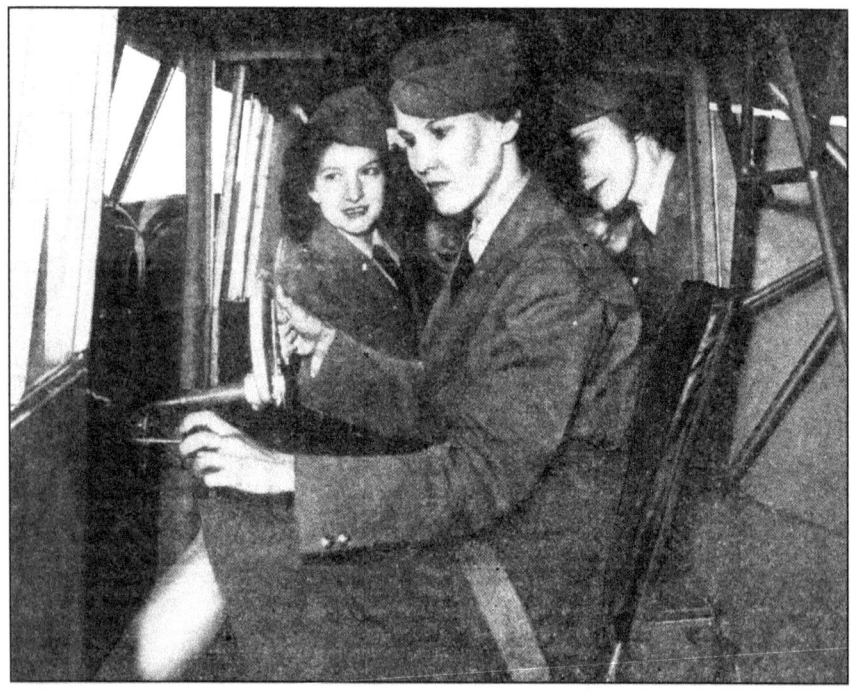

Figure 03.20. Geary investigates the airplane's controls from the pilot's seat as others look on, 1942.

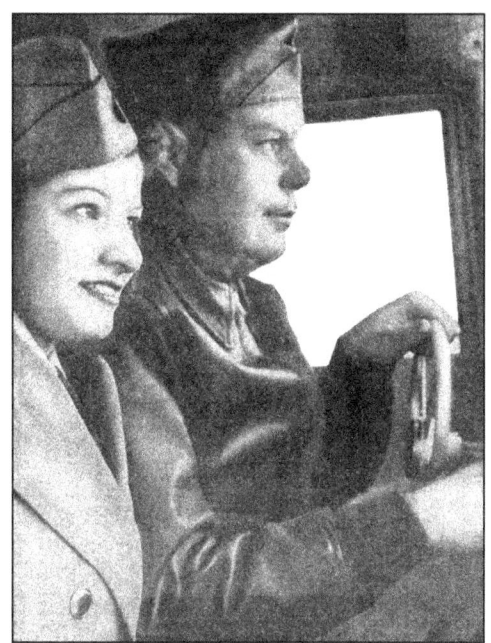

Figure 03.21. Member Mary Nell Goodman accompanies CAP Squadron Commander and Pilot Roy McGuire in the two-passenger Aeronca CAP ambulance plane, 1942.

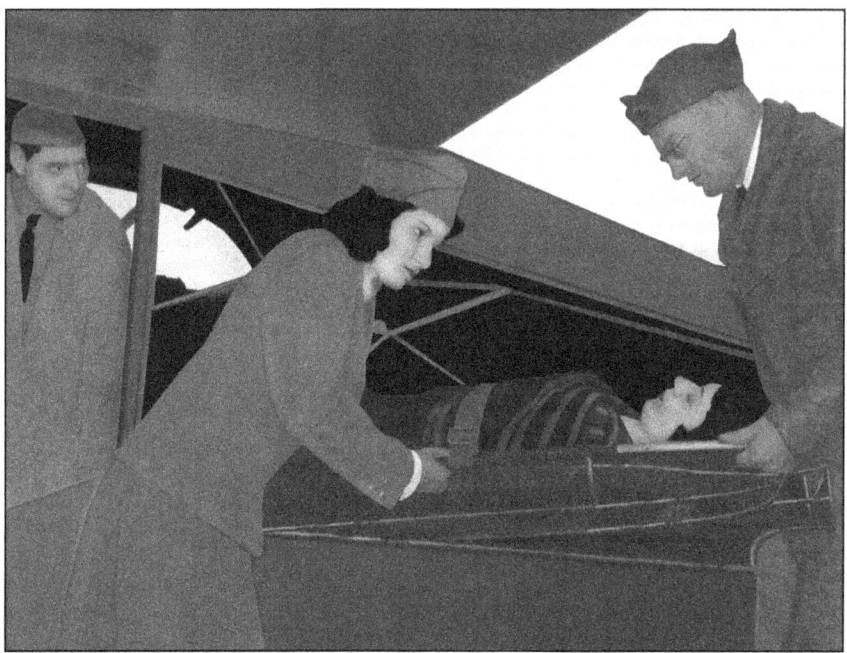

Figure 03.22. Goodman practices correct placement of the stretcher with CAP Pilots R.V. Clark, left, and R.B. Smith. Kathryn Finke poses as the patient, 1942. Colorized clipping, MMM Collection.

Chapter Three

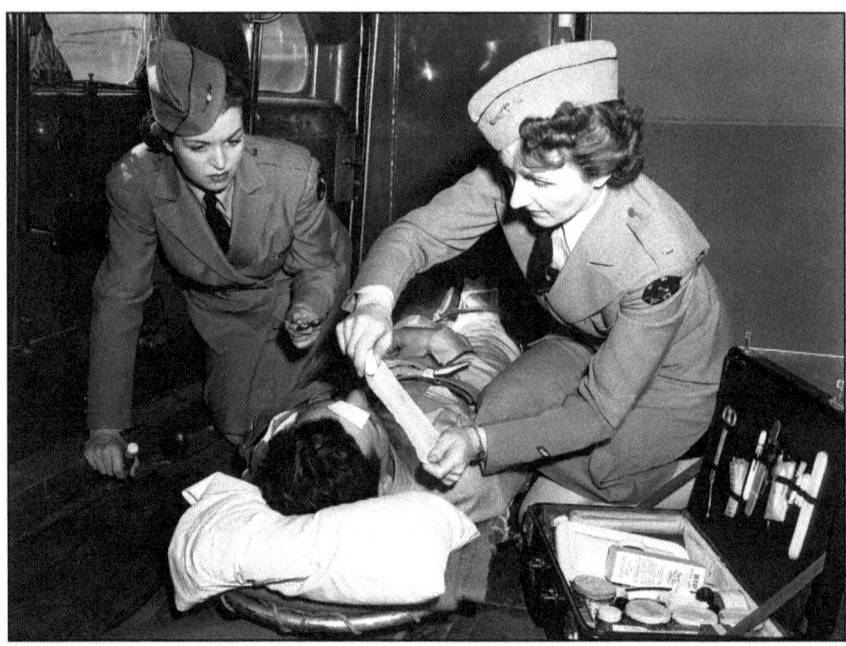

Figure 03.23. Tony Hoezart, RN, and First Aid Cadet Florence Heller of Company 1-A, demonstrating first aid to CAP, December 1941. BHS. Heller was a close friend of, and a movie stand-in for, Carole Landis. This photo could be the first ANCOA/AEC/CAP event as the members still wear the original patches and pins. CAP started in December 1941; ANCOA/AEC began using the CAP pin and arm patch in January 1942.

John Slevin, Medical Officer for the Army's Michigan Military, had told Stroup, "Within the next year, the call to active duty will deplete First Reserve Nurses. Your organization will lose many members." He was right. Schimmoler's Red Cross First Reserve requirement had an unplanned effect on the ANCOA: member depletion.

Weeks later, Stroup spoke to the Lansing Visiting Nurses Association on "Nursing and National Defense."[14] Many ANCOA nurses did join the military. Some non-nurses from the AEC also joined, but fewer because the war especially needed RNs. As CAP members, the AEC would keep the ANCOA alive—at least for a while.

Schimmoler wrote about successes to Stroup and Waples on 17 January 1942. The Sarasota Red Cross had placed the ANCOA in its headquarters. The Seattle Red Cross and the Defense Council turned over a high school near the airport for the ANCOA/AEC to use as a base hospital, and CAP gave them full charge of Boeing's Field and Plant. The Los Angeles group was the only personnel allowed at the National Guard airport; CAP offered them offices, hanger space, and a donated station wagon. The State Guard requested an RN be assigned duty at Griffith Park Airport to assist the Flight Surgeon. "I have been in uniform 18-20 hours daily," Schimmoler said. "I'm beginning to feel it."

Stroup wrote that Detroit's CAP had given them a "slap." They didn't want Company A-5's help. Schimmoler encouraged her, "One of these days, those fellows out at the City Airport are going to wake up."

By February, CAP was fully awake—they had accepted Company A-5 and even greatly needed their assistance. Stroup said:

> The roster of studies required by CAP is strikingly similar to the schedule of classes originated by the ANCOA. Our members are now qualified instructors with the Red Cross and have begun to teach First Aid to 400 or more pilots in the Detroit area now signed with the CAP, including the members of the Women's Squadron. They will also aid in teaching the Chemical Warfare Gases course.
>
> ANCOA members who are pilots are being assigned to the Women's Squadron in Detroit, Squadron #8, Group 2. [15]

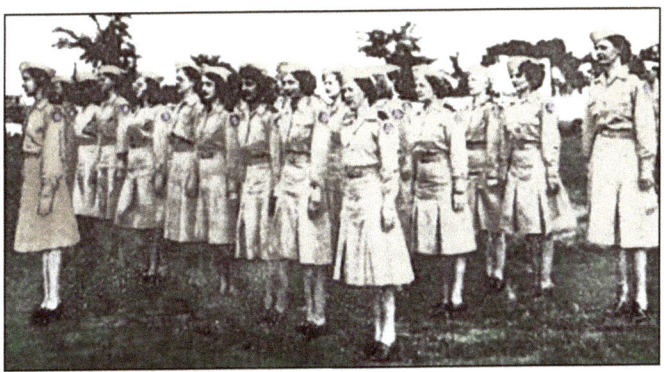

Figure 03.24. Women's CAP Squadron #8, Group 2, 1942. Leora Stroup Papers, AMEDD. The all-woman squadron had 41 pilots, including Stroup and other pilots from A-5. Alice Hammond, right, commanded the group.

Hammond competed in 16 transcontinental Air Races in the 1930s, placing in the top ten. She commanded the largest women's flying squadron in CAP during WWII and remained with CAP, Great Lakes, as a Lt. Colonel until 1961, moved to Philadelphia, and lastly to Illinois. She was the Ninety-Nines' President 1951-1953. President Kennedy honored her at the White House. [16-17]

Chapter Three

Stroup sent a detailed letter about the Los Angeles ANCOA's activities to the California Wing Commander and the U.S. Civil Air Patrol in March 1942—she had taken control as President Stroup. In her letter she referred to Schimmoler as the National Director. They had eliminated the ANCOA initiation fee but charged one dollar for the filing fee and the manuals. This same month Stroup accepted a position as the Director for Detroit's School of Practical Nurses.

Schimmoler wrote to Stroup and enclosed twenty dollars to ship the ANCOA flag to her (Stroup kept it in Detroit). She didn't specify why she needed the flag; Stroup didn't question her and sent it with the pole. Schimmoler soon told her she had signed a contract to be in a movie—they needed the flag as a prop.

Her work on the movie set, plus Schimmoler's CAP duties, might have overwhelmed her time, and she didn't write back to Stroup. In April, she asked Lida Dolan to contact Stroup on her behalf to say she would hear from her again after completing the movie. Stroup didn't reply.

On 11 May, Schimmoler wrote to Stroup on a U.S. CAP letterhead, asking her why she hadn't sent a report on CAP/ANCOA activities. She'd heard Stoup planned to enter the Army Nurse Corps and wondered who should take over the ANCOA duties in the Detroit area.

Finally, Stroup wrote back on 23 June. Schimmoler's quick reply on the 26th sounded as though she thought they might have had a split in their long friendship. Schimmoler said in her letter:

> I had not heard from you for so long that I began to think I would never hear from you again, and sincerely, Leora, I have never had anything to crush me as much as our break in friendship.

But their friendship had not broken. Stroup confirmed that she wished to preserve their friendship, and Schimmoler replied, "It has meant much to me…you will never know." [18]

Many reasons might have caused Stroup not to write: busy with her job as Director, CAP, plans to join the Army. Maybe she thought Schimmoler had neglected the ANCOA because of her film role. Did Stroup resent Schimmoler hadn't asked her to march in the movie with the others?

Regardless, neither archive contained additional letters concerning this issue. Stroup resigned and joined the Army a few months later. Schimmoler became President again and continued with the ANCOA.

The American Nurses Association hadn't sanctioned her air ambulance training, but they didn't control the military. Schimmoler hadn't given up that plan.

Although many ANCOA nurses had joined or would soon join various branches of the armed forces, she still hoped to have input in creating air ambulance training for the military. In July 1942, she wrote to Brigadier General David N. W. Grant, Air Surgeon for the Army Air Forces.

> Frankly, General, I have almost begun to think I am another Billy Mitchell. I have not, however, given up hope that somehow your department will create a school for nurses for air ambulance duty and that we might be accorded the consideration of doing our part in the operations of this school. I feel this department should be separate apart from the regular Army Nurse Corps and could be attached as a special unit of the Air Forces. [19]

The Army had tested an Air Ambulance plane in October 1940, but they hadn't considered training nurses for this purpose.[20] Now they did. Aerial evacuation was in the formative stages. Eventually, they would assign nurses with civilian aircraft experience from the Army Nurse Corps.

Grant encouraged ANCOA members to join. "Nurses are not recruited specifically for aerial duty but are being earmarked for this duty when the need arises."[21] The following month, he began implementing the air evacuation system.

The military hadn't previously considered nurses' air knowledge valuable, but that must have changed. The Red Cross added a check box about the ANCOA on its service application in 1942. Perhaps this was the earmark Grant referred to—they'd already discussed the idea with the Red Cross.

```
Are you now a member of the Aerial Nurse Corps of America?  Yes ☐   No ☐
Have you ever held a position as an air hostess?  Yes ☐   No ☐   How long?..............
FIRST RESERVE NURSES (Single and under 40 years)
    If not already serving with the armed forces, when and under what circumstances will you be available?............

        YOUR VALUE AS A RED CROSS RESERVE NURSE DEPENDS ON OUR ABILITY TO LOCATE YOU. THE NATIONAL
        EMERGENCY EMPHASIZES THIS FACT MORE THAN EVER. THANK YOU FOR FILLING IN THIS QUESTIONNAIRE
                                AND RETURNING IT TO US.

APR 6 1942
```

Figure 03.25. Red Cross Nursing Application clipping, 1942. National Archives.

Chapter Three

The highest highs and the lowest lows happened to Schimmoler in 1942, events she could not foresee. How did it happen that Hollywood came calling? War movies were the rising art. The economy, the style of dress, and life, in general, became centered on WWII, including the movies. The U.S. Treasury Department even used war-movie stars to sell war bonds. The Victory Caravan of stars traveled by train across the county and made stops, giving shows for the war effort. As Bob Hope said, "They had no trouble getting stars; who in Hollywood had the guts to tell the IRS he was going to be out of town?" [22]

Columbia Pictures hired Schimmoler as a technical expert for the war-movie *Parachute Nurse*. The plot centered on a group of nurses who had become bored working at Mitchel Reed Hospital and wanted to try something new. They joined a newly formed military group of nurses who would parachute into remote areas to render medical care. Danger, romance, a potential murder, and petty female arguments drove the plot.

The director thought Schimmoler fit the role of Captain Jane Morgan, the Commander of the Parachute Corps. Did her movie-star friend, Victor McLaglen, suggest her? The script described Morgan as "a very efficient, good-looking, plump, motherly woman, with a hardboiled exterior and a heart as big as her frame, which is ample." [23] Morgan waited in her Captain's Room, poised to whip into shape any nurse who might stray from the impeccable requirements. Naturally, one nurse did, which required Captain Morgan to force the nurse to resign. Morgan demanded:

> When I give the command ATTENTION, I want you to straighten up, stomachs in, chest out, chin up, shoulders back, eyes front, and no talking. And after a day of exhausting training drills—cheer up girls. Another week and you won't even know you have a muscle. [24]

Sixty-two members of the ANCOA color guard marched wearing their ANCOA/AEC uniforms. In the opening scene, they carried a flag with the Aviation Emergency Corps name and emblem—either a new AEC flag or a movie prop. In the closing scene march, however, they carried the ANCOA flag. Close examination of their cap pins indicates most marchers were AEC members.

The nurse actors and the show's stars wore the ANCOA uniform and first division arm patch but not the aerial nurse pocket patch. And although they were movie nurses, they used an AEC cap pin, not the ANCOA nurse cap pin. Schimmoler used both pins—sometimes, she wore the ANCOA nurse pin on her cap, and sometimes, the AEC pin. Naturally, she wore her commander pocket patch.

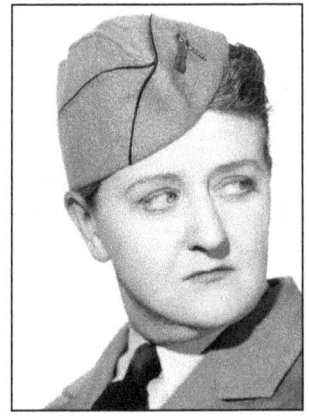 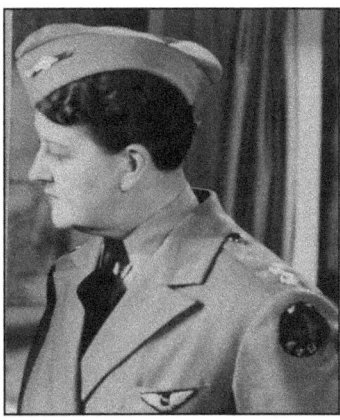

Figures 03.26. Schimmoler as Captain Jane Morgan, April 1942. Note the ANCOA cap pin on the left and the AEC pin on the right. BHS Collection.

The opening roll of the movie thanked the Aerial Nurses Corps of America and the Aviation Emergency Corps and dedicated it to military nurses:

> And to the women who realize that while this story is pure fiction, the idea is real and vital. To the Parachute Nurses preparing to play their parts in the defense of, and aid to, the United States. To the Paranurses who are ready for the fiction of today to become the reality of tomorrow, this picture is affectionately and respectfully dedicated. 25

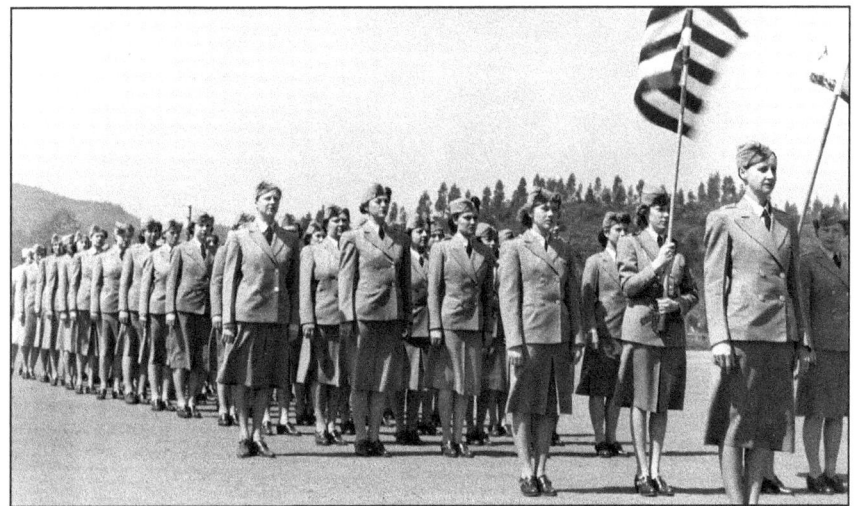

Figure 03.27. Los Angeles, West Los Angeles, and Glendale Platoons Color Guard marching in the movie *Parachute Nurse*, April 1942. MMM.

Schimmoler had considered the idea of parachute training for the ANCOA, but she said:

> It seems unnecessary for women nurses to run the risks of being dragged in rough terrain, being impaled in a tree, landing in water, or suffering other casualties...it seems to me that it will only be practical to train parachute nurses when there is an actual shortage of manpower. [26]

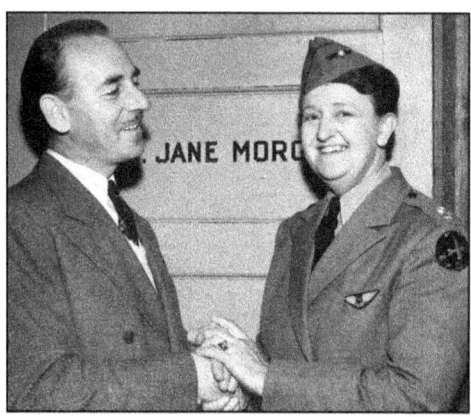

Figure 03.28. Schimmoler on the set of *Parachute Nurse*, standing in front of her Commander's Room, with William Wright, who played Lieutenant Woods—one of the few male roles in the movie. BHS Collection.

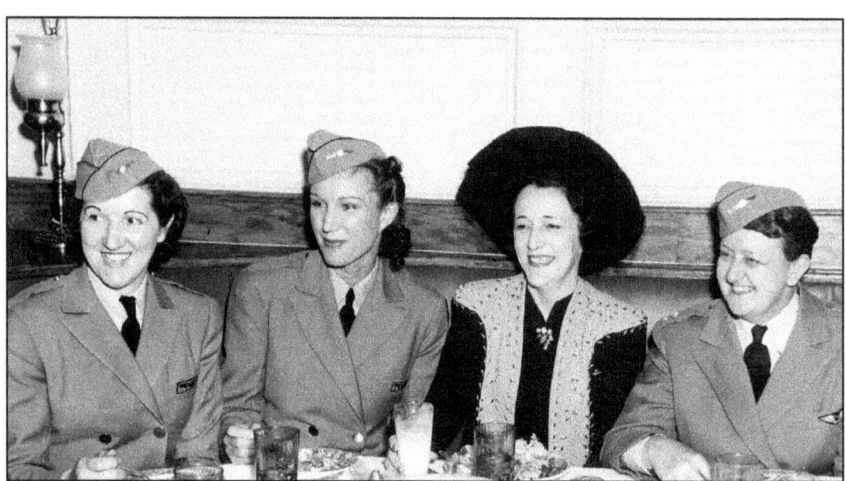

Figure 03.29. Dinner at the Brown Derby Restaurant in Los Angeles, 1942. Schimmoler invited several ANCOA members to dine at the famous Brown Derby Restaurant. In the hat is Juliette Sherman Toy, whom Schimmoler said was her "good friend and aid in organization." BHS Collection.

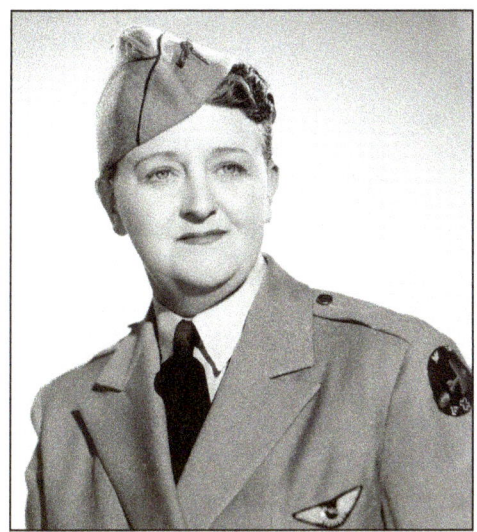

Figure 03.30. "One-Take Schimmoler," in *Parachute Nurse*, 1942. BHS.

The scenes in which Schimmoler appeared did not require retakes. Thus, she became known as "One-Take Schimmoler." The lure of Hollywood made her dream she could work as a character actress.[27] She procured a seven-year contract with the Jules C. Goldstone Agency, obliging a 10% commission. She paid dues to the Screen Actors Guild of Hollywood and waited for a follow-up movie. But like many other actors, Hollywood did not call again.

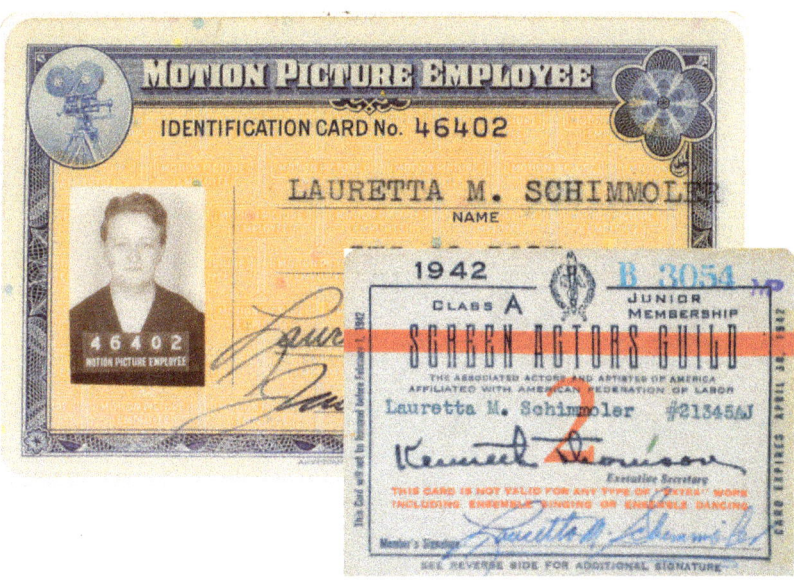

Figure 03.31. Schimmoler's Motion Picture and Screen Actors Guild cards. BHS.

Chapter Three

Although Schimmoler's activities with ANCOA decreased, she continued to receive accolades and awards:

- Station WGN, a very widely broadcast television channel from Chicago, saluted her with a "Bouquet of Honor Award" for recognition of her service in organizing and heading the ANCOA. [28]
- The historical aviation book *Women with Wings* and various others list her many accomplishments. [29]
- In 2011, the Air Force Association awarded its first "Schimmoler Award" for Aero Evacuation excellence. [30]
- Crawford County Veterans inducted her into its Hall of Fame.

Schimmoler's acting career hadn't progressed. Many ANCOA nurses had joined the armed forces. Some groups still invited her to present at meetings, but those requests were few and paid even less. The CAP and Civil Defense volunteer positions gave her no salary—she needed to pay her bills.

Schimmoler didn't accept an offered position in the Women's Auxiliary Army Corps (WAAC), because she was completing a course on aircraft engines. She hoped for a civilian role, not a military one. [31] She had a good reason—jobs in the civilian industry paid better. Unequal benefits with men, and poor attitudes within the Army about women, made the WAACs an undesirable choice. Few women joined. On 1 July 1943, the Army dropped the auxiliary status and renamed it the Women's Army Corps (WAC). The WACs were now part of the Army, giving women rank and privileges. [32]

She found successive posts with the Civil Aeronautics Administration. In August 1942, the CAA hired her as an Airport Traffic Controller Trainee, but she found a more exciting position after one year.

On 4 August 1943, she accepted a position with the U.S. Navy Bureau of Aeronautics as an Assistant Inspector of Engineering Materials, Aero, with the Inspector of Naval Aircraft, Vega Aircraft Corporation in Burbank. They assigned her a Grade of CAF-4 with a salary of $1,800 per annum ($31,806 in 2023). [33]

After working one year as an inspector, she decided to serve her county in some capacity. Later in her life, Schimmoler hinted she wished she'd studied nursing so she could be a flight nurse like her friends. She told Flight Nurse Colonel Kovach, "Would that it were possible to turn back the clock that I might qualify for active duty in such a rewarding way." [34]

Because experienced male pilots had enlisted for duty overseas, the U.S. faced a critical pilot shortage to deliver new planes from factories to local military bases. In 1942, the U.S. developed an experimental program to train female pilots to fly military aircraft—the Women's Air Force Service Pilots (WASP). More than 1,100 women flew B-26 bombers, B-29 bombers, and most every style of military aircraft.[35] With Schimmoler's knowledge of flying and airplane mechanics, she would have been perfect for that job and undoubtedly pleased to join. Unfortunately, the age limit for WASP duty was 35. Schimmoler was 42.

Schimmoler didn't indicate the date she ceased association with the ANCOA/AEC, but she left a simple statement:

> With the cessation of civilian flying and nurses entering the services, I have regretfully closed my offices in Burbank after placing my Los Angeles clerical staff with the War Operations in the Sheriff's Department. Devoted to the cause, which was my main interest in life, they established a fine record there.[36]

On 2 February 1944, a *Flashes* page cited rules and reporting directions for the War Operations Center—her last known ANCOA documentation.

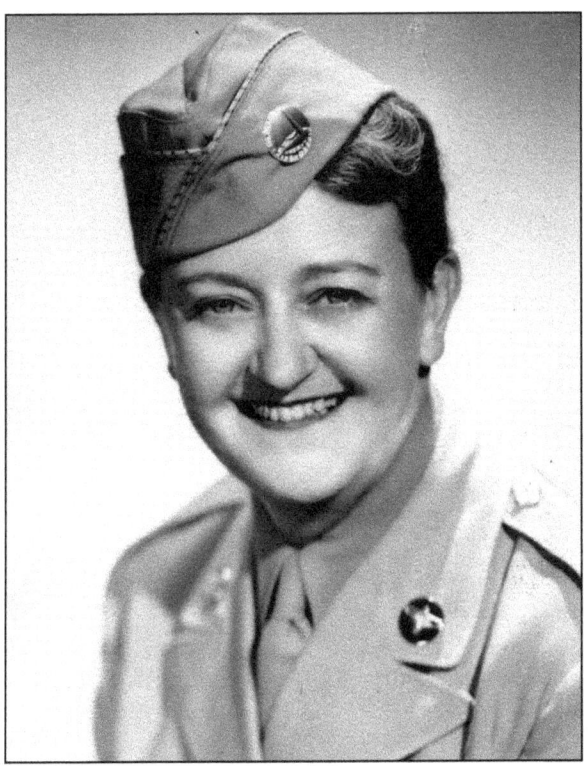

Figure 03.32. Schimmoler in her WAC uniform, 1944. BHS.

Chapter Three

Schimmoler requested leave from her civilian Navy position. On 22 July 1944, she enlisted in the WACs. She completed basic training at Fort De Moines, Iowa, on 12 September and reported to Fairfield-Suisun Air Force Base, California (renamed Travis Air Force Base in 1950) on 17 September. They assigned her to Aircraft Dispatch.

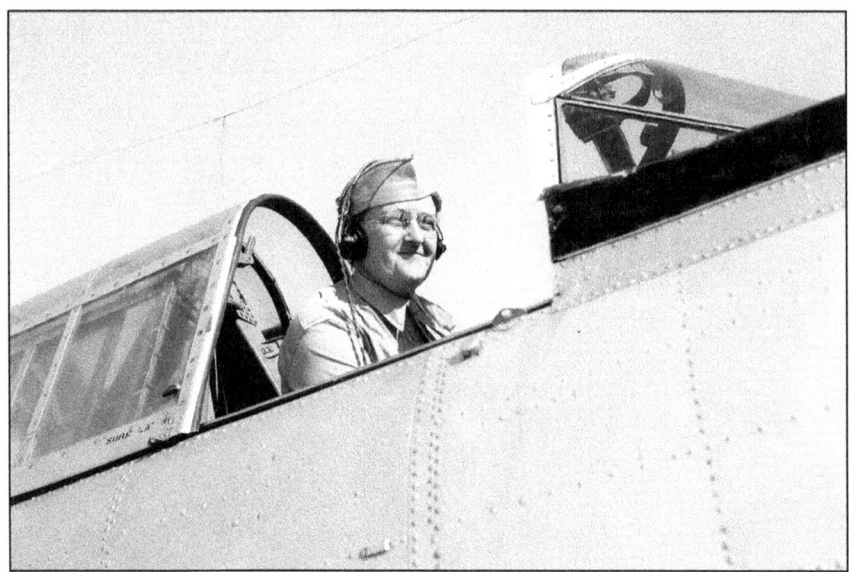

Figure 03.33. Schimmoler at Fairfield-Suisan Air Force Base, 1944. BHS.

Dispatcher wasn't the ideal job to commensurate with her knowledge of planes, but women only occupied one position in the Army Air Force—flight nurse. They couldn't even assign her to repair airplanes. At least Aircraft Dispatcher allowed her to work around aircraft. And it placed her in the perfect location for a most significant event that happened one night.

Although she didn't document the exact day, the remarkable event occurred at Fairfield. She recalled that night:

> Providence had seen to it that I should be the one, alone, on duty one night, in base operations to receive a message that a C-54 ambulance plane would land at Fairfield.
>
> The hospital had been notified, and the ground ambulances were dispatched to a waiting location on the field. Interest was high at the base, as we were about to see the first of many wounded men flown in by air ambulance from the Pacific, attended by flight nurses. This one carried its full capacity, flying direct from Guadalcanal in 36 hours.

We watched and waited. In less than 20 minutes from the time the message was received, the giant C-54, with its precious cargo aboard, gently set its wheels down on the runway. Aided by the alert crew, it was guided to a location directly in front of base operations, where I was on duty.

The Captain climbed down from the fifteen-foot ladder and walked to the office. He remarked that we were not well equipped to handle the unloading of patients from a C-54. There wasn't much I could say. We were not, for this was the first for me. Not until I had received the message from Hamilton Field advising of a change in flight plans due to fog in that area had I any knowledge of the forthcoming arrival of air ambulances.

The Captain went back to the airplane to supervise the unloading of the patients. Since we did not have available, at that time, the type of hoist that would reach the door of the C-54, the patients had to come down the long ladder, a slow process, particularly for the stretcher cases. They were placed in the waiting ambulance and taken to our base hospital for a rest, fresh dressings placed on their wounds, and such treatments as needed, and later to be flown in Air Evac planes to the hospitals nearest their homes.

When the first stretcher made its appearance in the open door of the plane, and they began to move slowly down the ladder, I was overcome by it for the moment. I said aloud, **AND THEY SAID IT WOULDN'T BE DONE.** There in the dark night, alone in the dispatch office doorway, I was witnessing a culmination of years of efforts and hopes that had at last become a reality. [37]

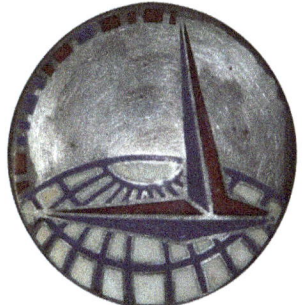 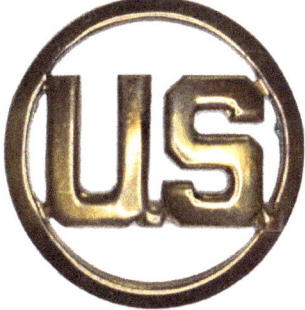

Figure 03.34. The WAC Air Transport Cap Pin for WWII.
Figure 03.35. Schimmoler's U.S. Lapel Pin for WWII, 1944.

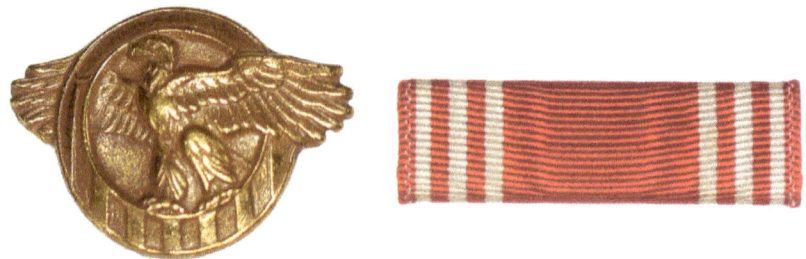

Figure 03.36. Schimmoler's honorable discharge pin, the "Ruptured Duck," 1945. The Army awarded veterans this pin upon leaving military service. Figure 03.37. Her WWII good conduct ribbon, 1945. Author photographed.

The Army released Schimmoler from service on 25 September 1945. She returned to her previous job at the Inspection Department of the U.S. Navy Bureau of Aeronautics but only remained for one year.

Pacific Airmotive Corporation (PAC) in Burbank hired her as an Assistant Dealer Sales Manager in 1946. PAC was an aircraft repair and overhaul company involved in many aspects of aero repair. They repaired large and small plane engines and sold parts. At one time, PAC employed over 1,500 people and was the world's most extensive overhaul and repair shop.[38] Schimmoler remained at PAC through 1949.

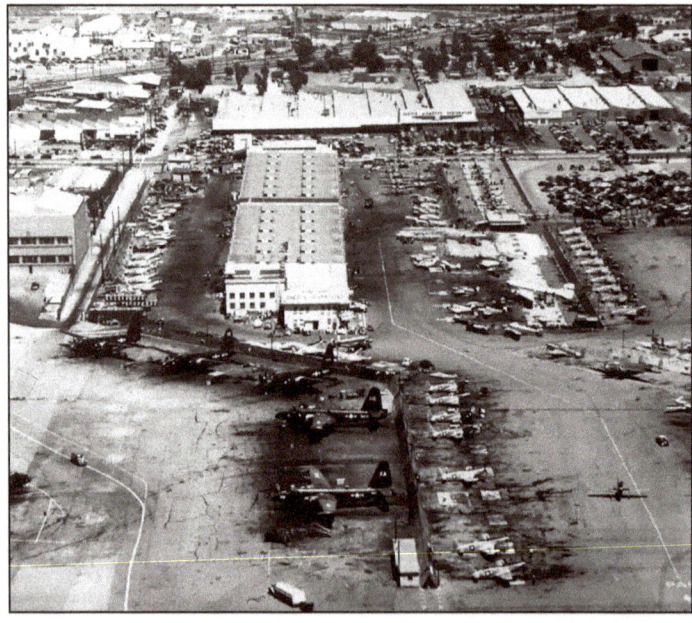

Figure 03.38 Pacific Airmotive Corporation in Burbank, California, 1946.

Schimmoler continued with her patriotic spirit. In 1946, she organized the American Legion Post 678 in Glendale, California, and dedicated it to the memory of her good friend Amelia Earhart. On 2 July 1937, at age 39, Earhart's plane was lost en route to Howland Island from Lae, New Guinea, in the Pacific Ocean.

The Post received its permanent charter on 24 October 1946. [39] With this charter, Schimmoler became the first woman to command an American Legion Post. She stayed active in Post 678 as a Life Member. They had initially named it the Women's Aviation Post 678 as it was the first aviation post for women, but three months after its organization they changed the name to the Amelia Earhart Post 678. [40-41]

Shortly after Post 678 opened, the Lockheed Corporation, an American aerospace company, commissioned artist Ralph C. Tripp from their illustration department to paint a portrait of Amelia Earhart to hang in Post 678. [42] They also presented the Post with a statuette. Lockheed had created the statuette several years before—they'd planned to give it to Earhart to commemorate her successful equatorial flight if she had completed that infamous journey. [43]

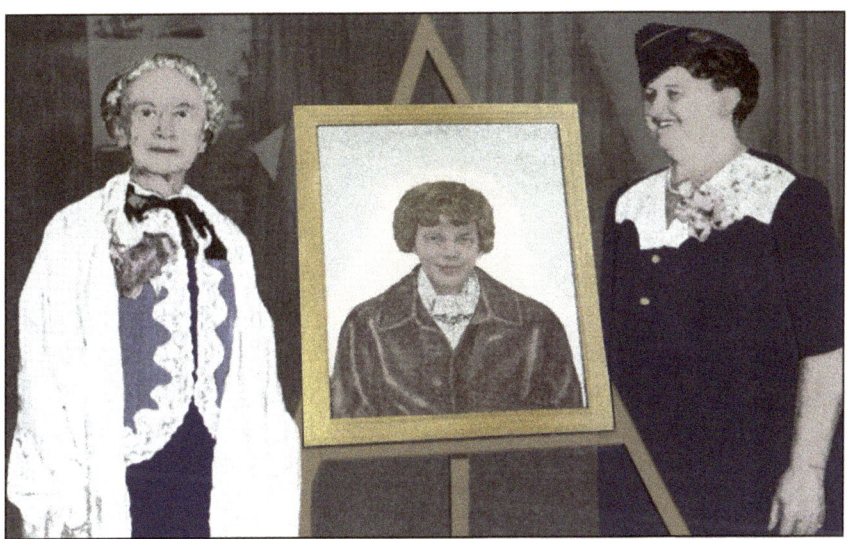

Figure 03.39. Amy Otis Earhart, Amelia Earhart's mother, at 79 years old, standing next to the painting of Amelia Earhart and Lauretta Schimmoler, taken at the dedication of American Legion Post 678 on 1 November 1946. Colorized clipping. Photograph by Paul R. Cramer, *Valley Times*.

At the ceremony her mother said, even nine years and four months later, she had never given up hope that her daughter would someday be found alive. [44]

Chapter Three

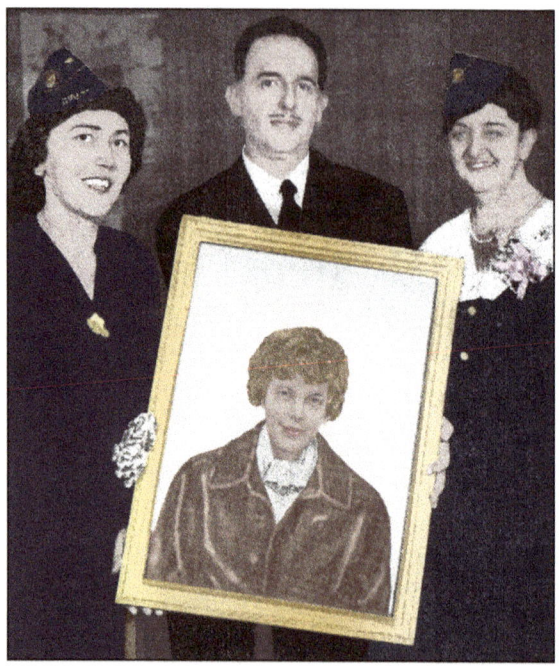

Figure 03.40. Mary Alexander, Vice Commander; Ralph C. Tripp, artist of the painting; and Lauretta Schimmoler, the Commander of Post 678, 1 November 1946. Colorized clipping, *Lockheed Star*.

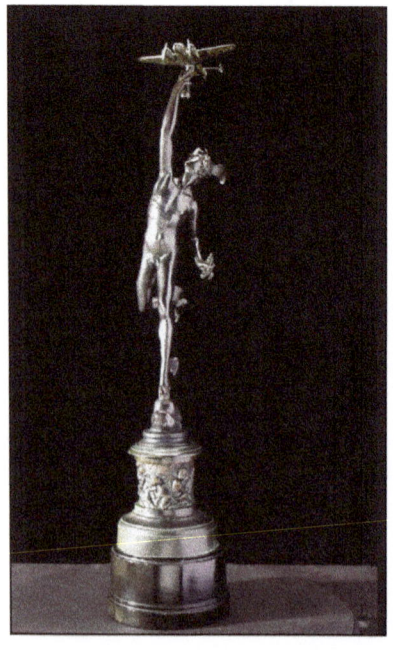

Figure 03.41. The Earhart Statuette, 1946. A pewter sculpture of the Roman God Mercury, holding a Lockheed Electra. Lockheed created the trophy for Earhart but gave it to Post 678 because Earhart didn't return from her flight. The Post gave it to the Ninety-Nines, and, eventually they donated it to the Smithsonian Museum. Photo by Eric Long, Courtesy of Smithsonian National Air and Space Museum.

The National Aviation Club resurrected the statue in 1996 and renamed it the Stinson Award to honor the Stinson sisters. The club awards the trophy annually for women's achievements in aviation and space. The Stinson sisters, Katherine and Marjorie, were the pilot trainers at their family's Stinson School of Flying beginning in 1912. Their stunt pilot father, Eddie, founded the Stinson Aircraft Company in 1920. Katherine became the 4th woman in the U.S. to obtain a pilot's license; she set many aerobatic flying records. Marjorie was the only women in the Aviation Reserve Corps; she trained WWI pilots.[45]

Before Earhart left on her fateful flight, she gave her 99 logo flying suit to Schimmoler and she placed the suit on display at Post 678. After the Post disbanded, someone gave the suit to former ANCOA Commander and Ninety-Nines Wisconsin club member Florence Fintak. The *99 Newsletter* reported Fintak had received it from "a friend of Amelia's." They didn't specify the friend was Schimmoler, but it seems likely. Fintak donated it to the Ninety-Nines; they displayed the suit in their headquarters in Oklahoma City in 1974.[46]

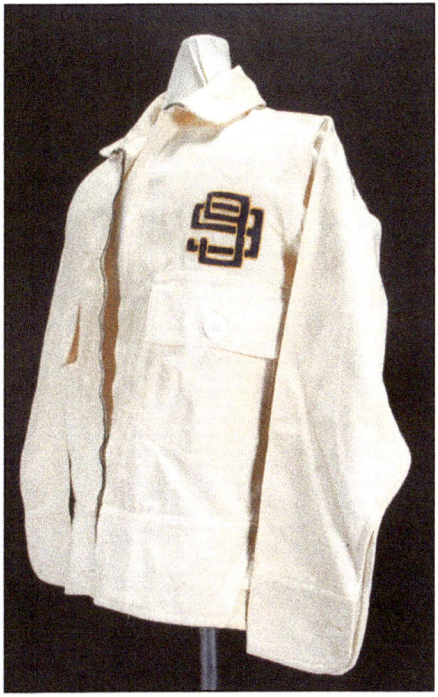

Figure 03.42. The 99 interlocking logos, two-piece, Amelia Earhart-designed suit she left with Schimmoler before her flight. Courtesy of the Smithsonian National Air and Space Museum.

Eventually, the Ninety-Nines donated the suit to the Smithsonian, credited as donated from American Legion Post 678. Earhart had designed the two-piece flying suit for the Ninety-Nines. Although the group never formally adopted the suit, the interlocking "9s" became their logo and they used the design for their membership pin in 1939.[47]

Chapter Three

Schimmoler was Commander during the 1st and the 17th years of Post 678. She also held other positions: Service Officer, 1946-1948; Chaplain; Executive Committee, 1963; Judge Advocate, 1966; and Historian.

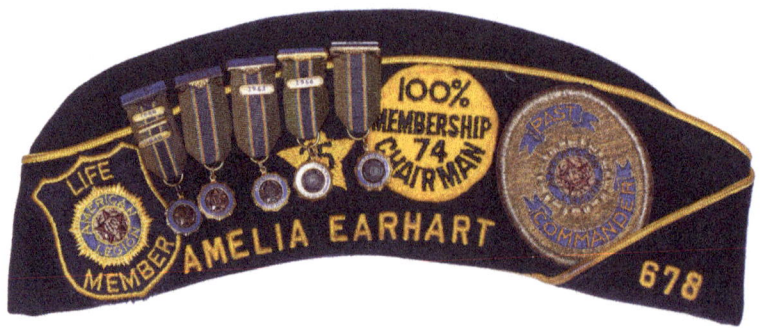

Figure 03.43. Schimmoler's American Legion cap with Past Officer's ribbon insignias. The Legion gave Past Officer's ribbon insignias to retiring officers to express gratitude and appreciation for services well rendered.

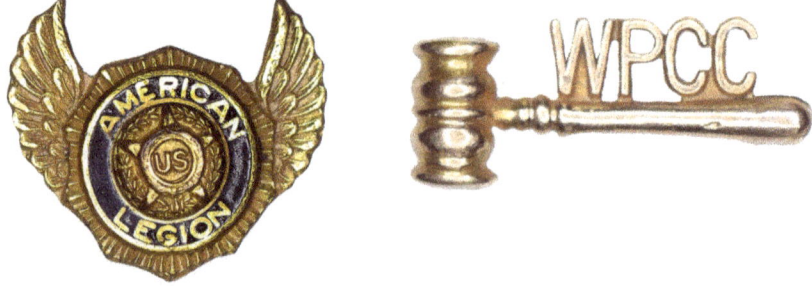

Figure 03.44. Schimmoler's American Legion dress pin for Post 678. Figure 03.45. Schimmoler's Women's Past Commanders Club of California pin. Author photographed at BHS.

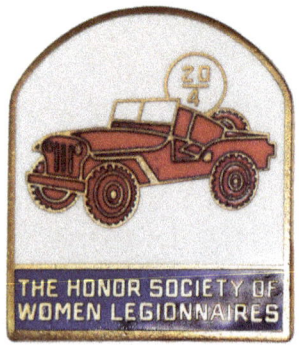

Figure 03.46. Schimmoler's National Honor Society pin, 20/4, the American Legion Echelon 1, California.

The Twenty and Four charters help women veterans in multiple ways. Members are women who served in U.S. military services during their designated wartime period. Membership recognizes the achievements of the American Legion women and is by invitation only.[48]

In 1933 the American Legion started an annual event called the Aerial Roundup or fly-in. These membership drives pitted all American Legion Posts in the United States against each other to see who could bring in the most new members for that year. New members would fill out cards with their names and additional information, and the roundup group would gather them in bundles.

The group would hop into a plane (primarily private) and race to the national headquarters at Weir Cook Airport in Indianapolis, Indiana. They flew in different size aircraft depending on the group size and availability. Seventy or more Post member planes would converge on the airport daily. In 1946 the enrollment of the American Legion neared 3,000,000. The 1946 roundup added 250,000 members.

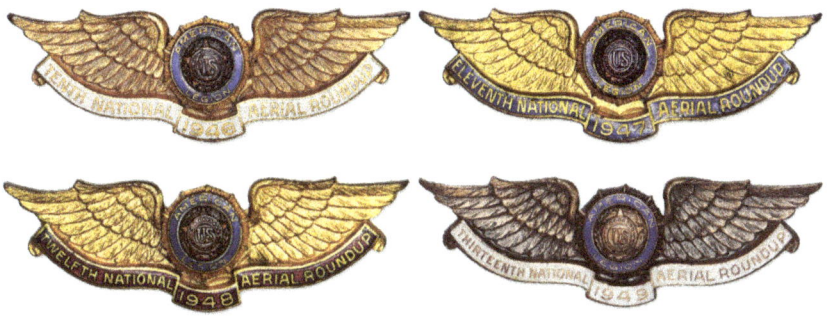

Figure 03.47. Schimmoler's American Legion Aerial Roundup Wings, 1946-1949. Authors photographed at BHS.

Naturally, they revised the event when WWII grounded private planes; during that time, they used airmail planes. After the war, they restarted the event.[49] They awarded prizes for competitions within the contest, as pilots often did in those days, such as the longest total distance traveled and other challenges. American Legion Officials awarded pins and trophies.

Schimmoler didn't leave a notation if she piloted the planes or accompanied a group, but she received four years of pins for the Amelia Earhart Post 678. The Aerial Roundups continued for 80 years.[50] As flight's silver age waned, drive-in replaced most fly-in roundups. Schimmoler remained an active member of 678 until it disbanded due to lack of membership. Post 678 transferred to Glendale Post 127 in 1975.[51]

After leaving the Pacific Airmotive Corporation job in 1949, Schimmoler switched focus and moved away from aeronautics entirely. The Sheriff's Department hired her as a detective in their anti-subversive division, investigating possible communist infiltrators during the 1950s cold war.[52]

Chapter Three

Perhaps the offer came from the long-time relationship she developed with the Sheriffs during her years in the ANCOA and the Civil Defense.

In 1945 Hubert Coleman, Ph.D., Professor of History at East Carolina College and a historian for the Army Air Force services during WWII, wrote to Schimmoler. He was gathering information for his book *Medical Support of the Army Air Forces in World War II*.

Coleman had searched the files of General Arnold. He found Schimmoler's letters explaining the tenants of ANCOA and her attempts to persuade the Red Cross and the Army of their potential value. He wrote to her:

> Your letter of October 19, 1940, to General Arnold is the last communication of yours that I have found in our files. I should like to have complete information about the Aerial Nurse Corps of America from that date to the present.
>
> Did the Nursing Divisions of the Red Cross and the Army ever recognize your organization? How many of your members are flight nurses in the Army today? I know that Captain Leora B. Stroup, once treasurer of the ANCOA, is on duty with the Air Evacuation Units. [53]

Schimmoler replied with a three-page letter explaining ANCOA history, her initial 1932 communication with the Director of the Red Cross, the first National Air Races in 1936 with a summary of other activities, the various manuals she had written and copyrighted, and the fees the nurses paid.

She continued her thoughts that its failure was because its President wasn't a nurse and the cessation of civilian flying due to the war. She mentioned the great reward of seeing the C-54 land with 26 patients and attendant flight nurses. She ended with her undeveloped but in-process idea to continue a peace-time program for the ANCOA. As to those numbers of ANCOA nurses in the military, she couldn't be sure:

> With reference to the number of ANCOA members now serving as Army Flight Nurses in Air Evacuation Units, I do not have a list available here to acknowledge this question inasmuch as I have lost track of some of them since their going into the service. I could, however, if it were possible to see a Roster of the Flight Nurses, and check the ones who were originally members of the ANCOA. [54]

No one ever sent her a roster of the Flight Nurses. Schimmoler and others estimated 400 ANCOA nurses joined various military forces during WWII.

While a count of ANCOA nurses who joined all the military forces was not possible, the known ANCOA nurses to Flight Nurses were Margaret Gudobba, Leora Stroup, Mary E. Newbeck, Mitilda Grinevich, Florence Fintak, Ellen Church, Josephene Sansone, and Wanda Fill later in Korea.

One curious paragraph stood out in Schimmoler's letter to Coleman. She didn't explain it or give the person's name, but it caused her enough stress that she mentioned it to him in an obscure manner. She said:

> In the interim, it developed a certain nurse endeavored to secure, in an appealing manner, information concerning ANCOA. I surmised an effort was being made to obtain what I had striven for many years to acquire without giving recognition to the organization or myself, consequently, I became very hesitant in my acknowledgments. 55

Schimmoler once had an issue with non-nurse pilot Ruth Nichols, who developed the aerial nurse program Relief Wings. Perhaps she wanted to disguise Nichols' identity and said she was a nurse. Stroup took credit one time for the idea of nurse-trained aero evacuation. After she entered the Army, she told a reporter:

> It was about six years ago that I foresaw the need for air ambulances, and from that time on, I spent every spare moment studying air transport and the possibilities of treating wounded in the air. My study was not in vain, because most of what I learned is now being drilled into Army nurses in air evacuation nursing. 56

But Stroup would not have needed to secure information "in an appealing manner" as she had helped start the group—she knew its internal workings.

Stroup once wrote to Schimmoler about a Detroit nurse who tried to take charge. This incident was partly Schimmoler's fault. When Stroup hadn't written to Schimmoler for months, she became anxious about Stroup's commitment as she wanted to keep Detroit's ANCOA going. Schimmoler asked this Detroit nurse to "get the other girls together." The nurse thought she'd been put in charge and went rogue. Stoup and Schimmoler agreed to "read her the rules."

Whoever the "certain nurse" was that Schimmoler referred to in her letter to Coleman, it was not trivial to her. She couldn't forget it. 57

Coleman wrote back he had found more correspondence of hers between the Red Cross and the Office of the Surgeon General. He finished with, "It must be a source of satisfaction to see your idea in full fruition today." [58] Finally! A written acceptance that her concept led to the formation of the Flight Nurses in the Air Evacuation Units. When the Department of the Air Force eventually published the widely read *Medical Support of the Army Air Forces in World War II*, nine years later in 1954, Coleman had written four pages that told her story.

He gave credit to Schimmoler for the idea, even though he did preface his credit with the obligatory word "appears." He said, "It appears credit for the original idea of a flight nurse belongs to Miss Lauretta Schimmoler." Now more than a handful of people knew about her idea; they had to accept it—the Office of the Surgeon General had published the book.

She stayed employed as a Los Angeles County Sheriff's Detective until 1964, the longest job she'd ever held. She might have stayed longer but retired, she said, because of failing eyesight. At 64, she had reached a well-deserved retirement age.

Although Schimmoler had since lost contact with most ANCOA nurses, she remained friends with Mickie Grinevich. Grinevich had met Schimmoler in the 1930s and organized the New York unit. During WWII she joined the Army Air Force as a flight nurse.

Grinevich thought the military should acknowledge Schimmoler as the flight nurse originator. Once while on Air Evacuation duty, she bestowed an unexpected honor to Schimmoler: she removed her Flight Nurse wings and gave them to her. As she pinned her wings on Schimmoler, she told her, "I want you to have these as a memento of our pioneering days together." Schimmoler hesitated to accept them; she knew they stood for graduation from Grinevich's rigorous Flight Nurse training. [59]

For years Grinevich tried to convince the Air Force brass to acknowledge Schimmoler's role formally. No one listened. Nevertheless, she persisted. Eventually, they agreed. Colonel Joseph L. Stromme wrote Grinevich a letter when he heard the news.

Stromme had previously served as the Assistant Secretary of the War Office; he must have stayed in contact with Schimmoler through the years. In the letter to Grinevich, he did not restrain his joy at hearing the news:

> I cannot recall when I received better news than I received yesterday when Loretta called me to tell me the good news—made possible by your constant effort to see that real recognition should be made to her for her great contribution to the "Flying Nurses."

Those of us who knew her knew her zeal to have the sick and wounded given speedy transportation to the hospital best qualified to treat the case in hand, which, in many cases, would be by air.

> Colonel Stromme had urged General Arnold, many times, to give Schimmoler the recognition for her part in the development of the flight nurses. He never did.

He said he'd spoken to General Arnold many times; he urged him to give Schimmoler recognition for her part in developing the flight nurses. Arnold had said he would, but he never did. Stromme told Grinevich:

> General Arnold never even sent her a letter. Through your efforts, you have made life much brighter for Loretta, she is so grateful…we thank you from the bottom of our hearts.

With the letter to Grinevich, he included an excerpt of a poem from 1915, which was widely quoted at the time, "Do It Now," by Berton Braley. He altered many words and changed he to she, but still maintained the author's general sentiment:

> If, with pleasure you are viewing
> The work someone is doing, tell her now.
> Don't withhold your approbation
> 'Till the Parson makes oration
> And she lies with lilies on her brow.
> For no matter how you shout it,
> She won't care a thing about it
> For she cannot read her tombstone when she's dead. [60]

Now, Grinevich had to create a ceremony to honor her. She wrote to the 1965 Chairman of the Flight Nurse Section, Lieutenant Colonel Agnes Arrington, hoping to include a presentation at the annual Flight Nurse Meeting in September 1966 in Las Vegas, Nevada. Arrington had spoken to the Ad Hoc Committee about Schimmoler. She doubted she could get national recognition and said they couldn't pay Schimmoler's expenses for the trip. But they could "invite her to be one of the honored guests at the head table during the luncheon."

They planned to introduce her with a short biographical sketch. She could talk about her difficulties as the "Billy Mitchell of the Flight Nurses." [61] Billy Mitchell had been an advocate and visionary of air power. Mitchell became regarded as the "Father of the Air Force," as he had brought the

Chapter Three

need for air superiority to the forefront. He'd publicly attacked superiors in the Army, Navy, and even the White House because they did not see the need for air superiority. "Brave airmen are being sent to their deaths by armchair admirals who don't care about air safety." They weren't pleased with his public statement; in 1925, they had the audacity to court-martial him. Eventually, they learned he was correct—air superiority could win wars. Mitchell finally received honors. President Harry Truman even promoted him to Major General, unfortunately posthumously.[62]

The public had forgotten about Schimmoler and the Aerial Nurse Corps. Arrington thought other Flight Nurses would be surprised to learn of Schimmoler's efforts to gain their acceptance. "It will be an honor and a pleasure to have her as our guest," Arrington said.[63]

ANCOA member, Veola Claunch, accompanied her to Las Vegas on 20 April 1966. They held the luncheon in the Monaco Room of the Dunes Hotel and seated Schimmoler at the Flight Nurse table. Pale yellow and Air Force Blue dominated the color scheme. Floral arrangements and an oversized Flight Nurse wing decorated the table. More than 200 members and guests attended. Stromme and Colonel Bohannon presented her with the first Honorary Flight Nurse wing pin and an Honorary U.S. Air Force Flight Nurse Certificate.[64]

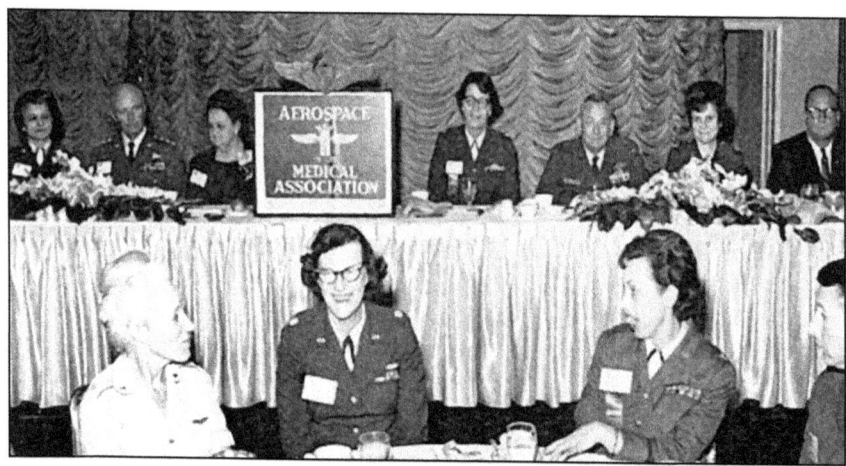

Figure 03.48. The Flight Nurse luncheon back table at the ceremony, left to right, Col. Ether Kovach, Air Force Chief Nurse; Lt. Gen. R. Bohannon, USAF Surgeon General; Lauretta Schimmoler; Lt. Col. Agnes Arrington, Section Chairman; Brig. Gen. F. Duff, Guest Speaker; Lt. Col. Anna May Hays, Asst. Chief Army Nurse Corps; and President Baxter. Unnamed attendees are at the front table, 20 April 1966. *Aerospace Medicine* photograph.

They introduced Schimmoler as "The Billy Mitchel of the Flight Nurses," and told the story of her struggle for the military to understand the importance of trained flight nurses, including how her many letters to the Red Cross, General Arnold, and General Grow were "thwarted by indifference." Bohannon lauded her for "her foresight, determination, and continued support for this vital element of aerospace medicine."

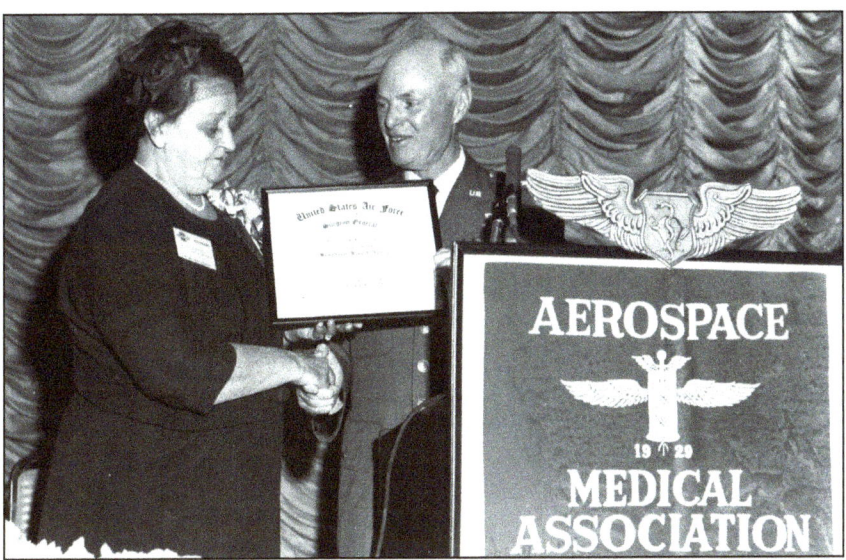

Figure 03.49. Colonel Bohannon awarding Schimmoler the first Honorary U.S. Air Force Flight Nurse certificate and wings pin, 1966. Courtesy of Special Collections & Archives, Wright State University.

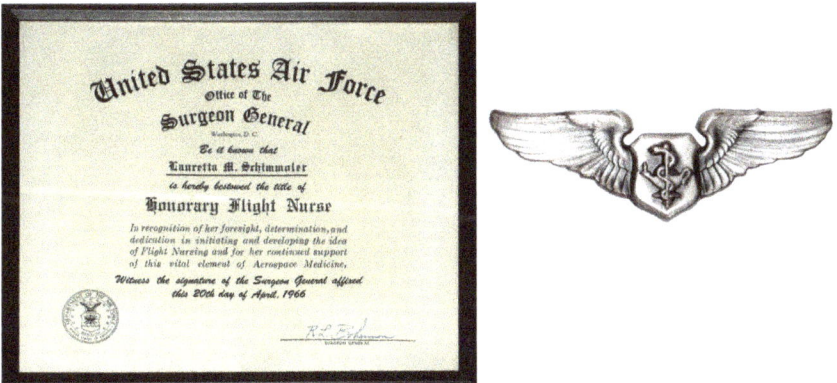

Figures 03.50. and 03.51. The certificate and honorary Flight Nurse wings given to Schimmoler at the Flight Nurse luncheon. Author photographed.

Chapter Three

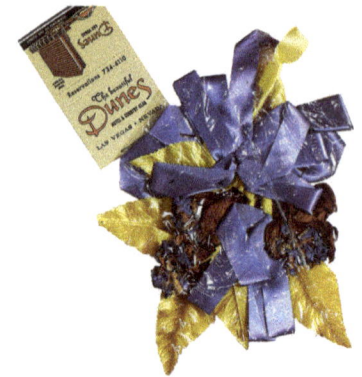

Figure 03.52. Schimmoler's corsage and the matchbook she preserved from the ceremony. Author photographed.

Grinevich presented Schimmoler with a large framed poster drawn by an Air Force artist at Langley base. The drawing depicts Schimmoler wearing her ANCOA cap, uniform, and cap pin. In the background, nurses load patients from a ground ambulance to an air ambulance. "The Billy Mitchell of the USAF Nurse Corps" is written at the lower right.

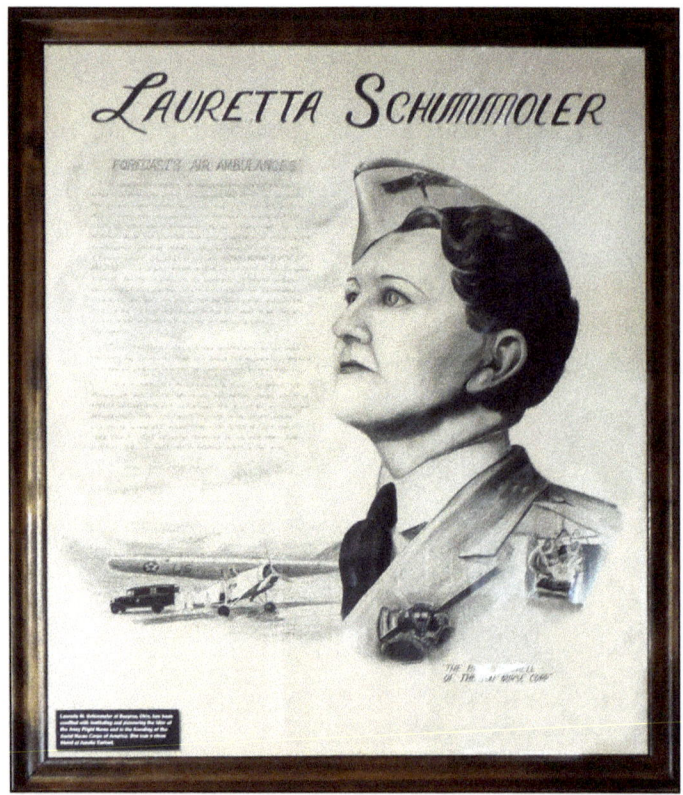

Figure 03.53. Forecasts Air Ambulances poster, 1966. BHS.

FORECASTS AIR AMBULANCES

She envisioned modern air ambulances. Many, even the Red Cross officials in Washington at that time, doubted her, as much as stated, 'We do not believe nurses will ever fly.' This did not daunt Miss Schimmoler's spirits. Quietly she pursued her project, and from December 1932 to September 1936, she devoted her time to research work and education. She availed herself of opportunities to prepare herself for the task of directing the national aviation activities of the now Aerial Nurse Corps of America. She spent nearly a year and a half at the Lockheed Aircraft factory to learn the rudiments of modern aircraft manufacturing. She became private secretary to the Commanding Officer of the Army Air Mail operations, Route 4, with headquarters at Union Air Terminal. Following this, she spent nearly four months in the U.S. Weather Bureau office on a special assignment.

Since September 1936, she devoted her entire time to the development of the Aerial Nurse Corps of America. She served without salary or compensation of any kind. This courageous woman set out to prove the feasibility and practicability of the Aerial Nurse Corps of America before publicly announcing the activities of such an organization. Her intelligent planning is no doubt easily understood when one knows that her motto is 'Act first-then talk.'

Afterward, Schimmoler told *The Beam*, a newsletter for the Amelia Earhart Post 678, she "left the wings pinned on her dress just the way they were put there." [65] Then she wrapped up the Flight Nurse wings Grinevich had given her years before and mailed them back to Grinevich. She was surprised to receive them—she had not asked for them back.

Figure 03.54. A note from Grinevich to Schimmoler for the return of her Air Force Flight Nurse wings, 1966. BHS.

> Dear Friend,
>
> Forgive me, forgive me - for the delay in writing. Have been so busy - could not get down to the Post Office. Had to call and have them hold it for me and then found out it was the package from you - with my wings. Really, Lauretta, you could have held on to them - don't like being an Indian giver. You deserved a pair of your own - for lo! these many years. Just, *"Mickie"*

Chapter Three

But the flight nurses were not finished honoring Schimmoler. In January 1968, at the 25th Anniversary meeting, at Lackland Air Force Base in San Antonio, Texas, they invited her to celebrate with them again.

Schimmoler presented "Flight Nursing: A Vision" during a course entitled "Operational Aeromedical Nursing." The Brooks Air Force Base opened its Museum of Flight Medicine that week. Schimmoler had sent forty-five pounds of her ANCOA memorabilia to the museum curator, including her ANCOA uniform. Many of her items were on display in an exhibit. [66]

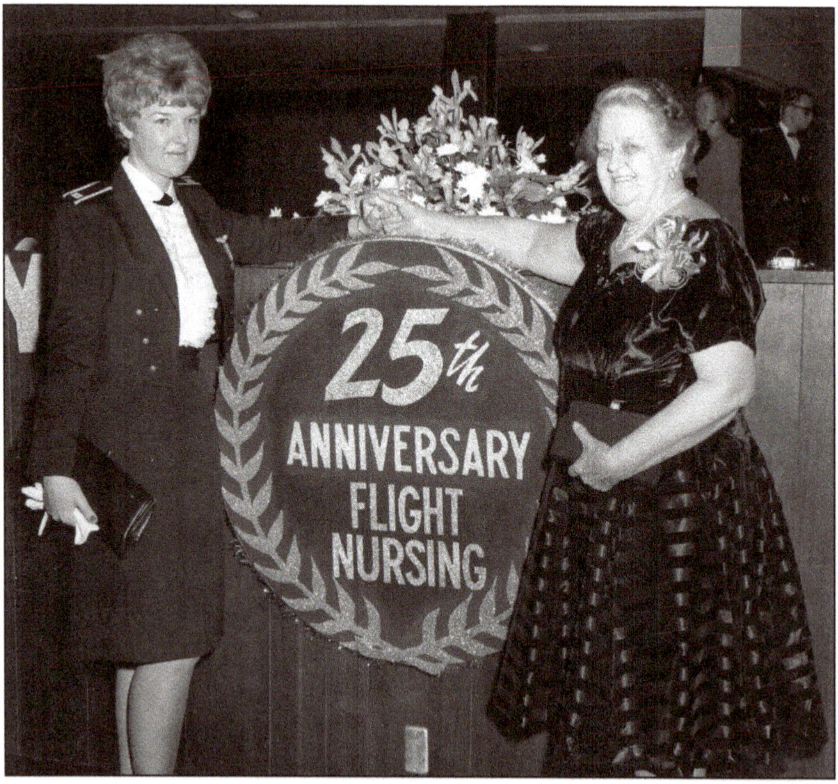

Figure 03.55. Captain Nancy Barran and Lauretta Schimmoler at the 25th Anniversary of Flight Nursing meeting. The School of Aerospace Medicine simultaneously celebrated its 50th Anniversary. Barran was the first RN graduate from the Air Force School of Aerospace Medicine's, Aerospace Nursing Residency Course. USAF photo.

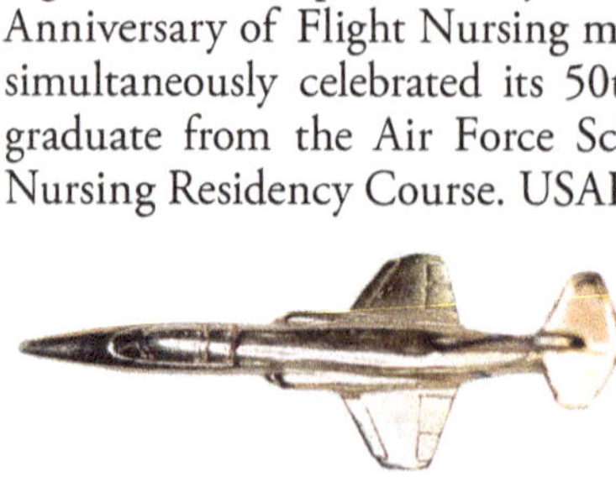

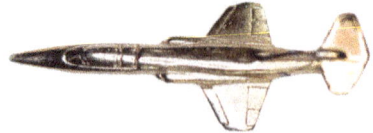

Figure 03.56. Schimmoler's conference gift pin January, 1968. A Lockheed F-104 Starfighter, Air Force. Author photographed at BHS.

144

Looking back over her life, Schimmoler thought of the events that were most meaningful and wrote them down.

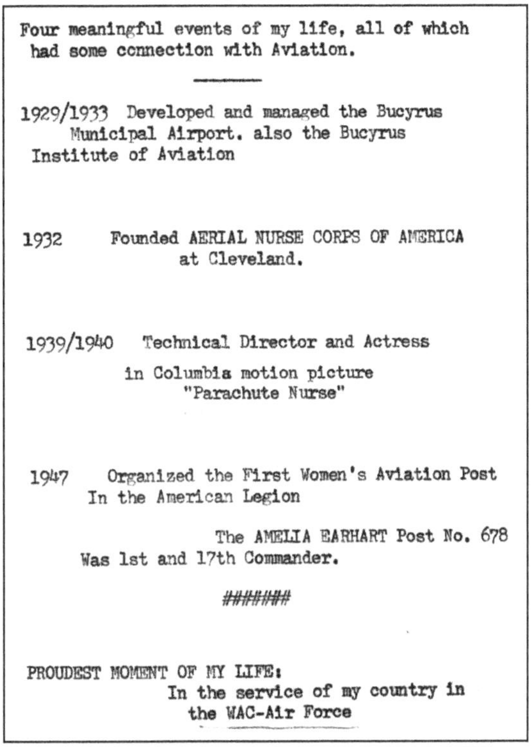

Figure 03.57. The "Four Meaningful Events," and the "Proudest Moment in My Life," note from Schimmoler, 1970.

```
Four meaningful events of my life, all of which
had some connection with Aviation.
                        ───────

1929/1933  Developed and managed the Bucyrus
           Municipal Airport. also the Bucyrus
           Institute of Aviation


1932       Founded AERIAL NURSE CORPS OF AMERICA
                    at Cleveland.


1939/1940  Technical Director and Actress
              in Columbia motion picture
                   "Parachute Nurse"


1947       Organized the First Women's Aviation Post
           In the American Legion
                        The AMELIA EARHART Post No. 678
              Was 1st and 17th Commander.

                        ######


PROUDEST MOMENT OF MY LIFE:
           In the service of my country in
              the WAC-Air Force
```

In June 1970, Schimmoler packed the items and ephemera she'd preserved since her early flying days, her ANCOA items, and her American Legion Post memorabilia. She wrote a letter of appreciation to Bucyrus and marked her items for donation to the recently established Scroggs House Museum, Bucyrus Historical Society, in Bucyrus, Ohio. [67]

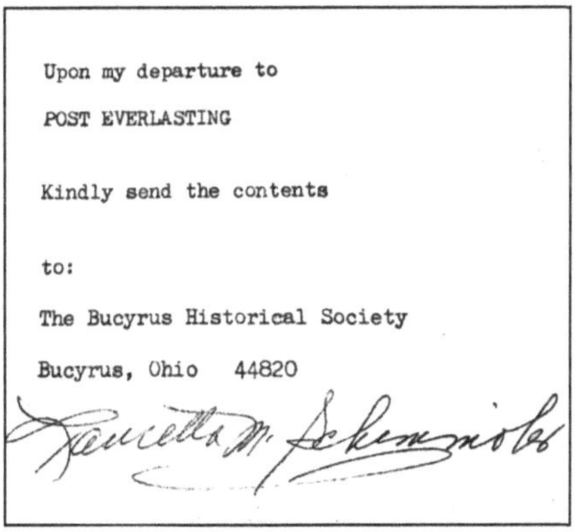

Figure 03.58. Her Post Everlasting note, 1970. She placed this signed note inside her memorabilia box, stating the contents should be sent to the Bucyrus Historical Society upon her death. [68] Post Everlasting is the final destination departed American Legion members will transfer to when the Supreme Commander calls them for duty.

```
Upon my departure to
POST EVERLASTING

Kindly send the contents

to:

The Bucyrus Historical Society

Bucyrus, Ohio   44820
```

Chapter Three

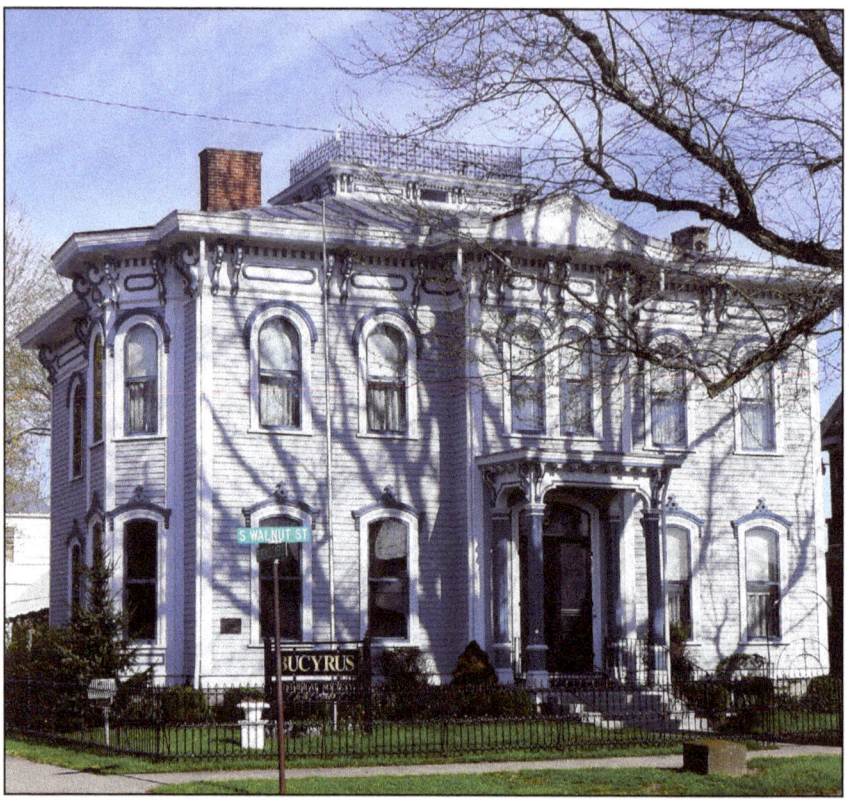

Figure 03.59. The Scroggs House Museum, home of the Bucyrus Historical Society in Bucyrus, Ohio, 2017. Author photographed.

She wrote a letter that revealed how precious the donated items were to her:

> …having begun my aviation career in Bucyrus in the development of Bucyrus Airport, I am pleased to present to the Bucyrus Historical Society the items and records that have been so much a part of my life. It is understandable that among these items entrusted to your care for posterity are some irreplaceable.

The last time Grinevich visited Schimmoler, she recalled she had removed a formal dress from her closet and said she wanted it to be her burial dress.[69] In October 1980, Schimmoler had an ischemic attack and a stroke. They transferred her to Glen Oaks Convalescent Hospital in Glendale. She died three months later, on 21 January 1981. They returned her body to Bucyrus, Ohio, and buried her in the cemetery near the house where she first raised her chickens.

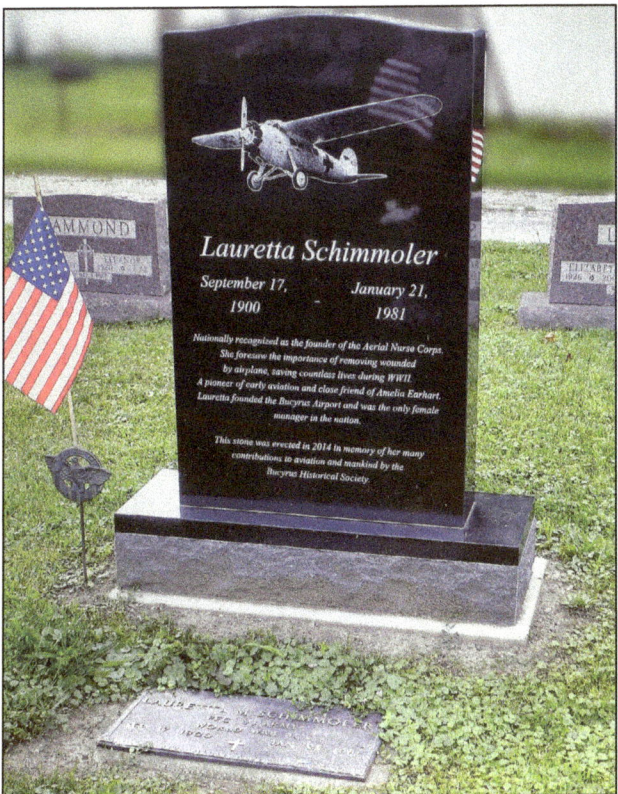

Figure 03.60. Schimmoler's Gravesite. The original 1981 headstone is in the foreground. The 2014 monument addition stands behind it. BHS.

While helping his daughter write her school paper, a Bucyrus Historical Society board member, Tim Musselman, found Schimmoler's memorabilia trunk. He learned about her achievements and visited her modest burial site at the Holy Trinity Cemetery.

He felt shocked to see that despite her contributions to society, only a small regulation military headstone marked her grave. He discussed his concern with the historical society. They agreed she deserved more and raised the money to fund a beautiful granite monument. The engraved epitaph states:

> Nationally recognized as the founder of the Aerial Nurse Corps. She foresaw the importance of removing wounded by airplane, saving countless lives during WWII. A pioneer of early aviation and a close friend of Amelia Earhart. Lauretta founded the Bucyrus Airport and was the only female manager in the nation.

On 7 September 2014, after the Bucyrus Historical Society installed the headstone, they hosted the dedication. The event included a song and a blessing. Members of the American Legion Colonel Crawford Post 181 gave a gun salute. Twelve Ohio residents of Schimmoler's extended family were present, although most didn't know about her accomplishments until the day of the ceremony. [70-71]

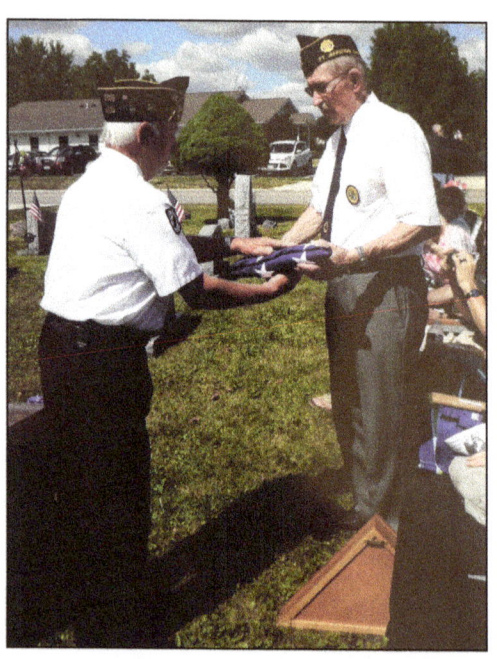

Figure 03.61. Two American Legion Post 181 members fold the flag during the dedication of Schimmoler's monument, 2014. BHS Collection.

The Ohio Women's Hall of Fame learned of Schimmoler in early 1985. They selected her for her achievements in science, technology, and non-traditional jobs. They inducted her posthumously into their hall of fame and invited her only living sister, Alberta Brown, to attend the reception honoring the 1985 winners and to accept Schimmoler's award. Brown then donated the plaque to the Bucyrus Historical Society. [72]

Figure 03.62. Alberta Brown, Schimmoler's sister, receiving the Ohio Women's Hall of Fame plaque from then-Governor Richard F. Celeste, 14 November 1985. BHS.

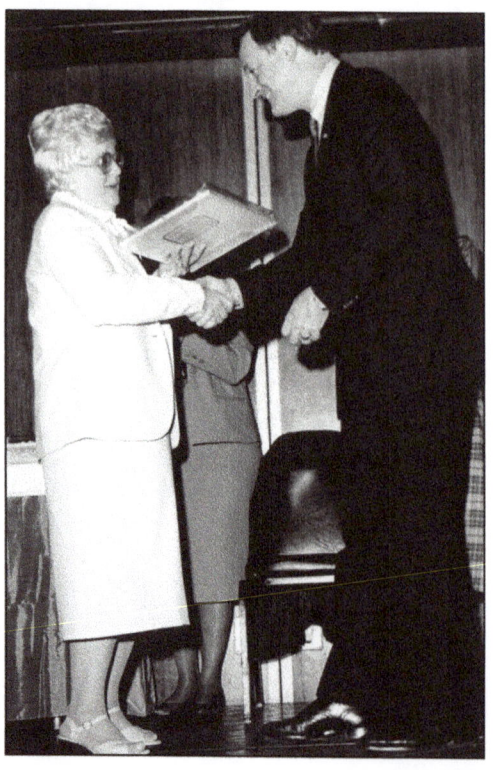

Figure 03.63. Schimmoler's Ohio Women's Hall of Fame plaque, 1985.

The city of Bucyrus continues to honor Schimmoler. The Bucyrus Airport Commission plans to remodel the administration building at Port Bucyrus (now named the Port Bucyrus-Crawford County Airport). Member Fred Fischer established a non-profit group, the Lauretta Schimmoler Museum Inc., in 2022. Although in its early stages, the group envisions a museum-style display in the new airport building and a monument to highlight her many accomplishments.

Figure 03.64. The Lauretta Schimmoler Museum logo, 2022. Image courtesy of laurettaschimmolermuseum.org.

Chapter Four
Major Leora Stroup

President; Director of Nurses; Quartermaster
Commander of Company A-5, Detroit, MI
Licensed Pilot; Flight Nurse

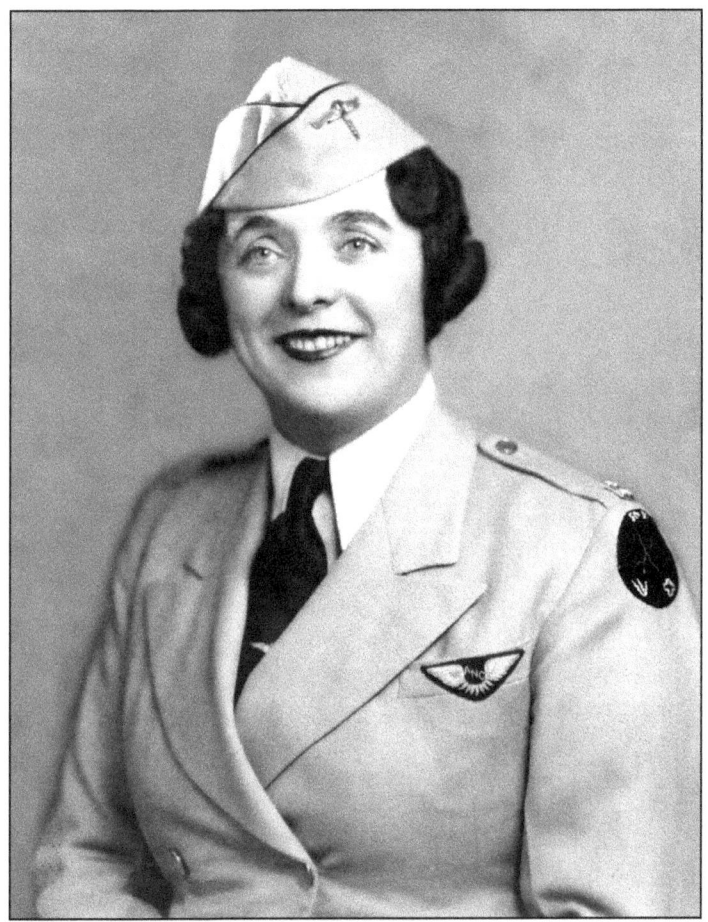

Figure 04.01. Official ANCOA photograph of Leora Belle Stroup, RN, 1939. She wears a commander patch on the pocket, double Captain's bars on the shoulder, a 5th Division patch on her arm, and a National Aeronautics Association pin on her tie. MMM Collection.

A favorite Stroup motto: "Never say you are too old to do anything you really want to do."

Leora would get things done. She was full of life. She would give her time, money and herself to causes she thought worthy, said one of her friends. She was full of vitality. I could understand why any kid would major in nursing after talking to her. You couldn't help but love Leora, everybody did, said another.[1]

Stroup was born in Windham, Ohio, Trumbal County, on 15 January 1901 as the middle sister between Edna Leona Stroup Wilfong and Olive Allen Stroup Hay. Their parents, Bertha and Elmer Stroup, were descendants of Trumbal's pioneer residents from the 1800s. Stroup decided to become a nurse in high school. She said, "…a lovely, extremely efficient nurse all dressed up in her crisp, starchy white uniform helped pull my father through a bad case of pneumonia."[2]

She had hoped to be a Red Cross nurse and participate in WWI, but she was only 17 when it ended in 1918—too young for nurses training.[3-4] She lived in Windham through high school, then attended Hiram College in Hiram, Ohio, while she waited to age. Finally, in 1923, she graduated from the Lakeside Hospital in Cleveland (now the prestigious Frances Payne Bolton School of Nursing, Case Western Reserve University) with a diploma in nursing. She secured her first nursing position at the esteemed Cleveland Clinic Hospital, where she specialized in caring for surgical cases.[5] When she left, only two years later, she was the head nurse in her ward.

In 1927, Stroup graduated from Ohio State University with a Bachelor of Science Degree in Education, a certificate in Public Health, and a Teacher's Certificate. She taught for the next ten years: as an instructor for the Health and Parent Education Association at the Cleveland Health Council; in Red Cross Home Hygiene, Care of the Sick; health education; and several first aid courses to varied groups in Ohio.[6]

She attended her first national air race in Cleveland in 1929. She knew she wanted to fly when she saw the female pilots land their planes in the cross-country derby. And she needed something new—her father died in 1928 and her mother in 1932.[7] She took her first flying lessons, soloed, and earned her pilot's license at the Cleveland Institute of Aviation in 1932.[8] Stroup said. "The airport had 1,000 acres, and I could throttle off anywhere and land."[9]

In 1933 she became engaged to a Canadian doctor, John MacCrimmon. Before they could marry, he was killed in a car accident while studying at Harvard University for eye, ear, nose, and throat specialty training. Stroup said, "He was tall, handsome, and intelligent. No one could compare with him." Her two sisters had married and moved. She was alone.

She needed new friends and activities, so she went to the Cleveland airport every Sunday—a gathering place for top flyers such as Jimmy Doolittle, Roscoe Turner, Blanche Noyes, Jacqueline Cochran, and Amelia Earhart. "We won many prizes at air races and shows," Stroup said about her friends' early flying days.[10] When she met Lauretta Schimmoler at the Cleveland airport in 1933, she told her she'd also envisioned starting a program to train aerial nurses.

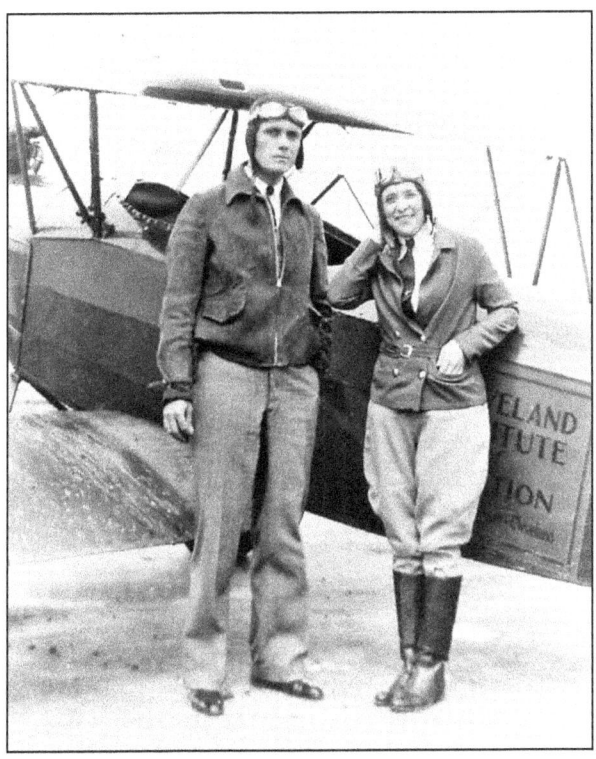

Figure 04.02. Stroup and her Flight Instructor at the Cleveland Institute of Aviation, 1932. Courtesy of Ellis County Historical Society.

She interspersed flying with more nursing education and work. Stroup never wasted an opportunity—in 1934, the Ninety-Nines hired her as a first aid instructor and considered her a prospective member. She joined the Ninety-Nines in February 1935, and by 1936 she was listed as a reporter for the North Central Ohio branch of the *Ninety-Nines Newsletter*.[11-12]

In 1939 she graduated with a Master of Arts Degree in Education from Western Reserve University. She moved to Detroit, Michigan, where she became the Educational Coordinator for the training program of practical nurses at Wayne University in Detroit.[13-14]

Chapter Four

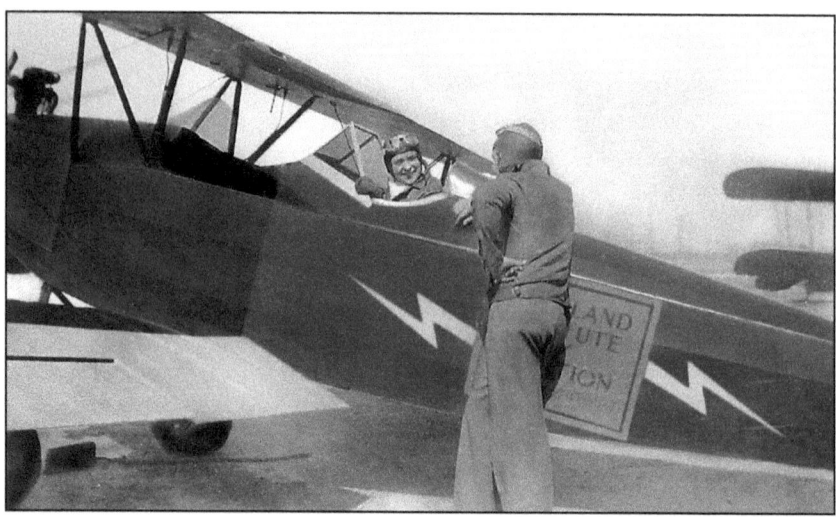

Figure 04.03. Stroup receiving a pep talk before a solo flight, 1932. Courtesy International Woman's Air & Space Museum (IWASM), Cleveland, Ohio.

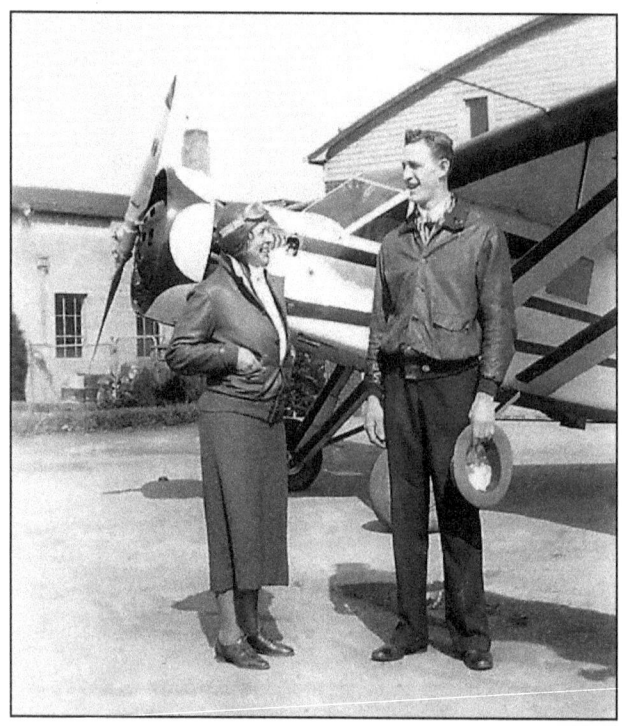

Figure 04.04. Stroup ready to pilot a different type of plane. Courtesy of the International Woman's Air & Space Museum (IWASM), Cleveland, Ohio.

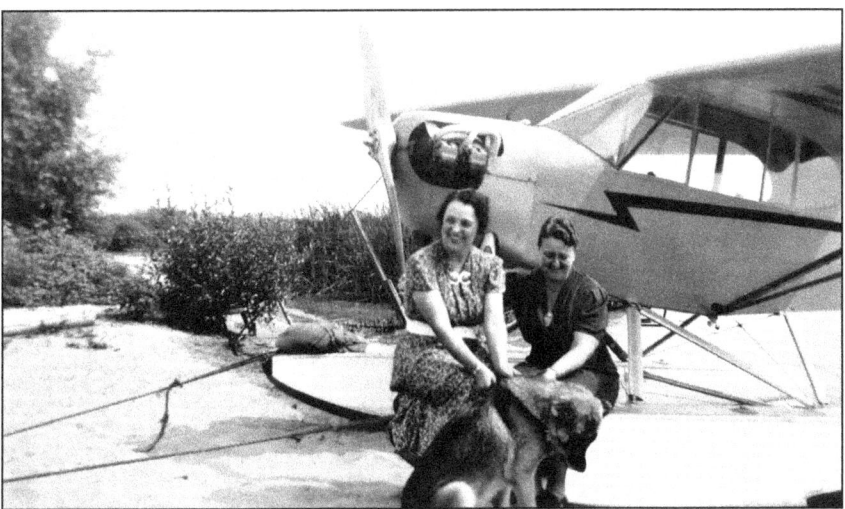

Figure 04.05. Stroup, Schimmoler, a dog, a plane. Was this dog related to the Superhero movie dog, Rin Tin Tin, Schimmoler reportedly once owned?[15]

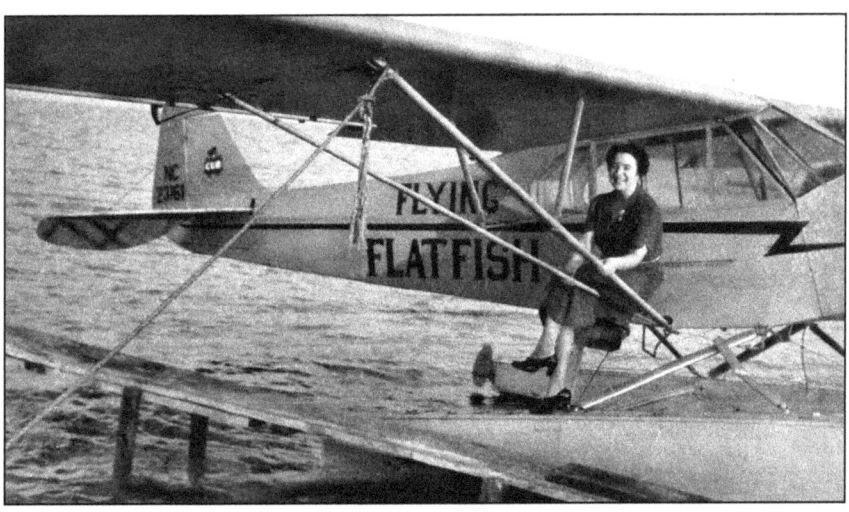

Figure 04.06. Stroup taking a break on the float of her airplane, c. 1939. U.S. Army Heritage and Education Center photo. This 1939 Piper Cub, J-3C-50, NC23161, is probably the plane in which Stroup maintained part ownership.

During hunting season, Stroup transported and administered first aid to injured hunters; a float-boat would've been helpful. Her sister Olive said, "No one in the family knew anything about these activities until Leora had surgery for an emergency appendectomy. While she was coming out of the ether, she began using the aviation signals that pilots use."[16]

Chapter Four

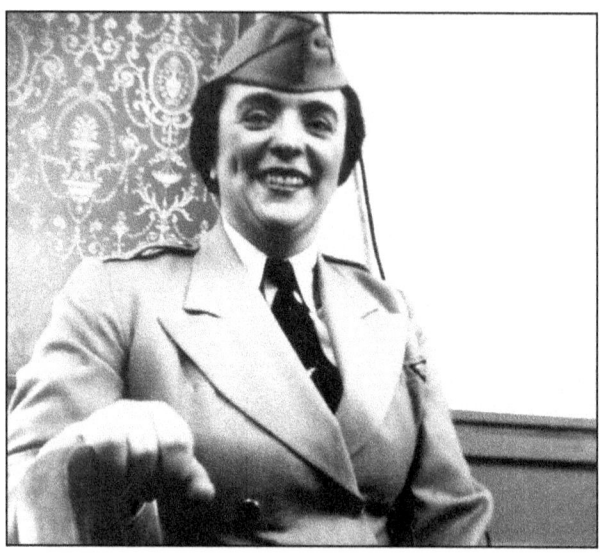

Figure 04.07. Stroup discussing the ANCOA at St. Joseph's Hospital in Detroit, 1939. MMM Collection.

In May 1938, she joined the ANCOA as member #93. When she arrived in Detroit the following year, she promptly organized the 5th Division. During her years with the ANCOA, she frequently traveled the state to discuss the new aerial nursing specialty and promote joining the group.[17]

During one presentation at St Joseph's Hospital, she told *Detroit Evening Times* that first aid was the principal training of the ANCOA nurses.

> Most of the nurses know little about first aid, as their entire training is devoted to the care of the sick in hospitals.

Detroit's ANCOA group A-5 assisted her during the hunting season, which attracted 50,000 hunters annually and resulted in numerous calls for speedy transportation of the injured to hospitals. She said:

> Not every nurse who joins as a cadet will complete the rigorous training, graduate as a flying nurse, and receive her wings. There is a special knack for taking a pulse or soothing the feverish brow while streaking above the clouds in the swaying cabin of an ambulance plane. But commercial airlines are recruiting ANCOA nurses. Detroit unit has already lost one member to an airline, and we will soon lose another.[18]

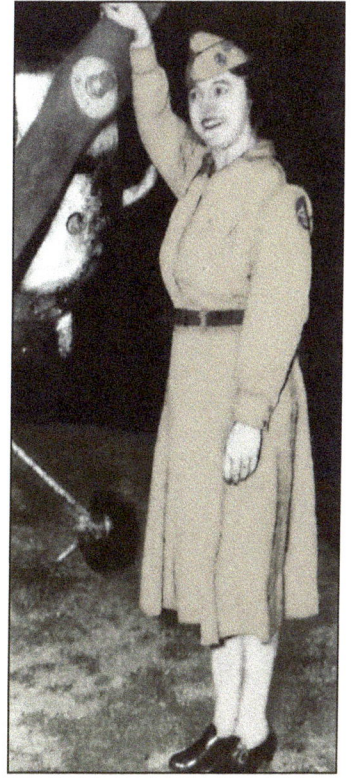

Figure 04.08. Stroup in the Civil Air Patrol, 10 October 1942. Stroup wore the CAP uniform, not the ANCOA like others did. Colorized clipping, MMM Collection.

By early 1942 the ANCOA had begun to diminish; her last known presentation about the ANCOA occurred in January. An article covering her discussion about the Civil Air Patrol described her as the former President of the Aerial Nurse Corps of America. [19]

Her public talks now centered on nurses in national defense. She taught first aid workshops with the College Women's Volunteer Service (CWVS). [20] Her civilian public speaking events didn't last long though—she answered the nation's call and entered the Army Nurses Corps (ANC) on 17 October 1942. She jotted down the memorable aspects of her journey to the ANC in a journal:

> ... shortened vacation & tore to Wash D.C. Went to see Julia Flikke, ANC. Sent to Walter Reed Hosp. & passed exam. Waited. Tense. Answer yes... go home & wait... sold big car. Got small car. Tried to pack. Couldn't... Bye to Cleveland.

Stroup studied her ANC training at Walter Reed General Hospital in Bethesda, Maryland. After completing it, the Army promoted her to first lieutenant and transferred her to Bowman Field in Louisville, Kentucky.

Although some writings downplay the importance of Stroup's prior years in the ANCOA as preparation for her flight nurse training, she must have thought those years were significant. During an interview she told reporter Jack Vriha:

> It was about six years ago that I foresaw the need for air ambulances, and from that time on, I spent every spare moment studying air transport and the possibilities of treating wounded in the air. My study was not in vain because most of what I learned is now being drilled into Army Nurses in air evacuation nursing.

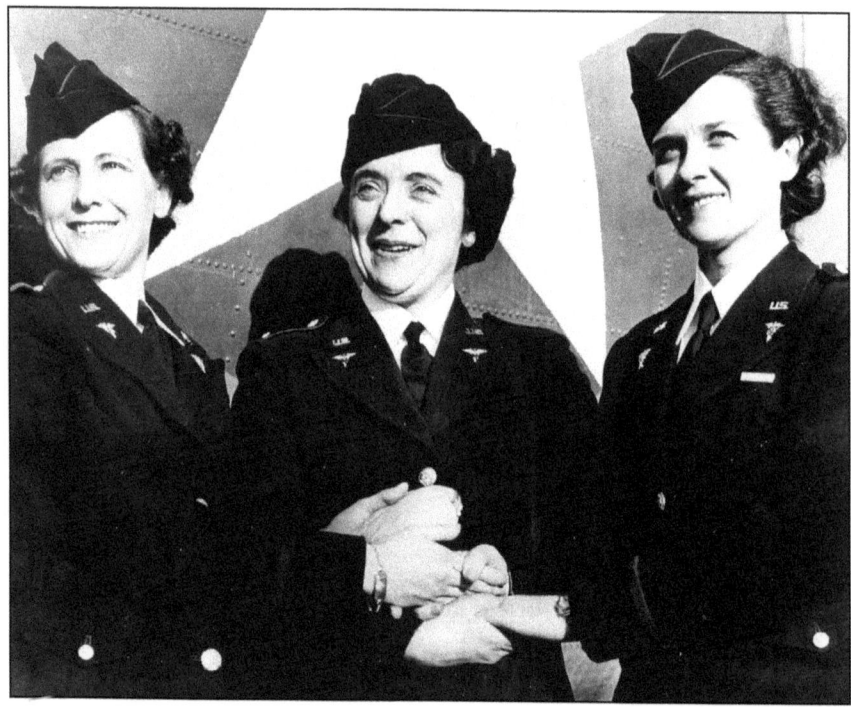

Figure 04.09. Three ANCOA friends, Eileen Newbeck, Leora Stroup, and Margaret Gudobba, reunite at Bowman Field, 1943. AMEDD photograph.

Stroup arrived at Bowman on 20 December 1942. To her delight, ANCOA nurse Eileen Newbeck appeared in January.[21] Newbeck had helped Stroup start the 5th Division Michigan Chapter and assumed the commander role after Stroup became the President.

"And now, if Margaret could be here," Stroup told Newbeck. Margaret Gudobba had also helped Stroup form the ANCOA Michigan Chapter. Then, on February 12th, it happened—Gudobba arrived at Bowman Field from Fort Brag. Gudobba had joined the Army several years before but had just transferred to Bowman. The reunion celebration of three aerial nurse pioneers began.[22] They must have discussed their great fortune to be in both pioneering groups of aerial nurses: private air ambulance nurses with the ANCOA and Flight Nurses for military air evacuation.

Stroup completed training. They assigned her to the 349th Air Evacuation as a Plans and Training Officer—the first and only woman to train flight nurses, with eleven male Air Force officers, in the Dept. of Aviation Medicine and Nursing. She worked hard but also enjoyed meeting the celebrities who visited like Don Ameche, Jackie Coogan, and Eleanor Rooseevelt.[23]

Because of her history with the Detroit Civil Air Patrol, Stroup invited thirteen of the female pilots from CAP to visit Bowman. Captain Alice Hammond said the Detroit CAP Squadron was the largest all-woman CAP unit. Two other visiting pilots, Lieutenant Maude Rufus, age 63, and Sergeant Marguerite Huff, age 58, were dubbed the "flying grandmothers." Rufus told Stroup she had written a book, *Flying Grandma or Going Like Sixty,* and bought a plane with the royalties. [24]

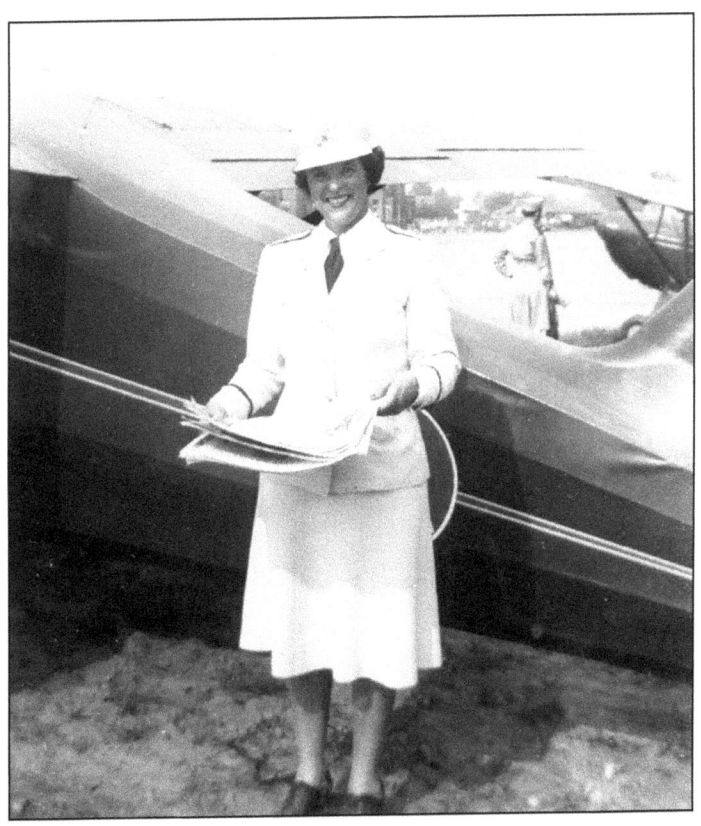

Figure 04.10. Stroup at Bowman, 1943. Ellis Historical Society.

During a five-day leave, Stroup studied the process of administering blood plasma at a Red Cross plant in Detroit. She learned that when a soldier is critically wounded, the most significant concern is the loss of fluids, which results in low blood pressure, shock, and death. Professionals can prevent shock with transfusions of plasma. The plasma doesn't contain red cells, blood typing is not required without the red cells, and rejection is not a life-threatening issue. Charles Drew, MD, developed the technique, in 1939, to separate plasma from the red cells and store it—just a few years before the U.S. entrance into WWII.[25] She told the *Detroit Free Press:*

I'm a nurse, a pilot, and a teacher, and I helped organize the Aerial Nurse Corps before joining the Army. Air evacuation, blood plasma, and the sulfa drug are responsible for the low casualty list of the war. The wounded are taken to an evacuation hospital near the forward zone; airplanes then transport them to base hospitals at the back of the lines.[26]

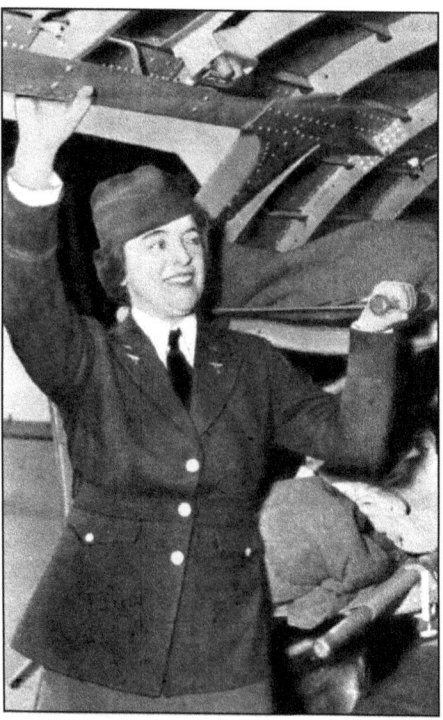

Figure 04.11. Lieutenant Stroup in an Army air evacuation plane at Bowman Field, 1943. USAF photo.

Cargo planes were equipped with hooks from which held stretchers, four deep. We could carry 42 patients on each trip, plus a nurse and a technician—no doctor.

Our first squadron of 25 nurses, 25 technicians, and one flight surgeon completed their first mission to North Africa, way out in the desert, far from medical material and water, and flew the injured to a hospital at Casablanca, where the American troops had landed.

The nurses sat on boxes and slept on the floor. Instead of sending thousands of nurses to the theater of operations and limited medical care, the Army was able to use a few specially trained nurses to care for the wounded on the plane trip from the front lines to a larger general hospital where the patients could get the best medical science offered. Flight nurses made a major paradigm shift in the care of the wartime wounded.[27]

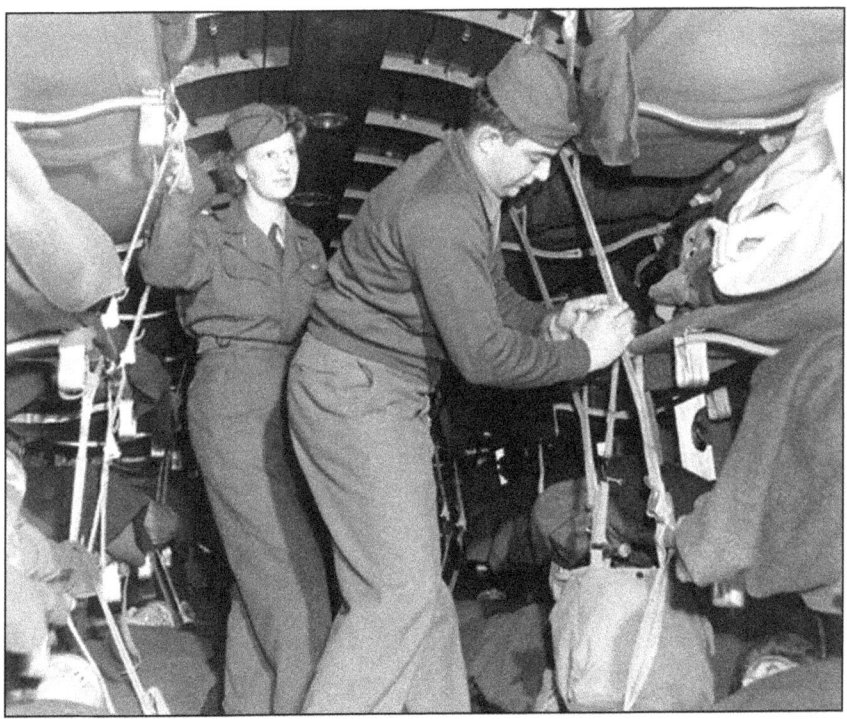

Figure 04.12. Lieutenant Anne Baran, RN, a technician, and patients on an evacuation plane at Bowman Field, 1943. The stretchers hang from hooks, as Stroup described. USAF photo.

Anne Baran was Stroup's best friend at Bowman. Baran became a Captain and Chief Nurse stationed at the Pentagon. Stroup said when they ordered her to the Pacific Command of the ATC Air Evacuation Unit, Baran told Stroup—jokingly but with serious intent—she would make sure that no nurse sent to the Pacific area would outrank Stroup. She didn't mention this again, but Stroup did maintain the highest rank.

When transporting ambulant patients, technicians or nurses could unfold the shelf-style bucket seats from the lower side of the airplane fuselage and quickly set them into place. Frequently each plane carried both types of patients, ambulatory and litter (stretchers).[28]

Chapter Four

The training curriculum for the flight nurses was incomplete when the first groups arrived at Bowman; the instructors, including Stroup, had to decide on the curriculum hurriedly.

The military assigned at least seven former ANCOA nurses to the first two Aeromedical Evacuation Squadrons, 801 and 802. As ANCOA members, they'd already studied one concept the Army considered vital: chemical warfare. Lieutenant Colonel Edward B. Vedder, a U.S. Army Medical Corps physician and researcher in military medicine, had written the book they used, *The Medical Aspects of Chemical Irritants*. Schimmoler, in her forward-thinking fashion, had begun this preparation for them.

The nurses were continually and emphatically reminded, "Gas will be used in the war." They must learn to recognize various gases, all aspects of them, and how to treat contaminated patients. Most importantly, they had to learn to don a gas mask quickly. [29]

Stroup said that she needed to impart something novel to students:

> They needed to learn the big, new idea to act as the doctor for just about everything—except operations—when flying from a battlefield with wounded fighters. But regardless of their importance, they still had menial duties. The school day is 8 to 4:30, except Saturday (time off at noon). Sunday is the day the nurses wash their shirts. [30]

Their training expanded. They learned to administer plasma, intravenous medications, and other skills. They couldn't graduate until they'd developed enough self-confidence to act. Although these skills are typical for modern nurses, it wasn't taught in the 1940s. Their education advanced again when the nurses' training moved from Bowman to the Army Air Force School of Aviation Medicine, which prepared flight surgeons and medical examiners.

Treating airborne patients involved understanding the two fundamental principles of reduced atmospheric pressure:

- oxygen saturation in the blood decreased at higher altitudes due to decreased pressure
- air or gas trapped in body cavities expanded

These principles applied to patients and nurses—the lower oxygen pressure reduced blood oxygen saturation from 96 percent to 86 percent. Pilots could fly under 10,000 feet if needed to prevent anoxia (oxygen deficiency). They carried supplemental oxygen to administer if required. These were a few of the independent decisions the Flight Nurses needed to master. [31]

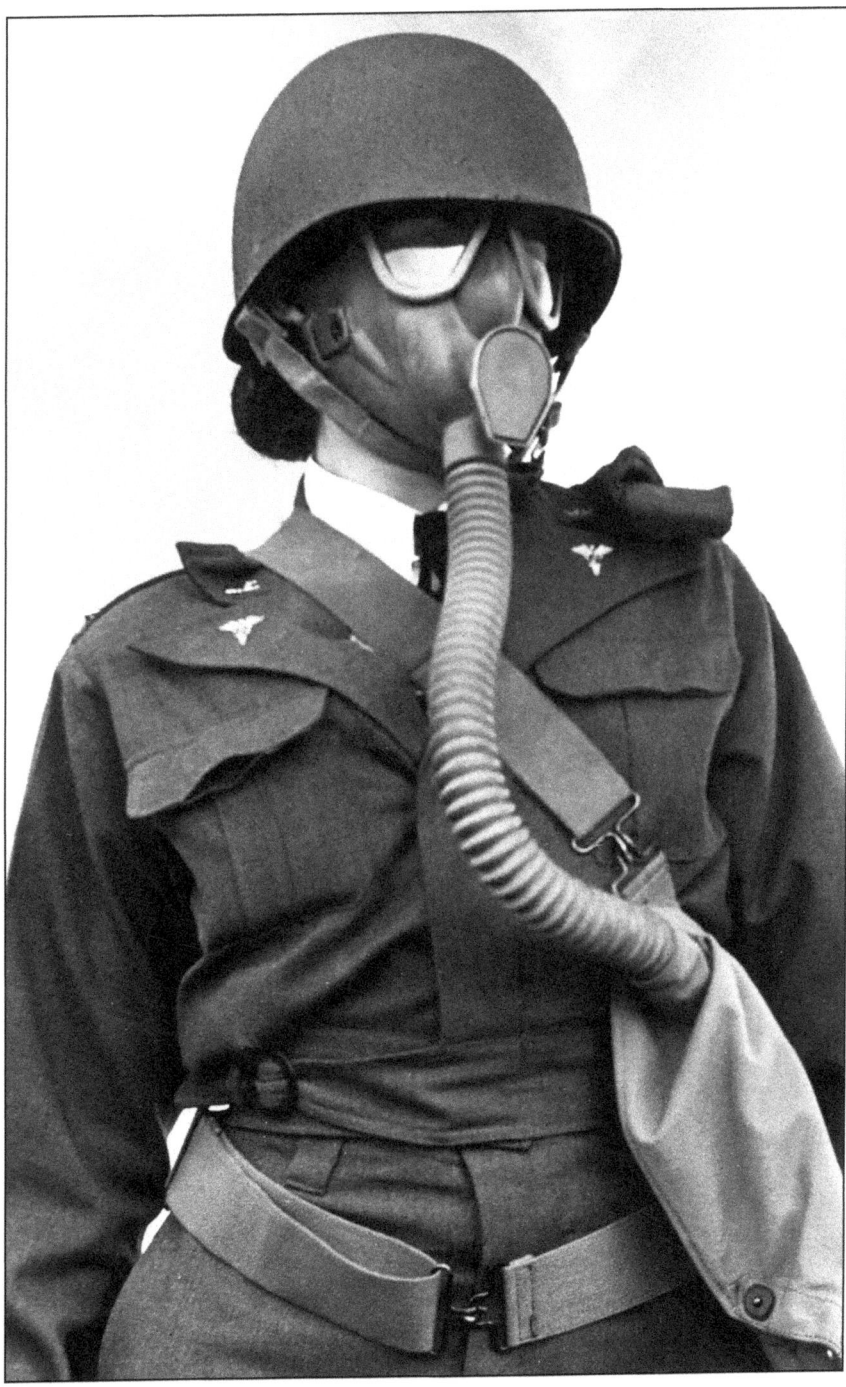

Figure 04.13. Stroup demonstrating the gas mask at Bowman. AMEDD.

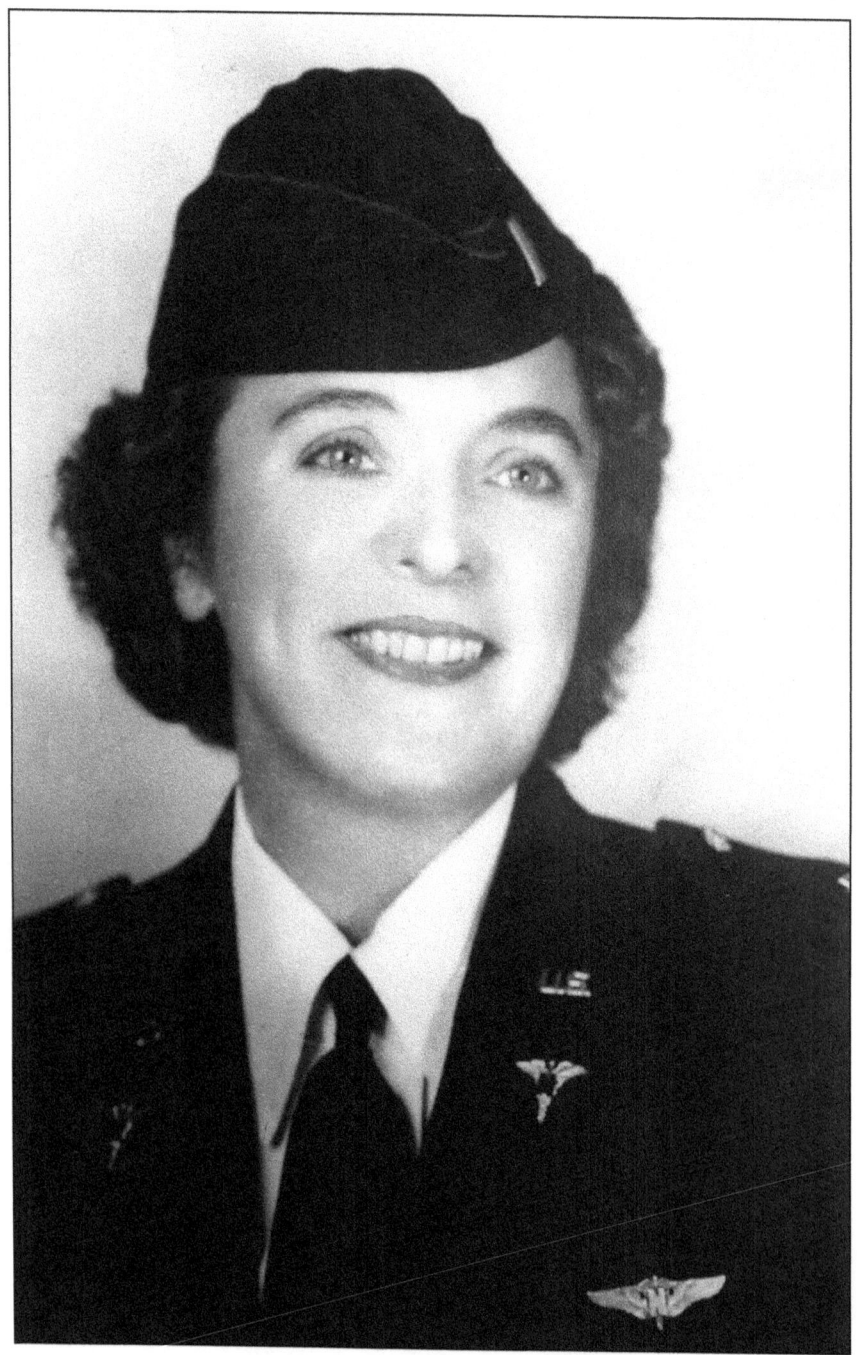

Figure 04.14. 1st Lieutenant Leora Stroup at Bowman Field, 1942. Her sister Olive Hay wrote on the reverse side, "This picture got her a Captaincy."

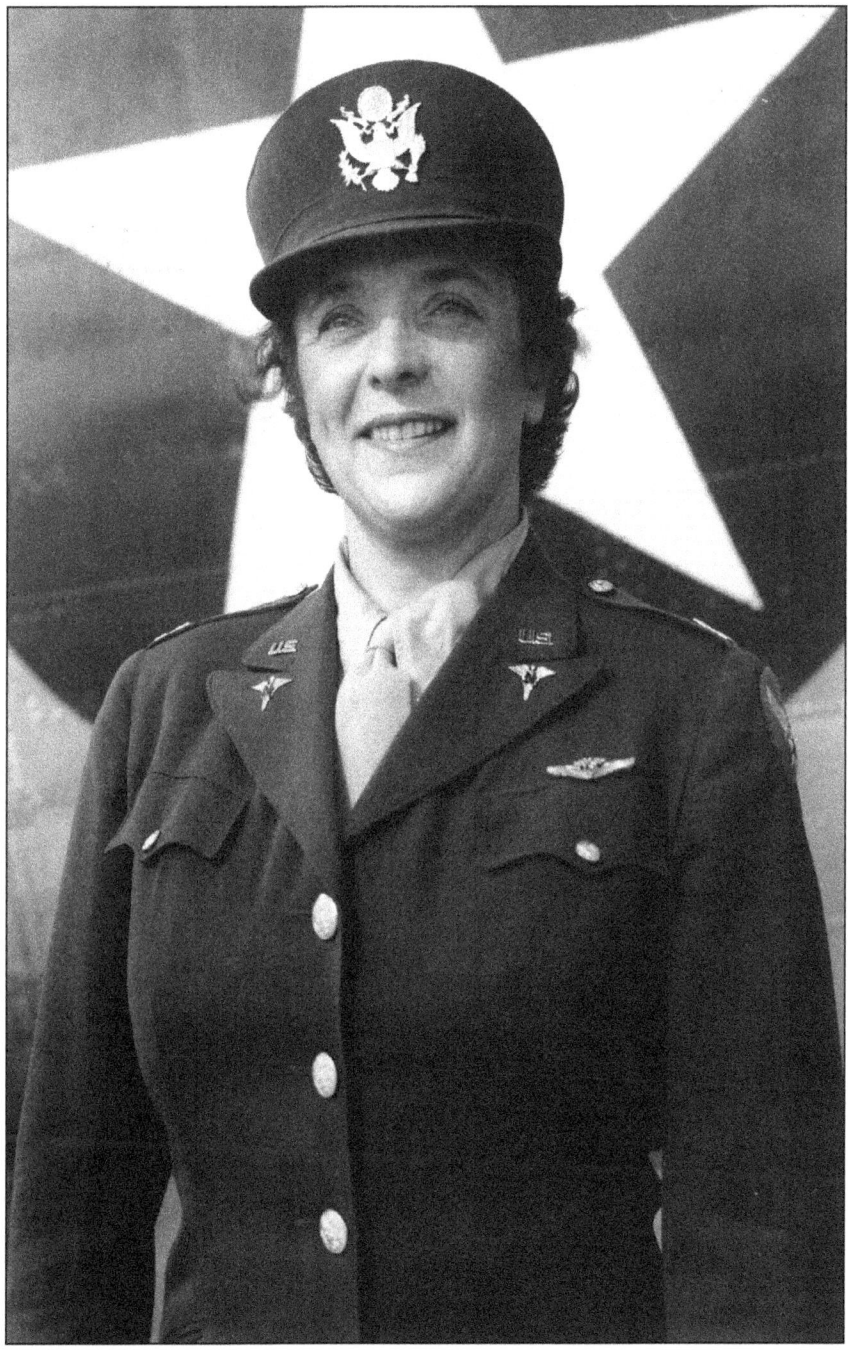

Figure 04.15. Captain Leora Stroup at Bowman Field standing in front of a transport plane, 1944. Leora Stroup Papers, AMEDD.

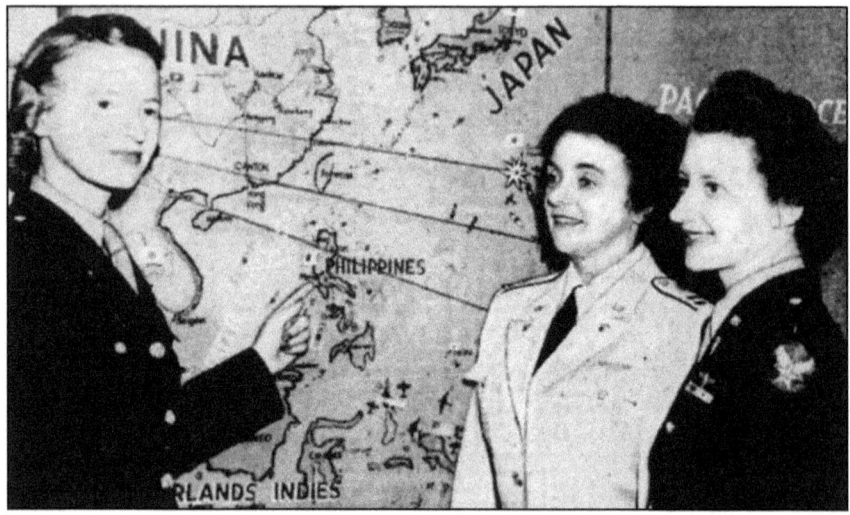

Figure 04.16. Stroup, center, with returned Flight Nurses Burnette Freedorn and Lucille Siuda, 1944. USAF photo. Stroup said of the nurses' return:

> I remember well that Christmas night when the girls left Louisville, the first group to help bring back the sick and wounded. You can imagine how I felt when they first started coming back to Bowman Field. It was a wonderful experience. We brought back 125,000 wounded soldiers, sailors, and marines across the Pacific, 42 at a time, by VJ Day. And we never lost a load. [32]

They selected Stroup as an instructor for her unique skills: more than ten years of teaching adults in healthcare, years as a pilot, years as a leader in the ANCOA, and her reputation for detail. She'd trained more than 1,000 flight nurses from 1942 to 1944 and accompanied them on the training missions. But she wanted the same opportunity her students had of deployment; she completed the upgraded flight training in March 1944, which she had deferred, and requested a change. [33]

In July 1944, she left as an Instructor and Flight Nurse in the 349th Evac Group and arrived as the Chief Nurse at Hickam Field, Honolulu. She supervised 350 nurses in the 828th MAES as Major Stroup—the highest-ranking nurse in the Pacific. She assigned herself to flights as needed. [34]

> I reign over a third of the world. My realm extends from the California coast to Okinawa, and soon it will stretch to China and the end of the line. I'm sure no woman anywhere is happier than I am.

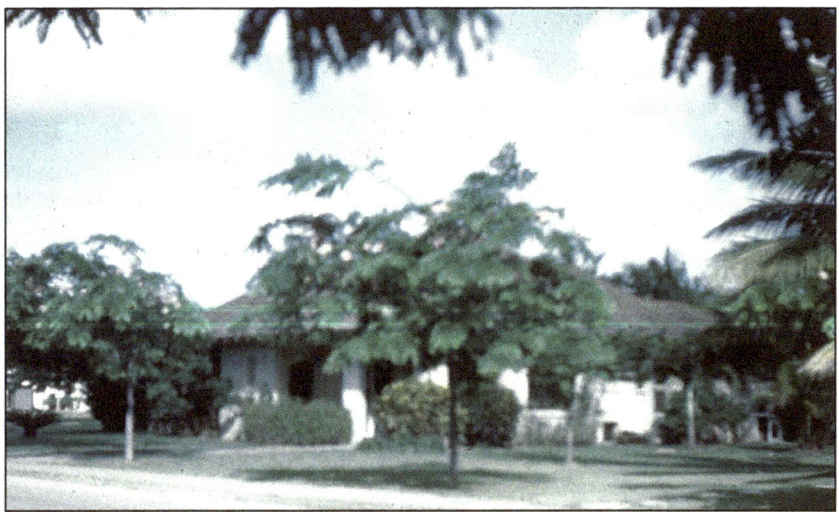

Figure 04.17. Stroup's house at Hickam Field in Honolulu, Hawaii, 1944. Courtesy of Ellis Historical Society.

> We can't understand why every girl doesn't want to be a nurse. I've always felt that way. And doing this Army work in the air makes our profession pretty wonderful. Besides, there's the romance element.
>
> Every little while, there's a wedding reception amid the flowers in my yard on the post at Hickam. A flight surgeon gives the bride away. I give the party.
>
> There's the five-day Honeymoon Cottage in an Army rest camp in the mountains, an hour from Hickam. Then back to duty. When I retire, I'm going to marry a hometown boy. I've had him picked out for quite a while.[35]

Stroup was living in Hawaii on VJ Day, 15 August 1945. She left for Tokyo three weeks after Japan's surrender on 2 September. She said:

> The Japanese people are always nice, and it amazes all of us, for they seem so sincere. They seem very humble in a natural sort of way and are very pleasant and courteous.
>
> Street vendors and department stores sell wares, but the stores are like stables—dirty, cold, and smelly places with nothing but brick-a-brac and baubles. And all the prices are out of this world.[36]

Chapter Four

Because she was the Chief Flight Nurse for the ANC, Stroup flew to the Philippines to accompany the return of the WWII prisoner of war nurses when they returned to the States in February 1945. Stroup said:

> Free the nurses was the cry of Americans during WWII. Everyone knew about the Army nurses. They wanted those nurses out. [37]

Stroup accompanied the nurses from Manila until the reunions with their families in San Francisco. She said it was her proudest moment. She left a heartfelt, handwritten account:

> They were taken by the Japanese military from the Island of Corregidor to Manila where they were held for over two years. They, with 4,000 other Americans were domiciled in the Saint Tomas University Buildings, surrounded by a high iron fence and Japanese guards at guard posts.
>
> One day an American plane dropped a note in the yard which said, 'We will see you Tuesday.' The next day they heard Army tanks and smelled gasoline. They said it was the best smell they ever experienced.
>
> The tanks broke down the iron gates and guard posts to the compound. The captives were overjoyed. Two Army trucks took the Army Nurses to a side highway outside the half-liberated city. A U.S. cargo airplane was waiting. The pilot, Mr. Johnson, flew his precious cargo to Leyte Island. There they rested and ate real food for five days.
>
> No one knew if they would need stretchers or chairs for the return trip. On arriving in Leyte, they were on their feet, anxious to leave. No stretchers or chairs for them. Each one was very thin and underweight. They were especially considerate of the Chief Nurse with them, who had white hair and weighed 90 pounds.
>
> The two planes stopped at islands for fuel and meals. At Kwajalein Island, every serviceman and woman was at the airport to meet the two planes. There were 'Welcome Home,' gifts, songs, and hugs by and for everybody.
>
> At Hickam Field, the rejoicing was terrific. These nurses wanted most to look well before their friends and families in San Francisco saw them. The PX was open for them only.

They could take for free whatever they wanted. They took perfume, combs, powder, rouge, lipstick, wristwatches. The supplies went dry. They were so happy. No television and no telephone calls to home were available.

Uniform caps and shoes were fitted to each one. The WACs came with ironing boards to their quarters and pressed the uniforms. The Hickam Army Nurses dressed them in the new Army Nurse Corps uniforms and insignia.

They wanted most to have their hair done. Every available hairdresser in Honolulu came to Hickam Field. They were to leave the next day for San Francisco.

That evening was a most remarkable one. A big reception was for all the Honolulu bases, including Pearl Harbor next door (likely 3,000 people). The Navy boys and VIPs were there. Brothers and sisters met. It was terrific. After speeches and honors etc., the band played the National Anthem. There was not a dry eye in the crowd. It was sung like it had never been sung before. It was dignified but oh so touching emotionally. Everyone was so happy. Pandemonium broke loose as everyone hugged and kissed.

The next day the two planes flew to San Francisco. I told them they had full back pay coming from the Army. They were so conscious of how they would look when they met their families and friends.

They were so proud. Each took her time walking down the airplane steps, including the little 90-pound, white-haired Chief Nurse. The cheer from the waiting crowd was a roar.

There were over 5,000 people at the airport. The fence that held them back almost broke down. I saw arriving generals wipe tears. Each one spotted her own family in the crowd, so went directly to them through the mob of people in the 'Ring Around the Rosy,' yelling, crying, and singing.

Watching the gaiety, each thought or said, 'Incredible, Thank God, Beautiful.' I am so happy to have been a part in bringing home these precious Americans who'd been prisoners of war for so long. It was a very great privilege. [38]

Leora Belle Stroup

Figure 04.18. A small paper flag of Kwajalein Atoll, an island the planes stopped to fuel on their trip home with the POW nurses. Stroup collected these flags from the places she landed when she worked in the Pacific region: New Guinea, Kusaie, Moresby, Lae, Luzon, Manila, Mindanao, Cavite, Peleliu, Bougainville, Okinawa, Guam, Tarawa, Guadalcanal, Canton, Kusaie, Midway, Honolulu, Molokai, Kahoolawe, Lanai, Hawaii, Maui, Waikiki, Oahu, Kauai, and Pearl Harbor.

Stroup flew on mail sacks to Okinawa, Iwo, Tokyo, and Shanghai with cargoes of blind, injured, paralyzed, and burned soldiers.[39] While caring for a shrapnel case and receiving radio instruction from Honolulu, they overheard her transmission as she fought to save a patient.[40] Soon after, Robert Ripley brought her to New York to appear on *Ripley's Believe It or Not!* radio series. She won $100 for setting a record: holding a bandage over a pilot's wound for seven hours while they flew to the hospital in Honolulu.[41]

The Air Transport Command called her to Washington and New York to speak. She reported on her inspections of Guadalcanal, Admiralties Islands, New Guinea, and her 20,000-mile tour of the Pacific area. When the Army released her on 13 March 1946, she had crossed the Pacific forty times on evacuation trips in the line of duty. Then she flew home to Detroit.[42]

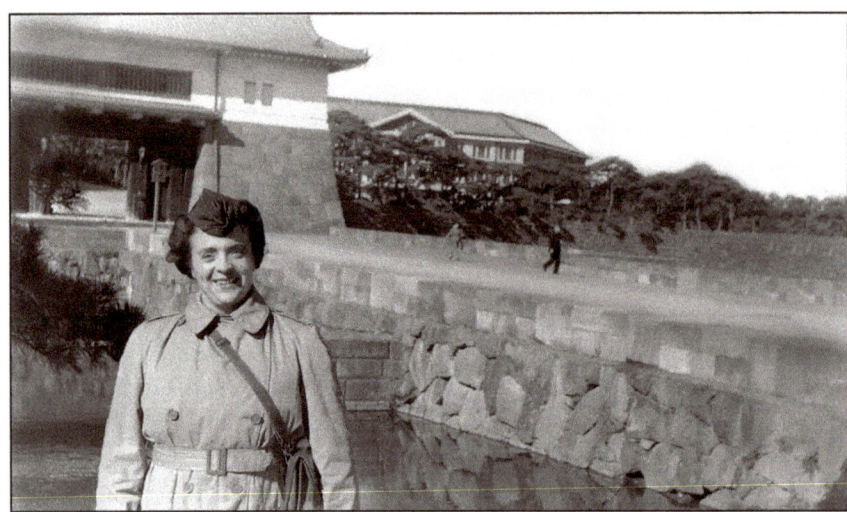

Figure 04.19. Stroup in Tokyo, Japan, in front of Emperor Hirohito's Palace, December 1, 1945. AMEDD

But Stroup didn't stay home; she flew to General McArthur's office in Tokyo to discuss her next plan. Two weeks later, she left for Korea to work as a civilian employee for the Department of Defense.[43]

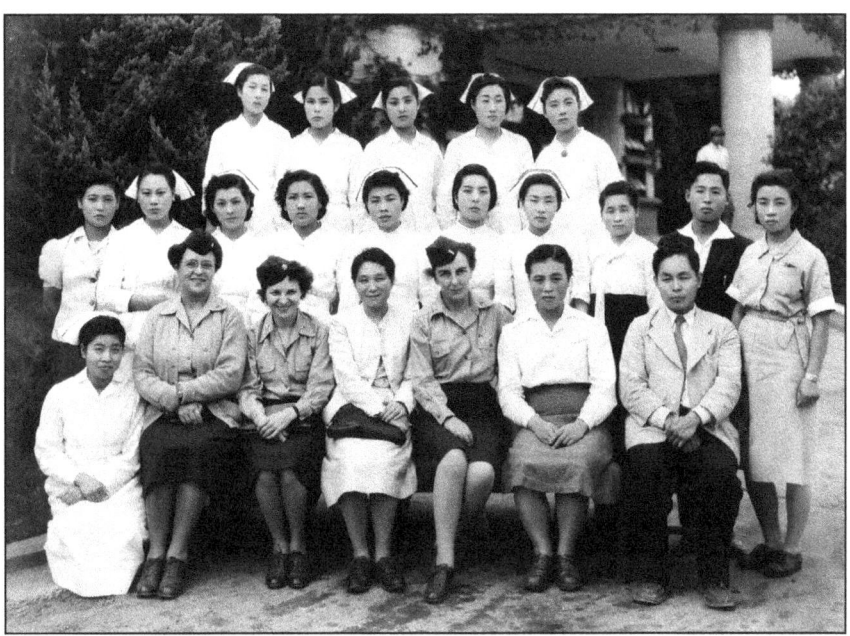

Figure 04.20. One of Stroup's nursing classes in Korea, She's sitting second from the left, c. 1947. Leora Stroup Papers, AMEDD.

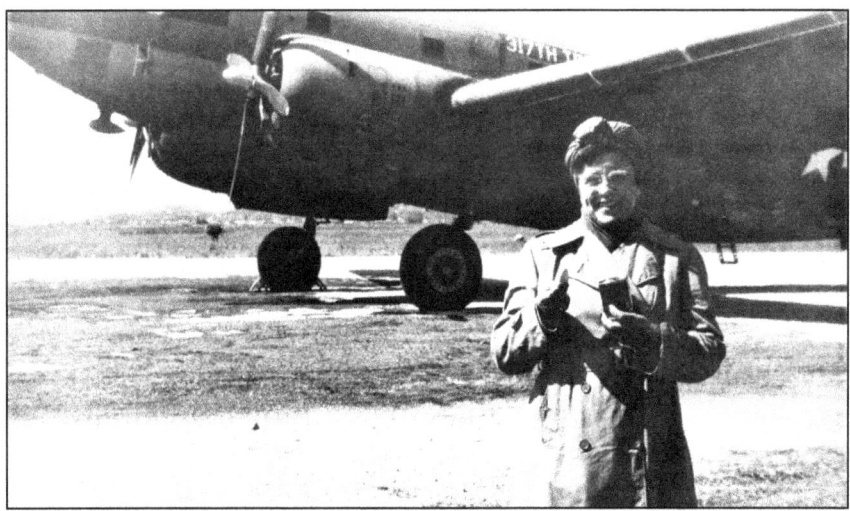

Figure 04.21. Stroup in Korea in front of a 317th Troop Carrier Squadron plane, c. 1947. Leora Stroup Papers, AMEDD.

Chapter Four

She was stationed in city of Busan, then called Pusan, as the Consultant in Nursing—the first female civilian employee, War Department, in Korea. She provided supervision in health and maternity care at refugee camps, supervised nurses in eight hospitals during a cholera epidemic, re-established the nursing services in the National Tuberculosis Hospital, and helped to re-establish the nursing schools and the National Korean Nurses Association.

The Army nurses functioned as advisors and consultants. But the job was immense. On a single day, they administered 2,500 vaccinations and 1,000 typhus injections. She described her living conditions:

> On one narrow street, practically downtown, the military government has taken over houses for us made of mud and logs. All are matting floors and no furniture. Everyone sits on the floors, which are warm from the stove flues under them. We leave our shoes at the door and walk in our socks. Ox carts are used for hauling, or people carry heavy loads on their backs.
>
> The crude houses are made of bamboo that are drafty and cold. A pot-bellied stove heats the houses, and the danger of fire is a constant one. Part of the providential hospital in Pusan burned after I started. Hardships were plentiful.
>
> Korean food is very expensive. Not enough vegetables and fruit, too many dried potatoes. After the Japanese left, Koreans went into homes, warehouses, and stores the Japanese formally owned and took whatever they wanted. They ate in six months an entire year's supply—now there's not enough rice. They cut down all the trees for firewood.

Stroup, a keen collector, skipped buying kimonos in Japan. Kimonos and Obis (the sash for a kimono) cost fifty American dollars. Too expensive. But in Korea, she could buy them for three or four dollars, so she did. She related her impressions of Koreans:

> Koreans are more healthy, robust, and virile looking than Japanese. The modern men wear Western clothes; the older men and women wear bright-colored costumes of silk.

She didn't, however, find Koreans as friendly as Japanese:

> They have no manners and never step aside on the street. They are sullen and don't like they have another nation imposed on them when they just got rid of the Japanese. [44]

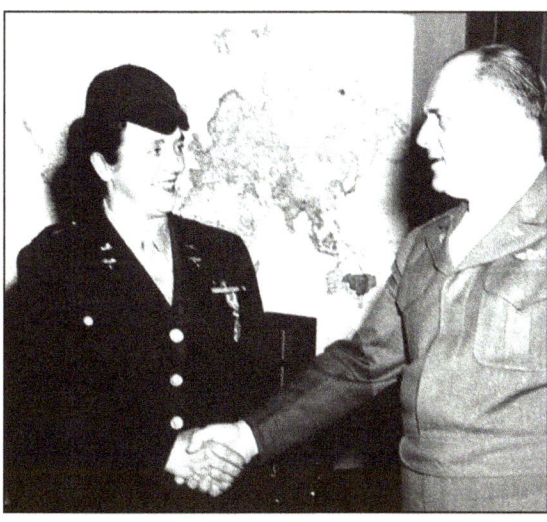 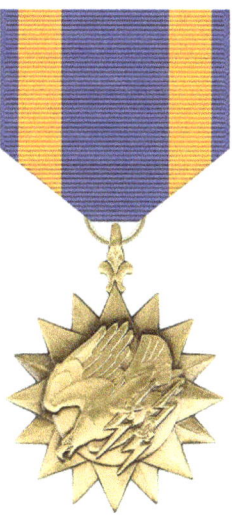

Figure 04.22. Stroup receiving her Air Medal award in 1947, AMEDD.
Figure 04.23. The Air Medal awarded for WWII. Author photographed.

She left civilian military work in March 1947. The Army awarded her the Air Medal for meritorious achievement while participating in aerial flights from December 1944 to December 1945. [45] She received many other WWII medals and collected over forty patches and various military medals.

Her work in Korea had severely degraded her strength—she'd planned to return after she fully recovered because of the country's desperate need, but her health wouldn't permit it. [46] She enrolled in a postgraduate course in Bellevue Hospital at Columbia University in New York, graduated with her second Master's Degree in Nursing Education, and then worked towards a doctorate. But Kansas called with a tempting offer; she left Columbia in 1952 with her doctorate completed, except for her dissertation. Fort Hays State College (FHSC) in Hays, Kansas, had recruited her to develop their first nursing program and serve as the Director. [47]

She wrote a carbon-copied letter to her friends when she arrived in Hays, telling them about her new life. She said she was "…happy and satisfied on the Great Plain." She told them:

> To me, after the insolent Army and the buffeting city life (with money to be spent at every turn), this is a veritable paradise. For the first time, I have a little free time for myself in the evenings and Saturday and Sunday. The college has its own oil well pumping night and day (while I spend it). The little hospital was given an estate with 58 oil wells

Chapter Four

which bring in $12,000 a week. Our college has its income from 4,000 acres of rich farm given to it by the government after the old Fort Hays closed.[48]

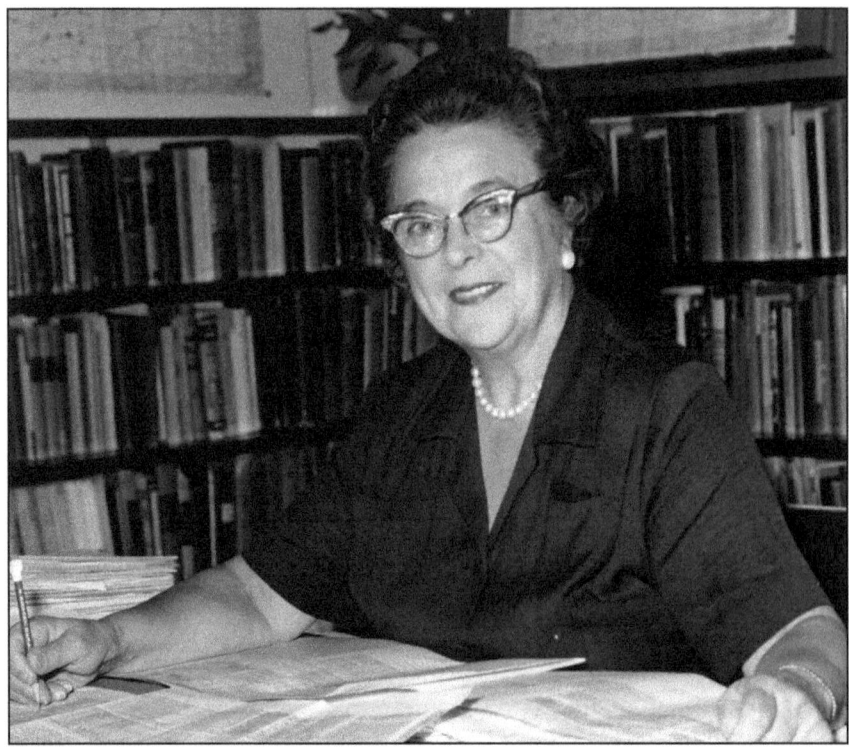

Figure 04.24. Stroup as the Director of Nursing Program, c. 1957. Forsyth Library Collections, Fort Hays State University (FHSU).

She encountered many obstacles during her attempt to make the program a success. But, as usual, Stroup rose to the challenge. The nursing program needed more local hospitals to fulfill their clinical practice. While they did have Hadley Regional Medical Center in Hays for general medicine, Hays had no space in the specialty wards for their training. Stroup arranged for hospitals outside of Hays and even some outside of Kansas.

Students trained at Denver Children's Hospital pediatrics ward, and the Chicago Lying-in Hospital for obstetric rotations. The first class graduated in 1955.[49] Still, the National League for Nursing wouldn't fully accredit the program until it offered psychiatric and public health nursing. Floyd Wagner from the city of Pratt donated $400,000 in 1968, which allowed Stroup to hire those specialty instructors and complete the full accreditation. Eventually, they trained at Topeka State Hospital for psychiatric clinicals.[50]

Wagner left the bulk of his estate to the Division of Nurse Education. The gift surprised everyone since his family had no known connection to the college. But Wagner had a particular regard for the nursing profession.

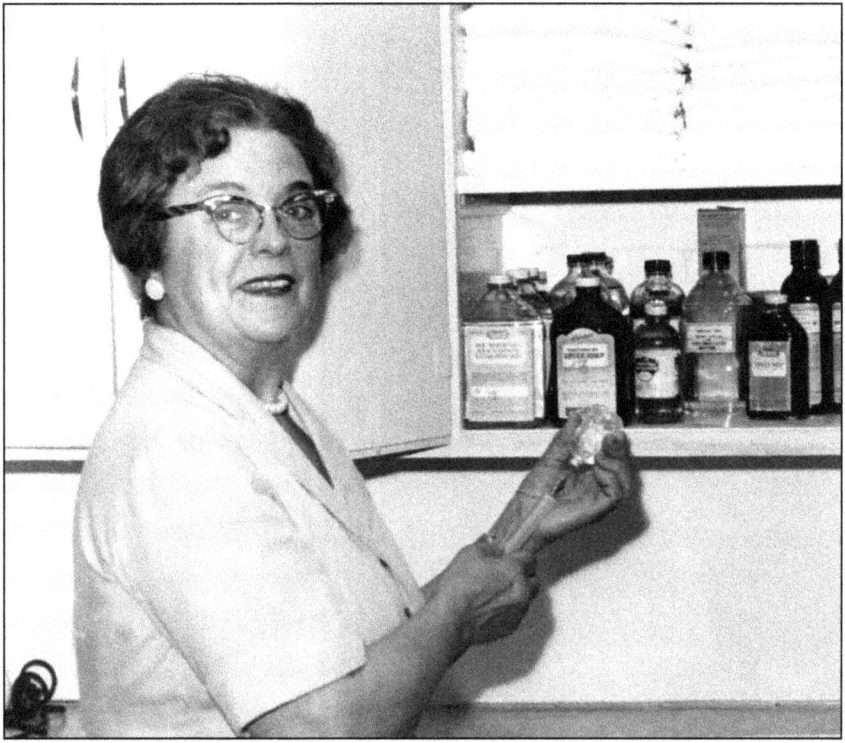

Figure 04.25. Stroup preparing an injection at the medicine cabinet with a glass syringe and a steel needle, c. 1957. Forsyth Library Collections, FHSU.

Even before the attorney settled the estate, he allowed a draw of $20,000 to endow the first chair in nurse education. Stroup said:

> Our program always had state accreditation. We have had a diploma program, but now the program has finally been approved for a change to the baccalaureate program with a degree in nursing.[51]
>
> But there is the very important problem of scholarships for student nurses. Most work at one or two jobs waiting tables, or on the telephone switchboards. The $104 tuition a semester is too big for some of them to handle without help. If only the public knew how desperately they need it. Each and every dollar is important to the students trying

to become nurses. Some will need to drop out if they do not receive help. [52]

The city of Hays was known for the Tommy Drum Saloon, a historical watering hole for soldiers from Fort Hays and the British Colonists from Victoria. Famous personages like Wild Bill Hickok, Buffalo Bill Cody, and General George Custer were customers. The building was still intact during Stoup's Kansas years. In 1961 they held a special event to recreate the old Tommy Drum Saloon. Women dressed as old-time dancers and performed musical numbers as "The Buffalo Girls." Stroup joined in and performed an old-fashioned reading titled, "The Broken Mirror."

Earnings from the event helped purchase nursing scholarships at Fort Hays State College. Other clubs, and the firemen, raised additional money for student nurses' fees. [53-54]

Stroup was an active Business and Professional Women's Club member in Hays. State nurses elected her twice as President of the Ninth District Kansas Nurses Association. [56]

She held memberships in many professional societies:

- International Council of Nurses, American Nurses Association
- Kansas State Nurses Association
- District 9
- National League for Nursing-Baccalaureate Group
- Kansas League for Nursing
- Sponsor for Kansas State Student Nurses' Association, District 9
- National Education Association
- Kansas State Teachers Association
- Phi Kappa Phi
- American Association of University Women
- Kansas Anthropological Association
- Kansas Mental Health Association [57]

Newspapers featured bits about Stroup as she spoke on various education and health topics. They printed news of the many parties she organized; she often decorated her home lavishly for them. "Her parties were famous," said one of her friends.

After the military, she continued to enjoy the life of an avid traveler, locally and internationally. She bought a new camper. She'd pack up on the spur of the moment and go to a lake for a week. [58] When she first arrived in Hays, she told friends she considered going to Denver for Thanksgiving but hated to spend the money:

> I am saving every penny for my 7th year for a sabbatical year of travel around the world, on half salary. Then I must return to teach two more years or return the money for the year. I won't be going on to NYC until a paid Board Trip in January. But I expect to come to Ohio and Michigan during the holiday time. [59]

She traveled to Italy, the Mediterranean, the Holy Land, the Caribbean, and cruised aboard the Delta Queen on the Mississippi River. An injury from a fall in 1978 robbed her and her sister Olive of their long-awaited Russian tour. [60] Frequent international travel was not customary for women then; that didn't stop Stroup.

In 1962 she was a guest of honor when Air Evacuation School personnel from Bowman in San Antonio, Texas, held a reunion in Hays. She lamented to a reporter, "…if I had remained in the service I'd be eligible for retirement now." But she also affirmed her return to teaching was the correct decision because of the great need for skilled nurses. [61]

In January 1968, the School of Aerospace Medicine, Brooks Air Force Base held its 50th Anniversary in Texas. Flight Nurses decided to celebrate their 25th Anniversary the same week. The Air Force had recognized Stroup's contribution every year, but this time it would be bigger, and they would include special tributes to her as a founder of the Air Evacuation Program.

They asked her to participate as a panelist on "Challenges in Aeromedical Evacuation in 1943." The nurses attended four days of meetings, including a live training demonstration using a mock-up training plane and occupants in life preservers thrown into a pool in inflated rubber boats to illustrate procedures of the various phases of rescue. Three Air Force Nurses training at Cape Kennedy with the astronauts were among the guests. "If a woman ever goes to the moon, the first will be these Air Force Nurses," declared Stroup. They also honored Schimmoler again at this meeting as the originator of the concept of the Flight Nurse.

Once home, she wrote a letter to Lt. Colonel Arrington about the week:

> I am still under the spell of the wonderful week we had. The majority of the World War II flight nurses I met there I had not seen since the day they left Bowman Field. We had lots of visiting to do and to catch up on their stories.
>
> Every hour of the Anniversary was happy hour. I am still reliving it as I go about College enrollment, capping new nurses, and all the rest. [62]

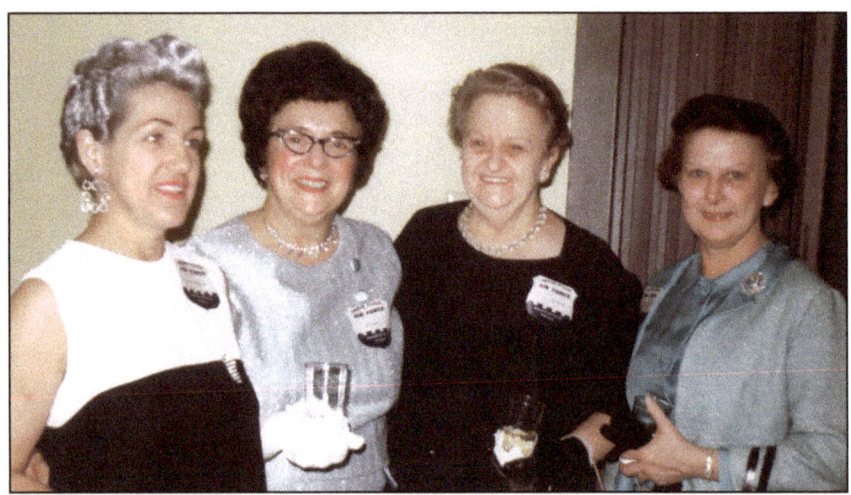

Figure 04.26. Former ANCOA members and Flight Nurses at their 25th Anniversary celebration: Mickie Grinevich, Leora Stroup, Lauretta Schimmoler, and Florence Fintak, 1968. Stroup referred to them as the "Four Horseman."

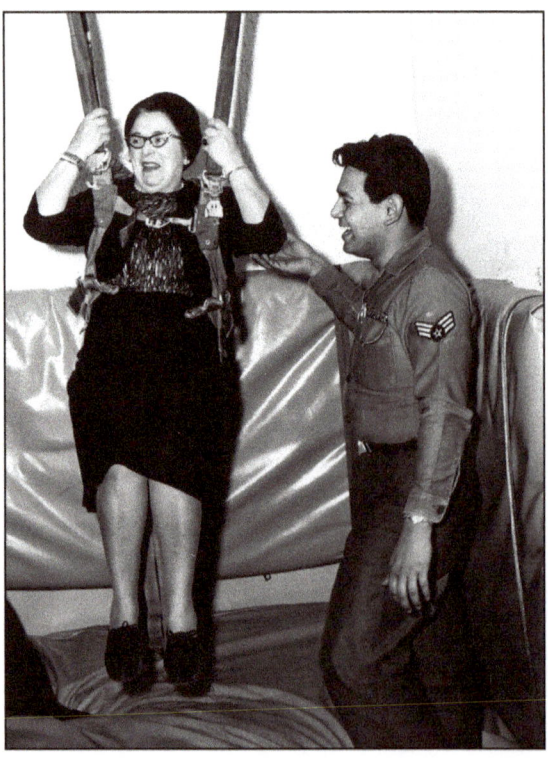

Figure 04.27. Stroup during a parachute demonstration, 1968. AMEDD.

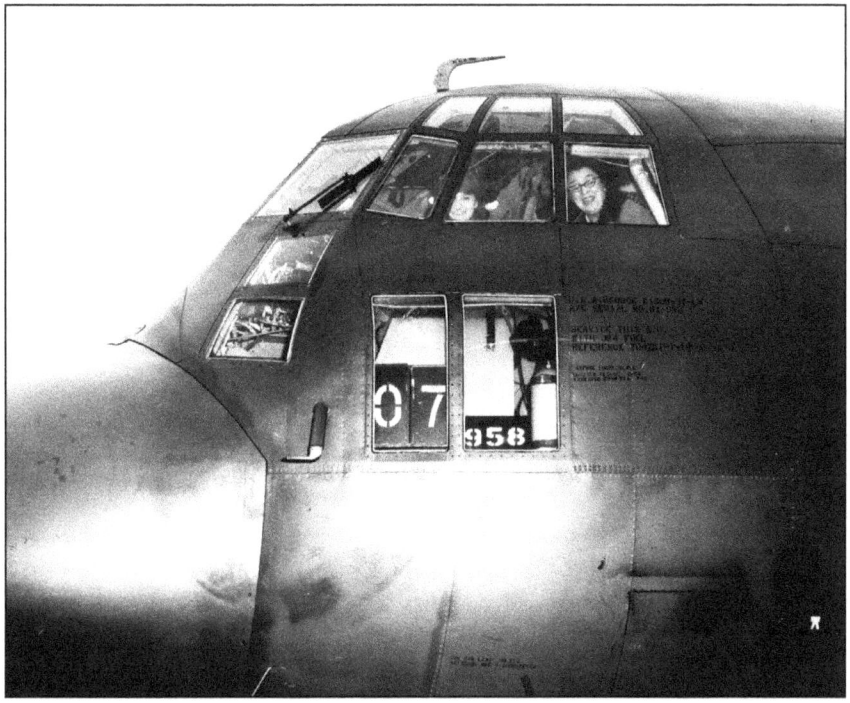

Figure 04.28. Stroup at the 25th Anniversary, in her element, in a massive military plane. This time with a woman in the pilot's seat, 1968. AMEDD.

She marked another milestone in 1968 for her nursing program—the graduation of the first male nurse from the program and his commission as a Lieutenant in the Army Nurse Corps.[63] In 1970, the nursing college employed a male instructor for the first time.

They had enrolled twelve men, mostly former military medical corpsmen. She hoped several would join a nationally promoted program as doctor assistants. The American Medical Association had suggested recruiting 100,000 registered nurses to train as assistant physicians to help in rural communities that had no doctor.[64]

Stroup said corpsmen possessed "…a wealth of training and experience, and can become the extended arm of the doctor in small communities." The program would involve a physician in the city and the assistant physician in the small community. The assistant would train six months with the physician before going into the community and stay in constant contact through "electronic equipment." Stroup thought the corpsmen were the obvious choice because of two desired qualifications: the general public preferred a man as a doctor, and the person must be licensed.[65]

Chapter Four

Stroup did not mention, or perhaps she was unaware of, Loretta Ford—a nursing professor at the University of Colorado who had created a nurse practitioner program (NP) in 1965, which sought to train nurses in the same primary care provider role. Neither military corpsmen nor exclusively male nurses were hallmarks of Ford's NP program. Duke University eventually created the first physician assistant (PA) program with four male ex-Navy corpsmen. They graduated in October 1967. [66]

Stroup retired from Fort Hays State College in May 1971. She returned later that year to award the first Bachelor of Science in Nursing degrees, which the college had started in 1968 after receiving the $400,000 estate gift.

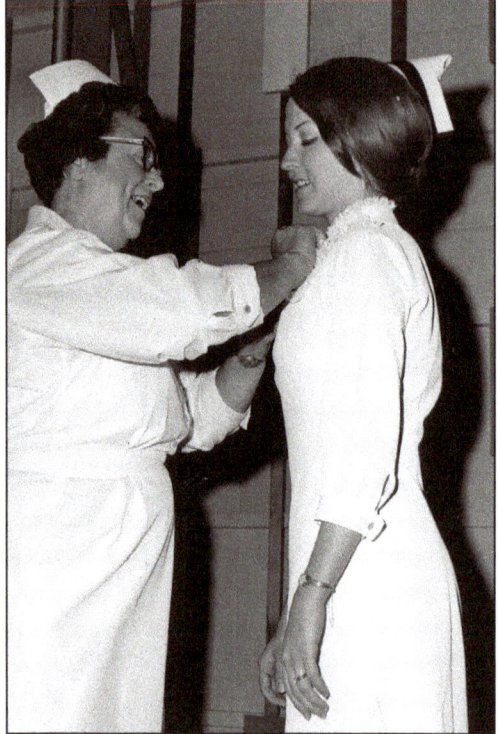

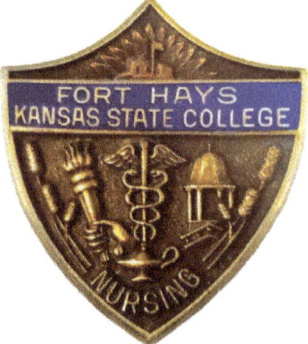

Figure 04.29. Stroup pinning the graduate nurse pin on a student. Forsyth Library Collections, FHSU.

Figure 04.30. The nurses' pin of the first graduate in 1958, Viola Vincent. The basic pin design hasn't changed except the word College to University in 1977. Photo by Samantha L. Harper.

Stroup had planned to write two books during her retirement. She told a reporter in 1966, "One day, I will write their story for Flight Nurses. When I retire, that will be my retirement project." [67] She had once begun a novel titled "The Belle of Pusan," the name they called her during her time in Korea—a play of words on her middle name, Belle. [68] She had wanted to complete both books but later said she was "just too busy."

On 4 June 1972, at 71, she married her longtime friend Raymond Eggen—Stroup's first marriage. Was he the hometown boy she spoke of so long ago, during those romantic days at her house in Hawaii? They'd met in 1942 when Stroup worked in the Civil Air Patrol. Eggen owned a Cessna Aircraft distribution company in Detroit; he moved to Hays when they married. Unfortunately, he died eight months later after a short illness. [69]

Despite this setback, she didn't rest—she volunteered at the Hays Senior Center and the Ellis Historical Society. In 1974 when Hays Senior Center needed more space, she became vice-chairman of the group and led a fundraiser to help them move to the Hadley Center in the west wing of Hadley Regional Medical Center. She became their first president. Another source states she led the charge to remodel the old James Motor Company building at 204 East 8th Street, south of Hadley Hospital, for the new center. The location within the Hadley Center may have been temporary or failed, as a 1977 announcement states the Senior Center was at 204 East 8th Street. [70-74]

She served as the nutrition program's Project and Activities Director at the Senior Center and then as Director for Northwest Kansas Meals, Inc. The Area Agencies on Aging honored her for service to elderly persons and for help in developing meal site councils in 22 communities at their Annual Kansas Conference on Aging. [75-76]

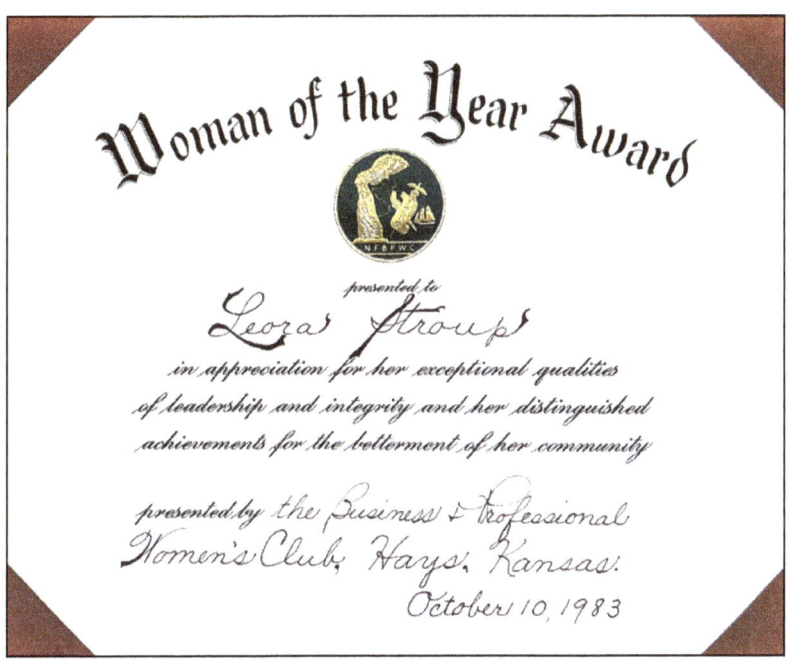

Figure 04.31. Stroup's Woman of the Year award from the Business and Professional Women's Club, Kansas Federation, 10 October 1983. The organization also awarded it to her in 1984. Leora Stroup Papers, AMEDD.

Stroup received numerous honors and certificates from various groups: the Kansas State Nurses' Association, Outstanding Faculty at FHSC, Delta Kappa Gamma Society, Medical Self-Help Training, Shelter Management, Kansas Health Mobilization Training, Kansas Public Health Association, Service to Older Kansans, Crime Prevention, Nutrition Program for the Elderly, Good Samaritan Society, Kansas Civil Defense, Kansas Heart Association, Ellis County Historical Society, The Memorial Union, Department of Earth Sciences, Certified Steam Calliopist, Blarney Stone Kisser, Jerusalem Pilgrim, and Crosser of the International Date Line.[77]

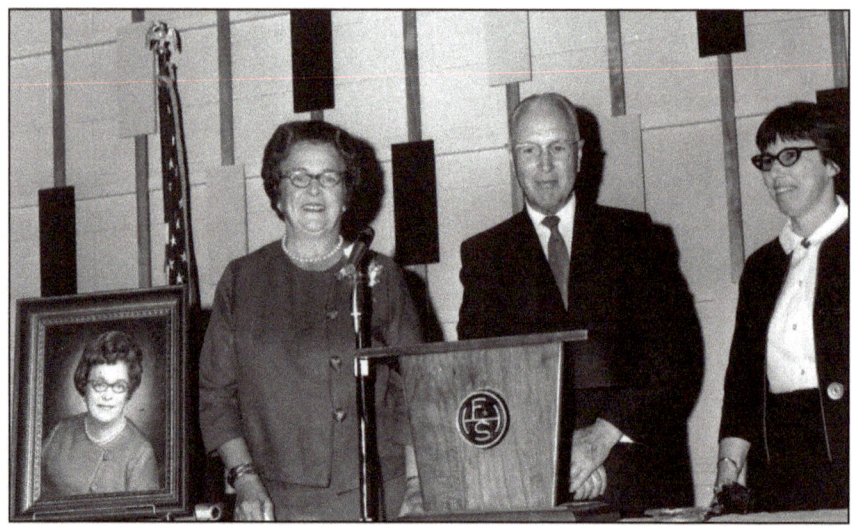

Figure. 04.32. Stroup Hall dedication ceremony, 1981. Stroup at left; other persons are unidentified. Stroup is wearing the identical outfit and glasses as the Stroup in the painting. Forsyth Library Collections, FHSU.

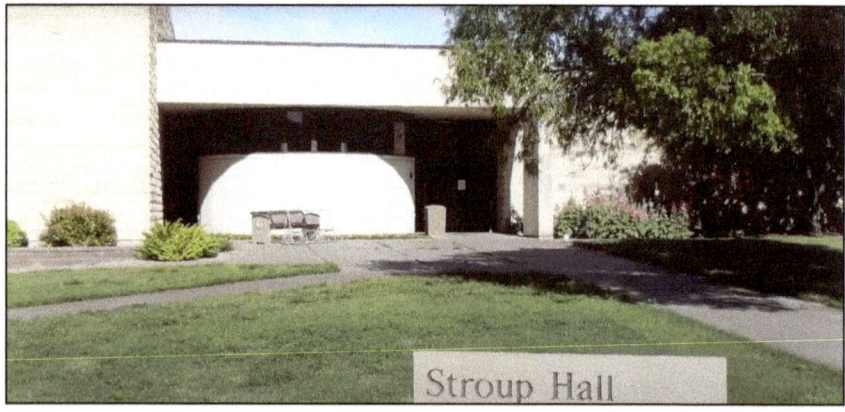

Figure 04.33. Stroup Hall, the 25,844 square foot building at FHSU, 2020.

On 13 June 1981, FHSU completed and dedicated a building in Stroup's honor. The Department of Nursing at Fort Hays State University is still located at Stroup Hall and now includes a doctoral degree program. FHSU also established the Leora B. Stroup Nursing Scholarship for outstanding clinical performance, community involvement, and academic achievement.

Stroup would certainly feel immense pride for the impressive growth of the program she started in 1952 with herself as the only instructor, sixteen students, two classrooms, and orange crates for bedside tables.

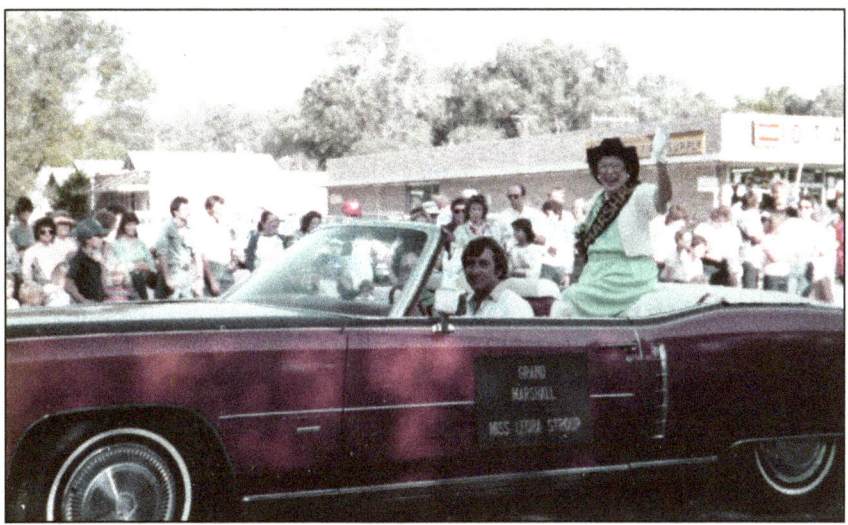

Figure 04.34. Stroup as Grand Marshall of the homecoming parade, 1983. Forsyth Library Collections, FHSU. Stroup returned to accept the honor as Grand Marshall of the Homecoming Parade.

Stroup was an avid collector. During her military years, she kept many items: scrapbooks, photographs, papers of flight nursing, Japanese kimonos, Kakemono scrolls, military pins, Japanese-occupied currency, and Korean pottery. She bought curios during her world travels: tea sets, bells, vases, glass birds, and tiny elephants. She ordered custom-made dolls of historical nursing figures to use in her nursing history class.[78]

Stoup had purchased Kakemono scrolls from Japanese citizens in Korea who sold them in a hurry—they needed to return quickly to Japan and could only carry a single suitcase. Stroup reportedly returned to Cleveland carrying the scrolls under her arm.[79]

She donated her impressive collection of Japanese scrolls to the Fort Hays State University's Art Department in 1983. At first, the Art Department lacked the financial resources to establish the collection's value, although John C. Thorns Jr., the art chair at that time, felt they were valuable.

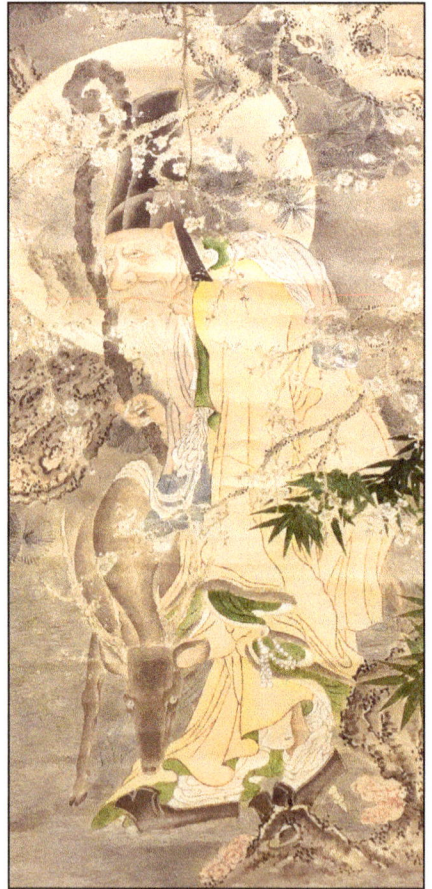 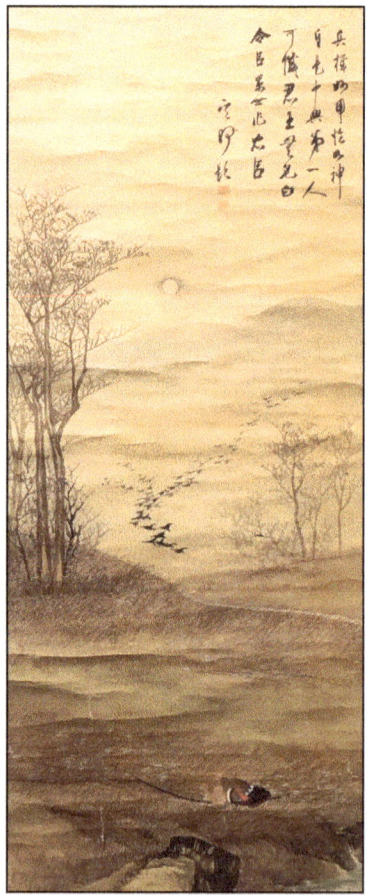

Figure 04.35. Jurojin, 1392-1573. Forsyth Library Collections, FHSU.

Figure 04.36. Dead Samurai Soldier, 1392-1573.

The Dead Samurai Soldier scroll illustrates the poem in the upper right corner. The artist chose not to emphasize the death of the samurai with a literal translation of death's agonies and violence but rather to suggest its presence by the samurai's abandoned helmet lying in the foreground and the poem's last line:[79]

> Samurai soldier dead
> Ducks are flying
> Moon is shining
> But life is not there

Jurojin, one of Seven Gods of Luck, incorporates symbols for longevity: plum, bamboo, pine, mushrooms, and a deer. In the Shinto religion, deer guard the sacred shrines and are considered messengers from the gods to priests in the shrines.

Finally, in 2005, a master's degree student in international studies, Linda J. Fleming, researched the scrolls. With the assistance of the Kampo Museum in Kyoto, Japan, she translated the inscriptions and interpreted the meaning of each scroll. They date between 1615 and 1868, placing them in the Edo period. The scrolls are mostly Japanese, but Fleming believed one is Korean and a few are Chinese. "Some of Stroup's pieces are equivalent to those in significant collections on display in large art museums," Thorns said.[80]

Stroup obtained Korean pottery during her years in Korea and donated the 16-piece collection to Fort Hays State College Museum (now the Sternberg Memorial Museum) in 1960. Stroup said the pottery pieces belonged to the Koryo Dynasty, 918-1392 AD. She learned about distinguishing marks on the bottom of the pottery left by three clay pellets on which the pieces rested while inside the kiln. "It is this variety which is the prize of the sophisticated collector and is uniquely Korean, without peer in the world," Stroup told the *Salina Journal*.[81]

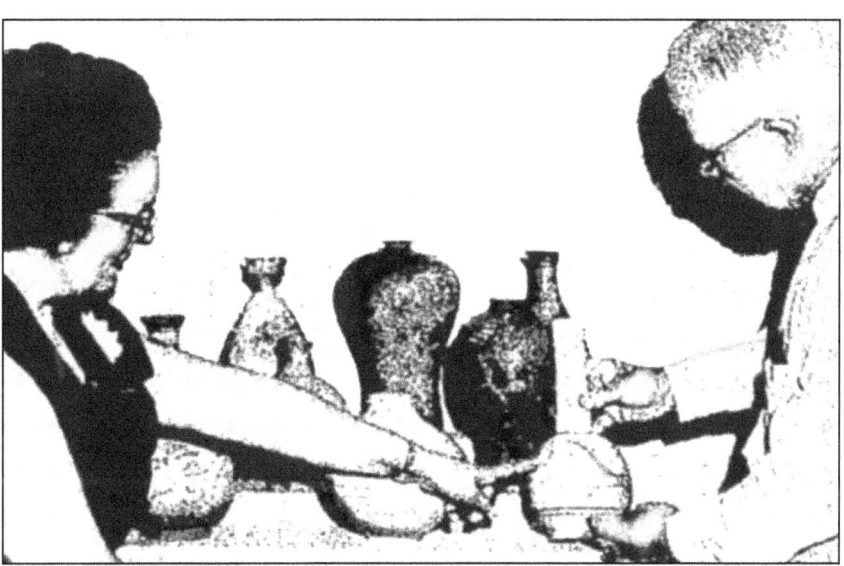

Figure 04.37. Stroup presenting her Korean pottery collection to the curator George Sternberg, c. 1960. Leora Stroup Papers, AMEDD. A form of the Korean inlay technique, *sanggam* decorates several pottery pieces. In others, the artist carved through the colored clay slip to reveal the vessel's body in a process called *barkji* (Korean for the Italian term *sgraffito*).[82]

Chapter Four

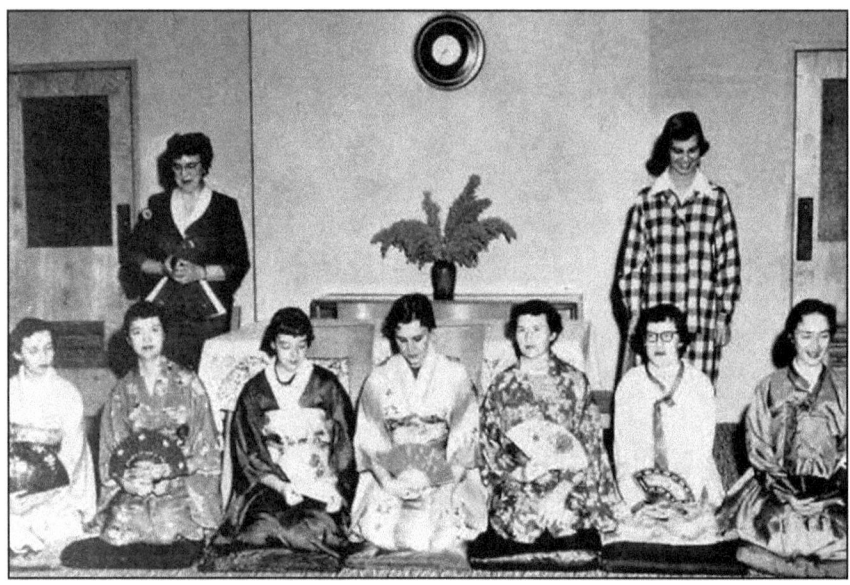

Figure 04.38. YMCA members model the various Japanese kimonos Stroup brought back from Korea, 1956. Stroup is standing at the left; the others are unidentified. Leora Stroup Papers, AMEDD.

Stroup often held Japanese tea ceremonies in her home. She attended a meeting of the college's Young Women's Christian Association (YMCA) and discussed the customs of Japan and Korea. The women donned Stroup's kimonos and knelt on pillows for a cultural-style photo. [83]

Stroup died on 13 February 1985 due to complications from diabetes. Her friends organized a well-attended memorial service at Hays Memorial Chapel in her lovely town.

During an interview in 1958, Stroup said she saw her life in three important phases: air evacuation, her work in Korea, and at Fort Hays State College. She lived twenty-seven years past that interview; she might have added her volunteer retirement work with seniors as phase four. [84]

Her longtime friend Calvin Harbin said, "She never got old in the sense that she resigned herself to quit and do nothing." [85]

"My goodness, what a gal," Bob Lowen said. "She was just full of vitality."

Katherine Rodgers said, "Leora Stroup was short in stature but stood tall among us for more than 30 years and has left an indelible imprint upon this community, which she regarded as home. We shall miss her." [86]

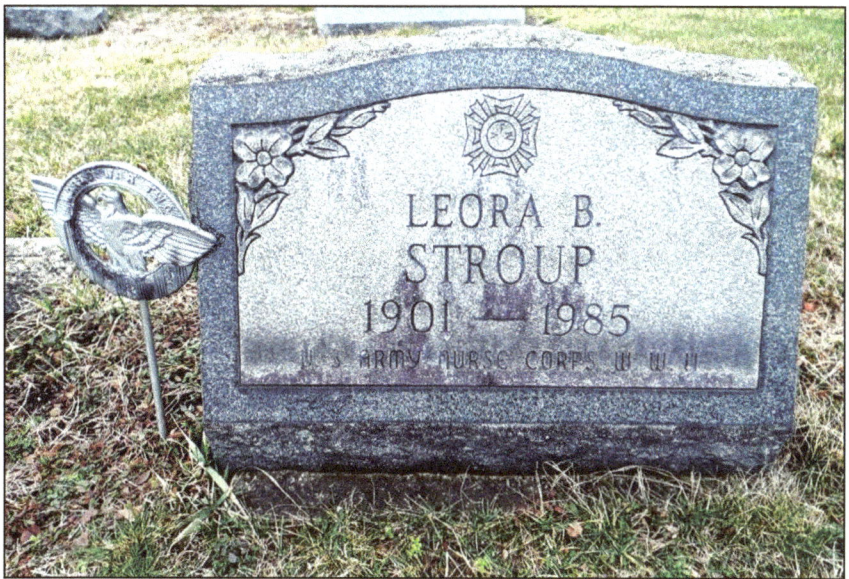

Figure 04.39. Stroup's headstone, Windham Cemetery, Ohio. The Windham American Legion Post 674 decorated her site with a WWII Ruptured Duck grave marker. Photo by Danny Burns, Windham, Ohio.

They returned her remains to her childhood home of Windham, Ohio, and buried her in the family cemetery. Her husband Raymond Eggen and her sister Olive Hay are beside her.

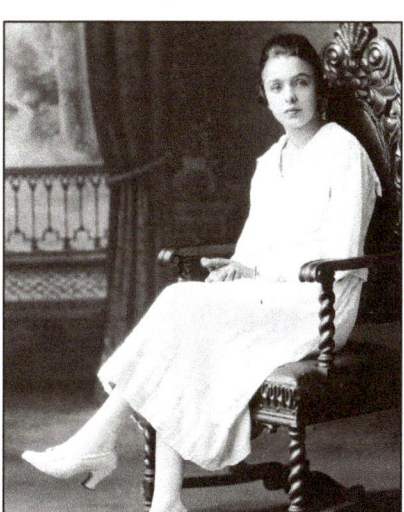 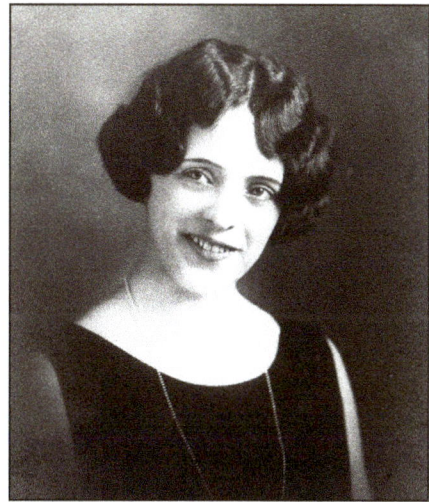

Figures 04.40. and 04.41. Stroup about 16 and 25 years old. Forsyth Library Collections, FHSU.

Chapter Five

The Companies

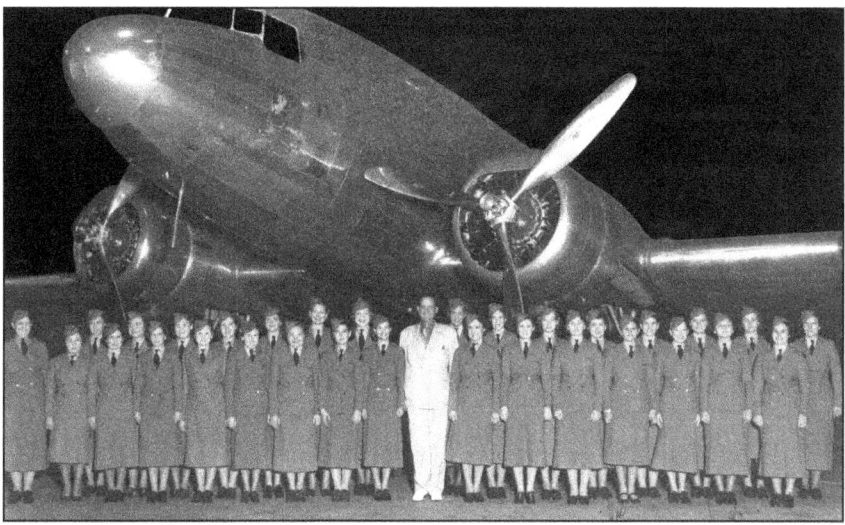

Figure 05.01. The 1st Division in front of a DC-3 during a Douglas Aircraft factory tour, Long Beach, California, 28 July 1938. Schimmoler stands at the far left. Visiting from Dayton, Ohio, is Captain Merle McGriff at the right of the man in white. MMM Collection.

They divided the Corps into three wings and the wings into nine divisions. The divisions split into companies. The number of companies in each division depended on the number of members in each location; major cities recruited many and small towns recruited fewer. Larger companies formed a locally based group of fifteen or fewer members called a squadron.

The National Commander, Lauretta Schimmoler, held the rank of Colonel and assigned rank commensurate with their earned positions. A Lieutenant Colonel commanded a wing, a Major commanded a division, and a Captain commanded a company. A Squadron Leader supervised under the direction of a Captain. Recruits held the rank of Cadet for six months of training, and then Schimmoler promoted them to First Lieutenant or Second Lieutenant.[1]

Company Commanders, and the other commissions, changed over time as members moved into higher commissions, resigned, or the commanders discharged them. Schimmoler ran a tight ship—recruits followed the rules, or consequences ensued. As she firmly pointed out, "All commissions are honorary and temporary."[2]

Chapter Five

A company consisted of the following positions:

- Captain as the Company Commander
- Adjutant as secretary
- Quartermaster as treasurer
- Public Relations
- Athletic
- Mess
- Photographer
- Recruiting
- Color Guard

Smaller geographic areas might not meet the required number of members to fill all the jobs. At the start of the ANCOA, Schimmoler wanted the full complement in a company; later, she allowed smaller groups to form even if they could not fill all the positions.

During peacetime, a company would ideally include the following number of commissioned and non-commissioned personnel:

- Thirty registered nurses
- Eighteen members as first aid workers, divided into assistants to nurses and clerical duties at a medical station
- Six radio operators

During a national emergency, a company would enlist dietitians to prepare the food for company personnel.

The companies fostered friendly competitions, called Competitive Interests, to create pep songs and company mascots. They designed the company's logo to be a favorite animal, a design representing a company member, or in memory of a famous individual in aviation.

While some songs and drawings might appear naive to modern standards, these types of rally songs and cartoonish logos were common among military groups of that era. The military often painted cartoon-style logos or pin-ups on the nose of the airplanes.

The ANCOA members showed immense pride in their company songs, mottos, mascots, logos, and the Aerial Nurse Corps of America flag. They composed a National Theme Song. The lyrics were original but used the tune of a well-known song, "Shipmates Stand Together," performed in the 1935 movie, *Shipmates Forever*. They used the movie's title for their song's title. Constantly vigilant, Schimmoler obtained permission from Romick Music Publishers to sing the ANCOA lyrics to the song's melody. [3]

SHIPMATES STAND TOGETHER SHIPMATES FOREVER

The National Theme Song, "Shipmates Forever"

Aer-i-al Nur-ses is our na-ame
    But we're more than that
Grow-ing is our fa-ame
    Banded for a pur-pose
We'll stand pat
    We'll glad-ly play the ga-ame
Watch us go to bat
    We're the guardians of the airway
And we do the do or dare way
    For our nation grand
Com-rades march to-gether
    Eyes upon the plane
Bad or sun-ny weath-er
    We've a mission, we'll surely gain
Now ho-rizons beckon
    For a thrill-ing trip
We don't have to stop a second
    We're trained for our ship.
With our first aid kits

Aer-i-al Nur-ses is our na-ame
    For a cause that's grand
Over trails un-light-ed
    We are marching forward
Hand in hand
    By du-ty we are guided
For you un-der-stand
    Be it ci-ty state or nat-ion
We will face the situation
    As only nur-ses can
Aer-i-al Nur-ses stand together
    With a first aid kit
Fair or stormy weather
    We're there to do our best
Our little bit
    Fri-ends and pals for-ever
And if you chance to meet disaster
    We will come a way that faster
With our first aid kits. [4]

Chapter Five

1st Wing

The 1st Division

1st Wing, Division Commanders: Lauretta Schimmoler, Edith Corns.

Company A-1, Los Angeles, California

Schimmoler listed the names on the Aerial Nurse Corps Roster by the active date. She started the list with the number two, apparently counting herself as number one. The 1st Division, Company A, began in August 1936 with the following ten RNs living in various areas of Los Angeles County. Other companies and divisions started as the number of members increased.

2. Emma Koenig, 8 Aug
3. Velma Maul, 8 Aug
4. Ora Brook, 15 Aug
5. Velma Cook, 15 Aug
6. Rose Cummings, 15 Aug
7. Edwardine Malone, 15 Aug
8. Cecelia Getsfred, 29 Aug
9. Edna Yarnell, 29 Aug
10. Nelda Anderson, 30 Aug
11. Dorothy Zimmerman, 30 Aug

The 1st Division Companies

- Company A in Los Angeles, California
- Company B in Pasadena/Glendale, California
- Company C in Santa Monica, California, and Phoenix, Arizona
- Company D in San Diego/La Jolla, California
- Company E in Bakersfield, California
- Company F in San Francisco, California
- Company K in Seattle/Tacoma, Washington
- Company L in Boise, Idaho

Company A-1 Officers

- Commanding Officers: Ora Brook, RN; Edith Corns, RN; Myrtle Martin, RN
- Adjutant: Nadine Hill, RN
- Quartermaster: Marie J. Wallace, RN
- Public Relations: Rose Marie Sternberg, RN
- Athletic: Joanne Frederickson, RN
- Mess: Lida Dolan, RN
- Photographic: Georgia Eckerd, RN
- Drill Officer: Joanne Frederickson, RN
- Color Guards: Laura Cheshire, RN, Gladys Bowen, RN, Patricia Estes, RN
- Operations: Lavinia Hopkins, RN

- Sports Editor: Margaret Doronia, RN
- Finance Officer: Pauline Busch
- *Flashes* Editors: Shirley Weidman, RN; Edith Corns, RN; Ailen Crain, RN; Florence Walden & Sue Ottig (assistant editors),
- Recruiting Officers: Squadron A, Ruby Bolch, RN; Squadron B, Novella Bowman, RN; Squadron C, Margaret Connell, RN
- Squadron Leaders: A-Los Angeles, Ruby Bolch, RN; B-Pasadena, Elizabeth Tintorri, RN; C-Santa Monica, Myrtle Martin, RN

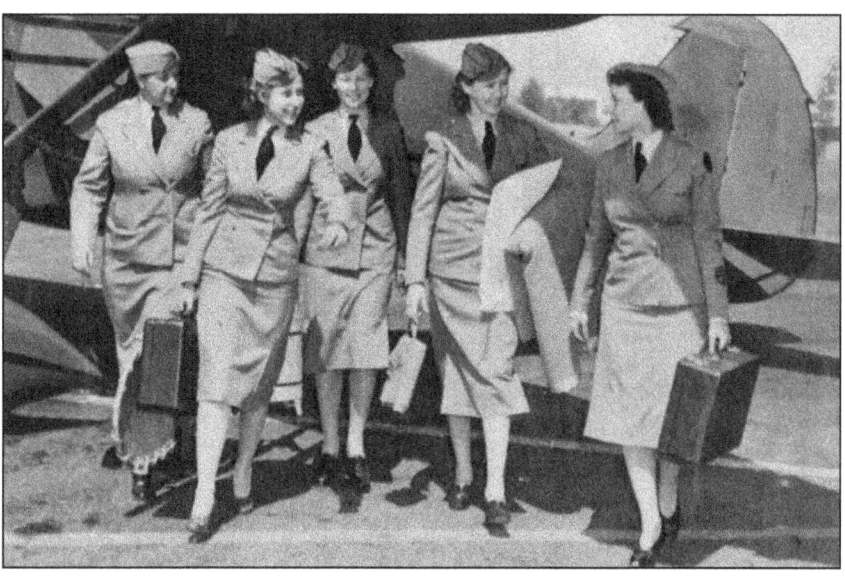

Figure 05.02. The Los Angeles ANCOA nurses on duty, elegant in their uniforms while performing a valuable service, 1939. MMM Collection.

Figure 05.03. A peek into a flight kit with the most common contents listed in the manual: alcohol, merthiolate, bandaids, scissors, rolls of adhesive, triangular bandages, sterile towels, gauze pads, boric acid or Collyrium for eye wash, ammonia, peroxide, aspirin, soda-mint tablets, ivory soap, pus basin, safety pins, hemostats, depressors, tourniquets. AMEDD.

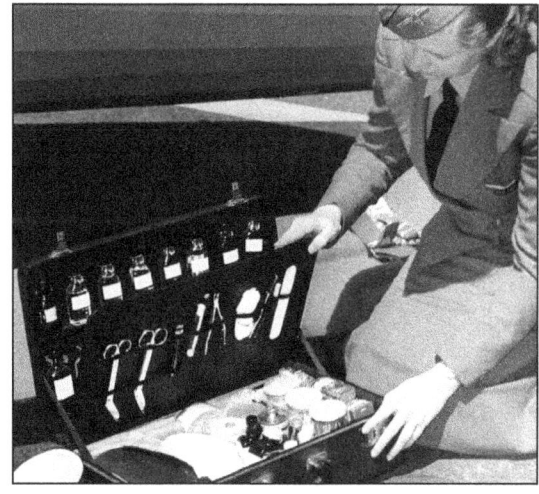

Chapter Five

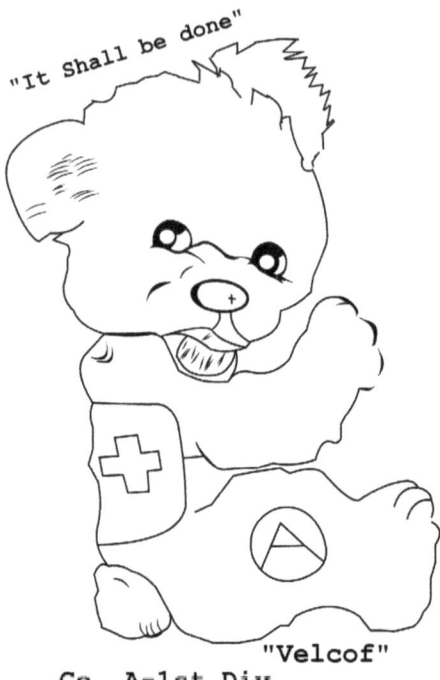

Figure 05.04. "Velcof," Company A-1 mascot logo. Re-created from a sketch in the *Flashes* newsletter.

- Motto: "It Shall Be Done."
- Mascot: A California grizzly bear named Velcof, based on the first letter in the names of the six senior members at the time of the name choosing, Velma, Edith, Lavinia, Cecelia, Ora, and Francis.

Company A-1 Pep Song

Company A stands first and fore-most
The best in all the land.
We're the cho-sen child-ren
Of the Corps that's famous
And that's grand.
We meet each week to-gether
Playing straight and fair.
Tho fun and frolic have their inning
Serious work marks our beginning,
Leading nurses in the air.

by Lieutenant M. Derenia [5]

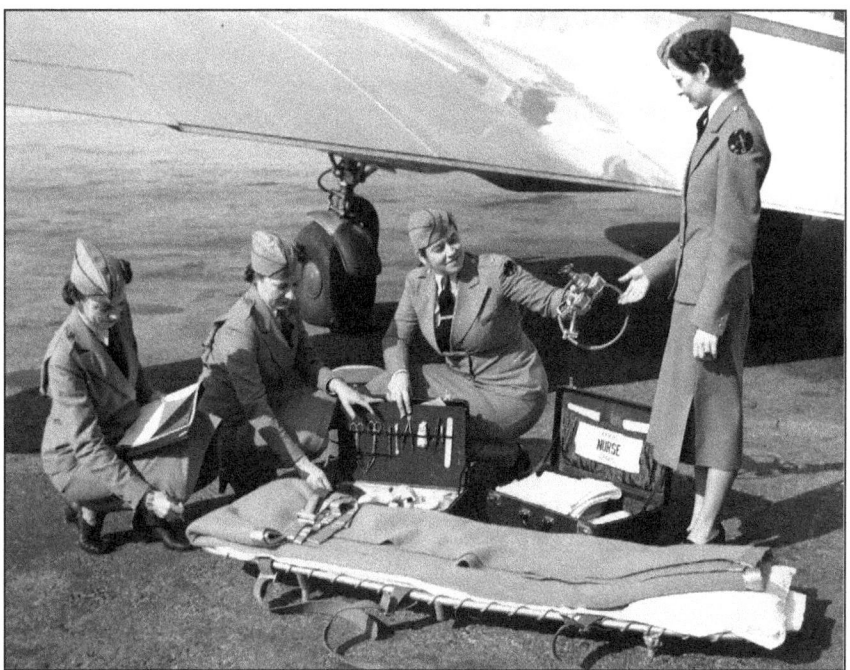

Figure 05.05. Members Florence Walden and Suzanne Otting, of the First Aid Department, check equipment after a flight with Aerial Nurses Margaret Helton and Lida Dola. MMM Collection.

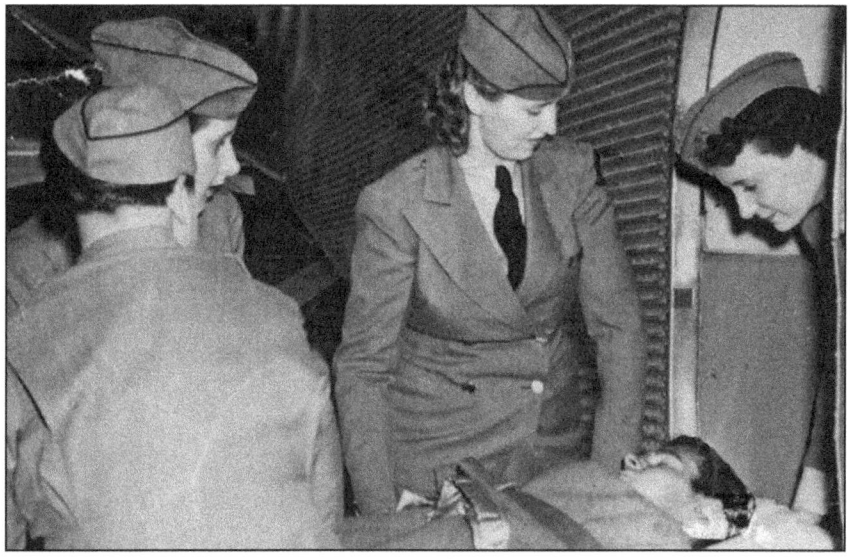

Figure 05.06. Los Angeles group loading a patient, 1939. MMM Collection.

Brothers Orville and Wilbur Wright built an airplane, the Wright Flyer; they documented the first sustained flight of an aircraft on 17 December 1903, in Flyer I (the Kitty Hawk), marking the start of the aviation era. Franklin Delano Roosevelt established National Aviation Day on 19 August 1939—Orville Wright's birthday. More than a century later, Orville's accomplishment continues to be honored: in 2017, a television show and its starship, *The Orville*, were named in remembrance of Wright.

Orville Wright was born in Dayton, Ohio; Schimmoler was also born in Ohio. She must have felt a pilot's kinship with him because in March 1939 the ANCOA named Orville an honorary member of the ANCOA.[6] On 25 March Company A-1 sponsored a fundraising dance in his honor, the "Bal des Avions," at the Ambassador Hotel in downtown Los Angeles. He was invited but was unable to attend.

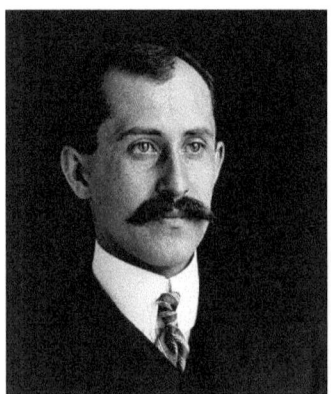 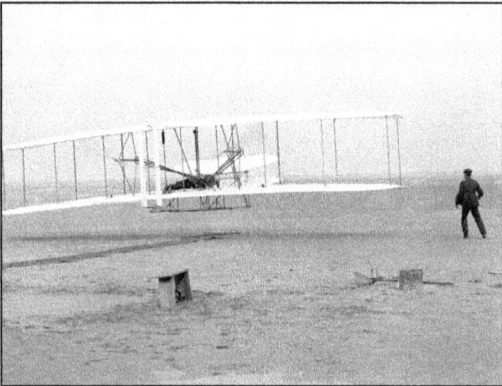

Figure 05.07. Orville Wright's portrait, 1907. Figure 05.08. First successful Wright brother's flight. Orville is in the pilot's seat, 17 December 1903.

Figure 05.09. A stewardess, Josephine Connor, buying tickets for "Bal des Avions" from ANCOA members Lida Dolan, Lillian Jensen, and Loretta Schimmoler, 24 March 1939. MMM.

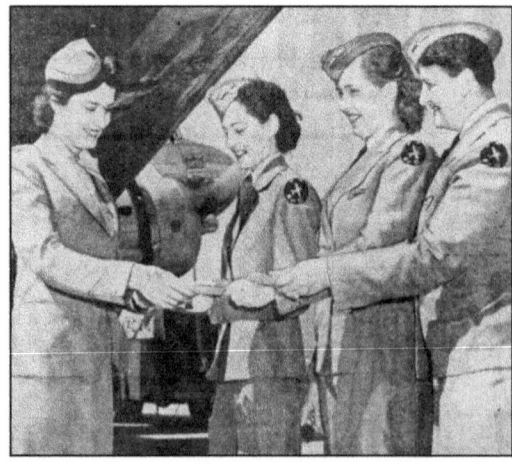

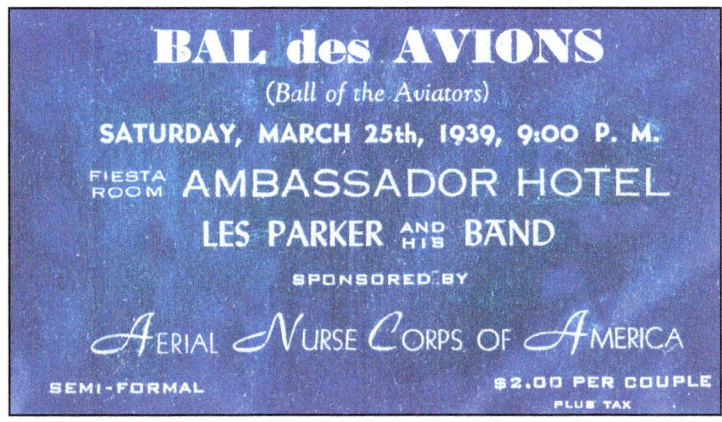

Figure 05.10. Ticket for the "Bal de Avions," 25 March 1939. MMM.

A long list of sponsors attended to hear the musical stylings of Les Parker and his Band. Members from several ANCOA companies attended; many flew in from faraway states for the big event.

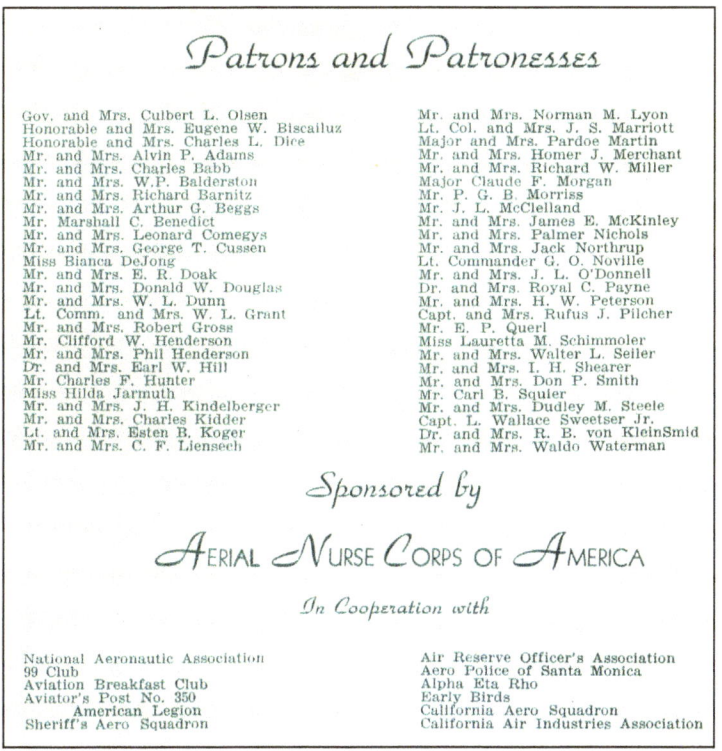

Figure 05.11. Patron list for the "Bal de Avions," 25 March 1939.

Chapter Five

Company B-1, Pasadena & Glendale, California

Company B-1 Officers

- Commanding Officer: Captain Lucille Hurst, RN
- Public Relations: Cadet Rachel Page, RN
- Squadron Officer: Ruby Bolch, RN
- Recruiting Officer: Novella Bowman, RN

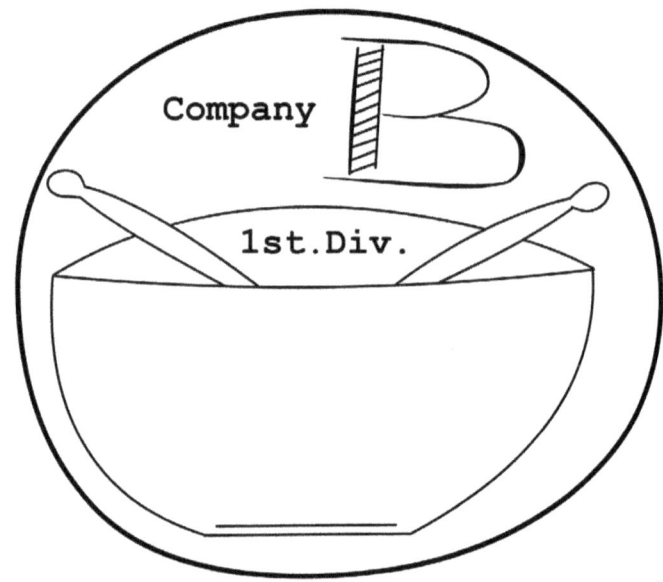

Figure 05.12. Company B-1 logo. Re-created from a sketch in *Flashes*.

Company B-1 Pep Song

Company B is coming for-ward
With her banners bright.
We're going to endeavor
To make this group a worthy one for flight.
We may be small in number
But you just watch our speed.
With a leader like our Major
We can climb and soon we'll wager
We'll be in the lead.

by Captain Lorraine Hurst

Company C-1, Santa Monica, California, & Phoenix, Arizona

Company C-1 Officers

- Squadron Officer: Myrtle Martin, RN
- Recruiting Officer: Margaret Connell, RN

- Lydia Gray, RN, was the only recruit listed in Phoenix

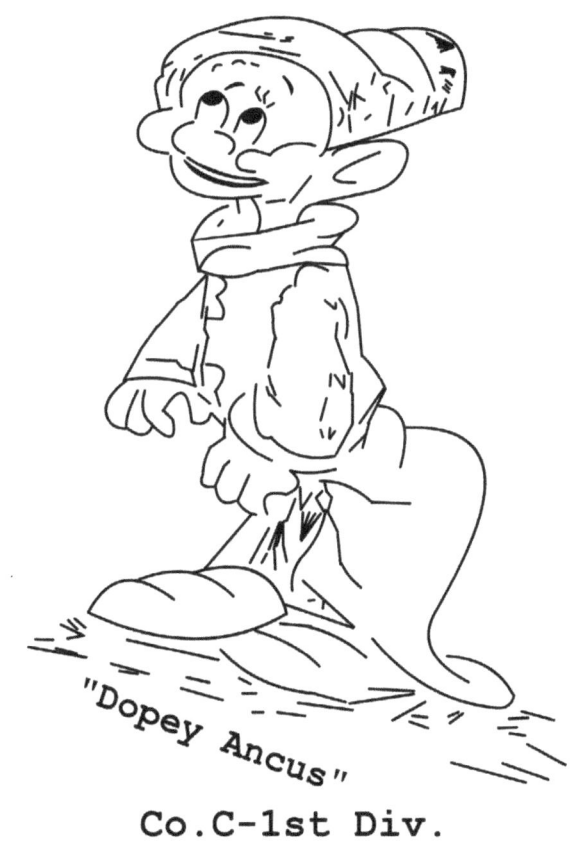

Figure 05.13. Company C-1 mascot logo, Dopey Ancus. Re-created from a sketch in *Flashes*

- Motto: "Upward and Onward"
- Mascot's Name: Dopey Ancus

Chapter Five

Company D-1, San Diego & La Jolla, California

Company D-1 Officers

- Company Commander: Bernice Minucci RN; Wanda Fill, RN
- Public Relations Officer: Grace Scharforth, RN

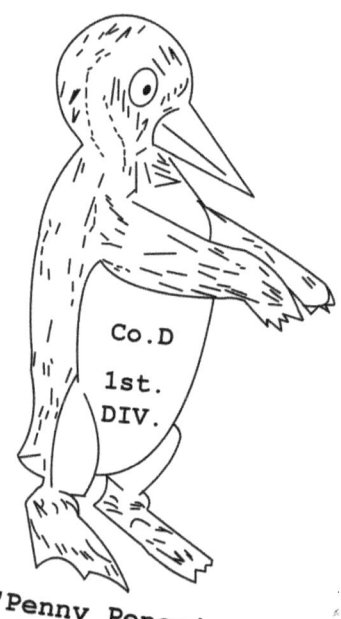

Figure 05.14. Penny the Penguin, Company D-1 mascot logo. Re-created from a sketch in *Flashes*.

- Motto: "Time and Tide Wait for No Man"
- Mascot's Name: Peggy Penguin

Company D-1 Pep Song

Company D of San Diego
AER-I-AL Mates to be.
The too-mod-est to say so
We're the best that ever saw the sea.
On-ward with the "Hay-Ho"
Straight to vic-tor-y.
Tho our emblem is a pen-quin
We have dressed him like a gen-man
The gang from Company "D".
                by Captain Bernice Minucci

Companies

Company K-1, Seattle & Tacoma, Washington

Company K-1 Officers

- Commanding Officer: Henrietta Palmer, RN; Alice Moyer, RN
- Adjutant: Amy Koenig, RN
- Quartermaster: Lorraine Phelps, RN
- Athletic: Helen Anders, RN
- Mess: Borghild Robertson, RN
- Photographic: Elsie Strandness, RN
- Recruiting Officer: Marjorie Good, RN
- Public Relations: Constance Rateliff, RN

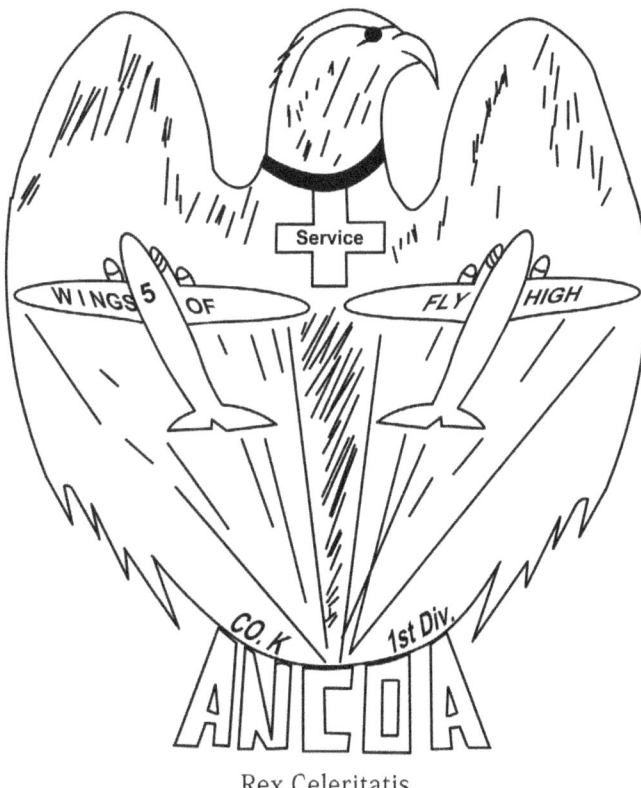

Figure 05.15. Rex Celeritatis Company K-1 mascot logo. Re-created from a sketch in *Flashes*

- Motto: "Fly High"
- Mascot's Name: A falcon named Rex Celeritatis (King of Speed). With wings outspread, he harbors the zooming of service, flying high over Company K-1.

Chapter Five

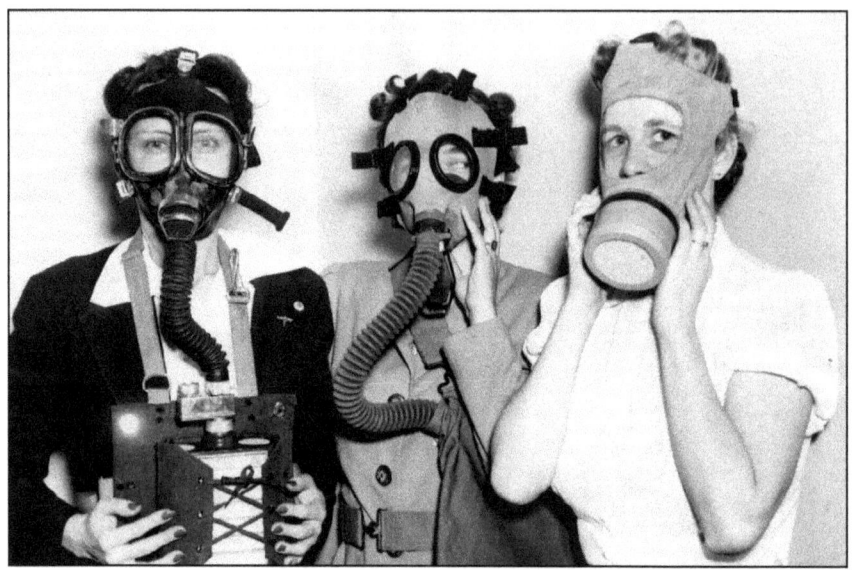

Figure 05.16. Seattle members demonstrate gas masks, 1941. Anita Owens, left, wears the type used by fireman and police. Edna Cox wears the latest in Army masks. Kitty Provo dons a mask used by British civilians. BHS.

Company K Pep Song

We're working together
We are all prepared
For no matter whether
Strife, disaster, or a war's declared
Our aim is to service
We're ready to comply
Company K is for a purpose
And are wing mates and
We'll always fly our banners high.

K members are now mastering the wireless code every Tuesday evening at the Amateur Radio Club House. The Course is the study of the Continental Code which will take several months to learn. Experience is acquired by using a practice table equipped with a buzzer. If the term of instruction is completed successfully, one is eligible to take an examination from the Seattle Federal Commission Office which includes questions of technical information and sending of messages at thirteen words per minute...Flashes.

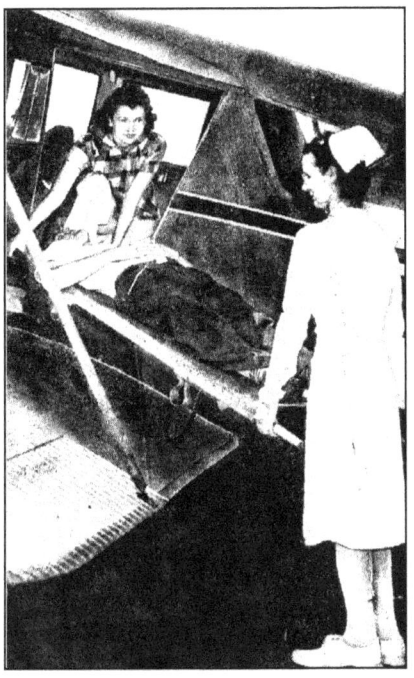

Figure 05.17. Seattle members Julie Loldhamer, in white uniform, and Elsie Hansen, loading a patient into a plane, 1940. *Flashes* photo.

Figure 05.18. A Seattle member, Rita Sutherland, learns the radio operations from Howard Hayes. *Flashes* photo.

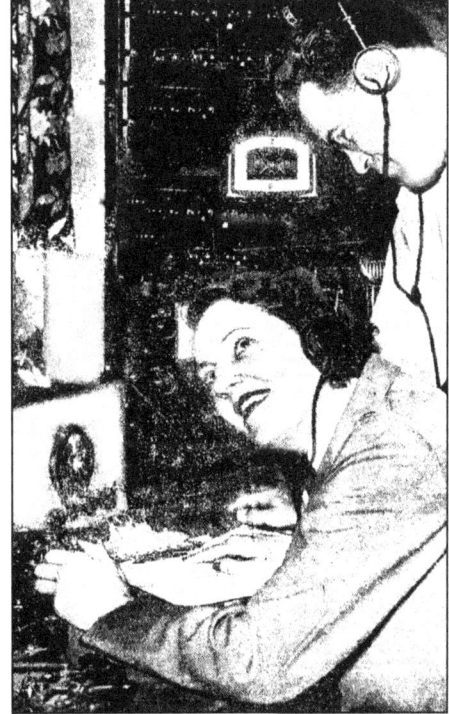

Chapter Five

3rd Wing

3rd Wing Commander: Merle McGriff

The 2nd Division

Company A-2, Denver, Colorado

Company A-2 began on 6 February 1941. *Flashes* lists several members but does not detail officers or activities concerning A-2.

The 3rd Division

Company A-3, Ingleside, Nebraska

Company A-3 began on 3 November 1940. *Flashes* lists several members but does not detail officers or activities concerning A-3.

The 4th Division

Company A-4 in Chicago, Illinois

Company A-4 Officers

- Company Commander: Dorothy Lathrop, RN
- Adjutant: Helen Molloy, RN
- Quartermaster: Thelma Macumbor, RN
- Public Relations: Virginia Schrodt, RN
- Athletic: Betty Roy, RN
- Mess: Florence Fintak, RN
- Photographer: Dorothy Alke, RN

Company B-4, Milwaukee, Wisconsin

Company B-4 Officers

- Company Commander: Florence Fintak, RN (transferred from A-4)
- Adjutant: Ellen E. Church, RN
- Quartermaster: Florence Lehmkuhl, RN
- Public Relations: Frances E. Stark, RN
- Photographer: Mary Agnes Leary, RN

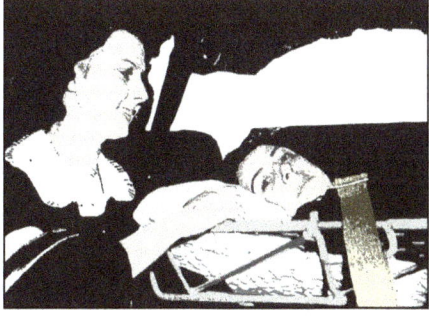
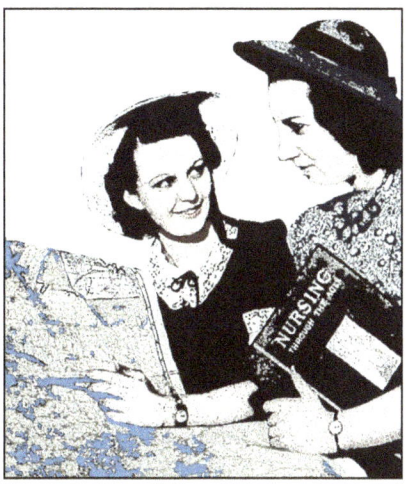

Figure 05.19. Florence Fintak, left, and Florence Lehmkuhl, Midwest Airways in Milwaukee, ground school training at the Wisconsin Avenue School.

Figure 05.20. Commander Florence Fintak, left, and Mary Agnes Leary during their first meeting of Company B-4 in Milwaukee, Wisconsin, July 1940. Colorized *Flashes* photos.[6]

Company C-4, Decatur, Illinois

C-4 began on 16 February 1939

- Company Commander: Genevieve Waples, RN
- Motto: "Pari Passu" (side by side)

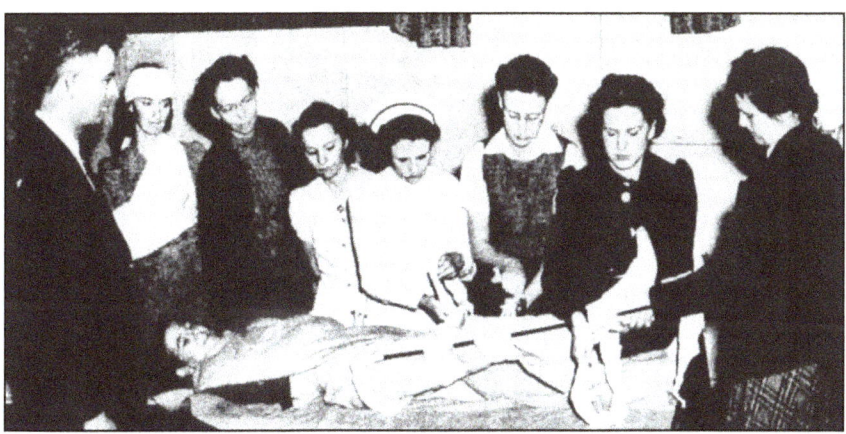

Figure 05.21. ANCOA members during a first aid demonstration for the newly formed Decatur company. Anne Frances Dorn, Genevieve Waples, Helen Bourne, Jewel Conway, Hazel Angle, Esther Tveldt, Lousie Ousley. Dortha Dean poses as the victim.[7] BHS.

Chapter Five

The 5th Division

Division Commander: Merle McGriff, RN

The 5th Division Companies

- Company A in Detroit, Michigan
- Company B in Cleveland, Ohio
- Company C in Dayton, Ohio
- Company D in Dayton, Ohio
- Company E in Toledo, Ohio
- Company F in Lancaster, Ohio
- Company G in Cincinnati, Ohio

Company A-5, Detroit, Michigan

A-5 began on 5 May 1938

Company A-5 Officers

- Company Commanders: Leora Stoup, RN; Eileen Newbeck, RN
- Public Relations: Margaret Gudobba, RN, Lauretta Van Antwerpt, RN
- Adjutant: Mary Anne Chomin, RN
- Quartermaster: Laura Dixon, RN
- Athletic: Lenore Bomholt, RN
- Mess: Louise Blair, RN
- Photographic: Gwendolyn Grimes, RN

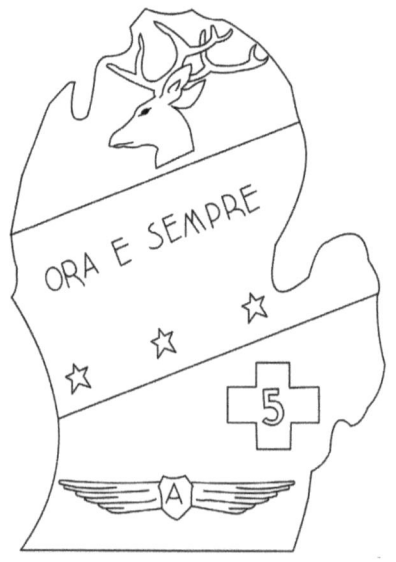

05.22. The logo "Ora E. Sempre" (Now and Forever). Company A-5's *Flashes* page, the "Great Lakes Breezes," used this logo of a deer mascot, three stars, a Greek Cross with the number 5, and wings with the letter A. Re-created from a sketch in *Flashes*.

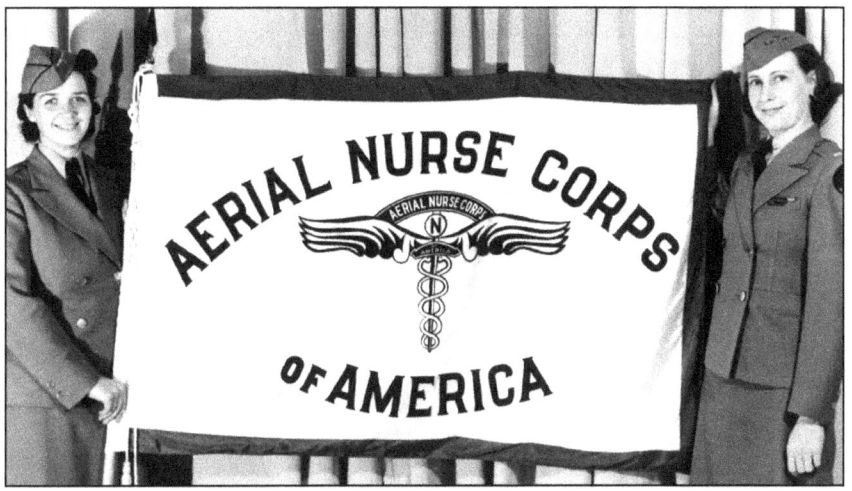

Figure 05.23. Company A-5 Members, Margaret Gudobba, left, and Eileen Newbeck, proudly display the ANCOA flag. Leora Stroup Papers, AMEDD.

Company A-5 had two mascots, an emblem, and two mottos—they enjoyed creating the symbols for their company.

- Mottos: "Ora E. Sempre" and "Whatever We Do We Do Well"
- Mascot's Name: Eddie the Dog. Named in honor of the pioneer flyer and founder of the Stinson Aircraft Company, Eddie Stinson. A-5 often called themselves the Eddie Stinson Company.

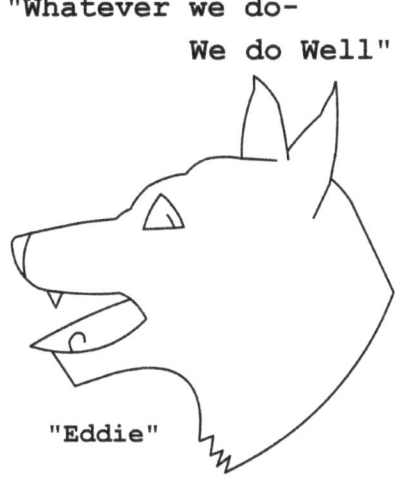

Figure 05.24. Eddie the Dog. Company A-5 logo #2. Re-created from *Flashes*.

Chapter Five

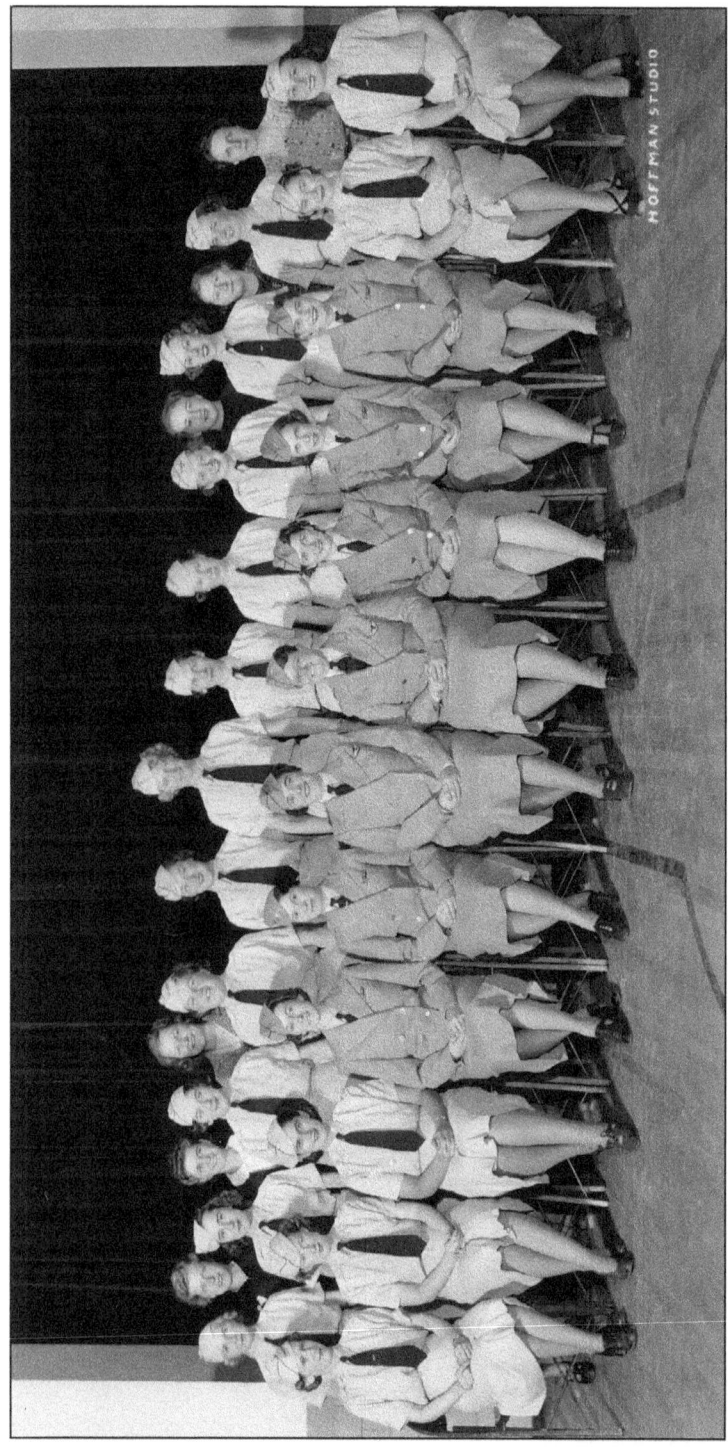

Figure 05.25. Company A-5, Detroit, Michigan, 1939. Leora Stroup sits sixth from left, and Lauretta Schimmoler sits seventh. Members are wearing a mixture of formal and summer/indoor uniforms. MMM Collection.

Companies

Company A-5 met for training classes each Wednesday night. They gathered at a local airport to fly with Stroup or Howard Hartung, an Army Reserve Officer who assisted the Corps on Sunday afternoons. By February 1939, the company included fifty-six members. Eight were pilots. Stroup told the *Detroit Evening News*:

> Membership has become more difficult to maintain as the Corps has become a recruiting agency for airline hostesses. The Detroit Unit has already lost one member to an airline and is about to lose another. [8]

Naturally, commercial airlines wanted ANCOA nurses; they were already air fitness tested. And, of course, the nurses would have wanted to become airline stewardesses as the job paid well, had prestige, and was less stressful than patient care. Plus, they could regularly experience the adventure of flying frequently—the reason many joined ANCOA in the first place.

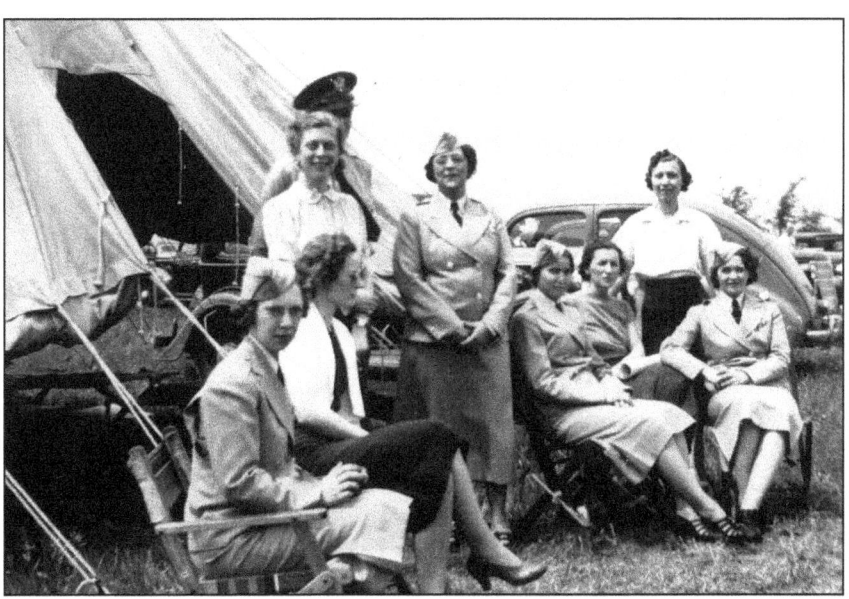

Figure 05.26. Company A-5 at the Erin Township Air Show, 1939. Members staffed the field hospital at Hartung-Gratiot Airport in Roseville, the site of the first commercial airport in Michigan. Leora Stroup is standing at center.

At the Spring Dance, later in the evening after the air show, the Detroit Company sponsored a raffle with a grand prize of a round-trip flight from Detroit to the 1939 World's Fair in New York. One lucky person won an excellent draw for the mere price of twenty-five cents. The raffle hopefuls, however, had to stay until the midnight drawing. MMM Collection.

Chapter Five

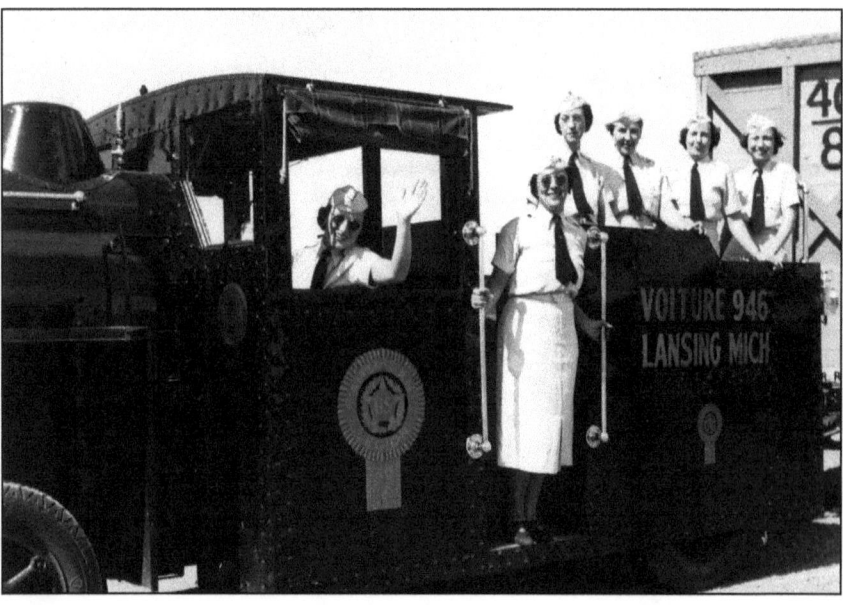

Figure 05.27. A raffle ticket for the Spring Dance, 15 April 1939.

Figure 05.28. A-5 members visiting the American Legion 40et8, in Lansing, Michigan. Leora Stroup is standing on the platform. MMM.

They derived the name Society of Forty Men and Eight Horses, (La Société des Quarante Hommes et Huit Chevaux), from the box cars they used to transport troops in France during WWI; it could transport forty men or eight horses. As a gesture of thanks, France sent forty-nine box cars to the United States, one for each state, laden with five tons of gifts donated by private French citizens. In 1960 the 40et8 separated from the American Legion and became an independent veteran's organization.

Twenty-five members of A-5 were guests of U. S. Army Air Corps officers at Selfridge Field in Michigan. Captain Allison and his lieutenants escorted A-5 through the hangers. The group inspected the equipment; all twenty-five members of Company A-5 squeezed into the C-33—the Army's new cargo aircraft designed as a hospital plane.

The group experimented with the recent military-adopted invention, the laryngophone (a throat microphone), when conversing with the radio tower inside the hanger. They watched many ships land from the vantage point of the radio observation tower. The group also inspected the Lockheed C-40 model, the Douglas Bomber B-18, and the Curtiss Pursuit P-36 plane. Following the tour, they stopped at the Seadrome Cottage on Lake St. Clair and took rides in the seaplane.[9]

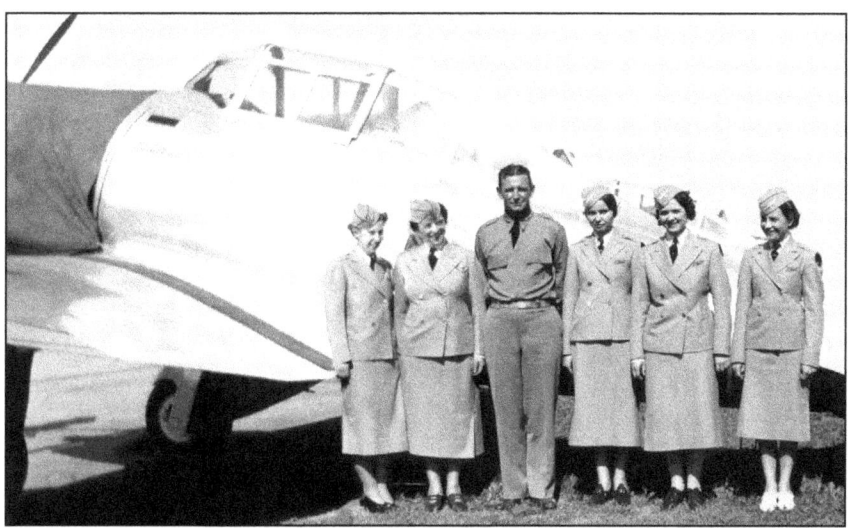

Figure 05.29. Company A-5 members standing before a Seversky P-35 Air Ship, 4 June 1939. Left to right, Laura Dickson, Leora Stroup, Captain Allison, Mary Chomin, Margaret Gudobba, Dorothy Laska. MMM.

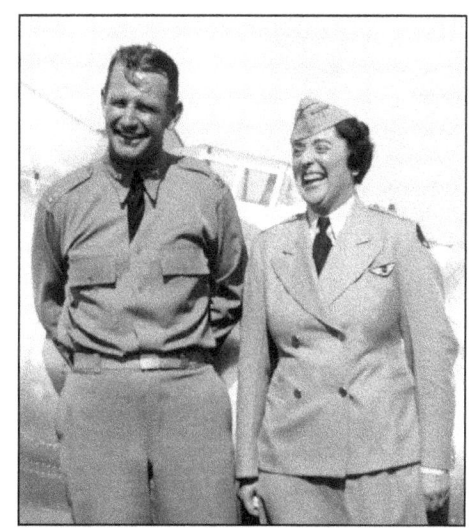

Figure 05.30. Captain Allison and Commander Stroup having a smashing good time during their tour of Selfridge Field on 4 June 1939. MMM.

Chapter Five

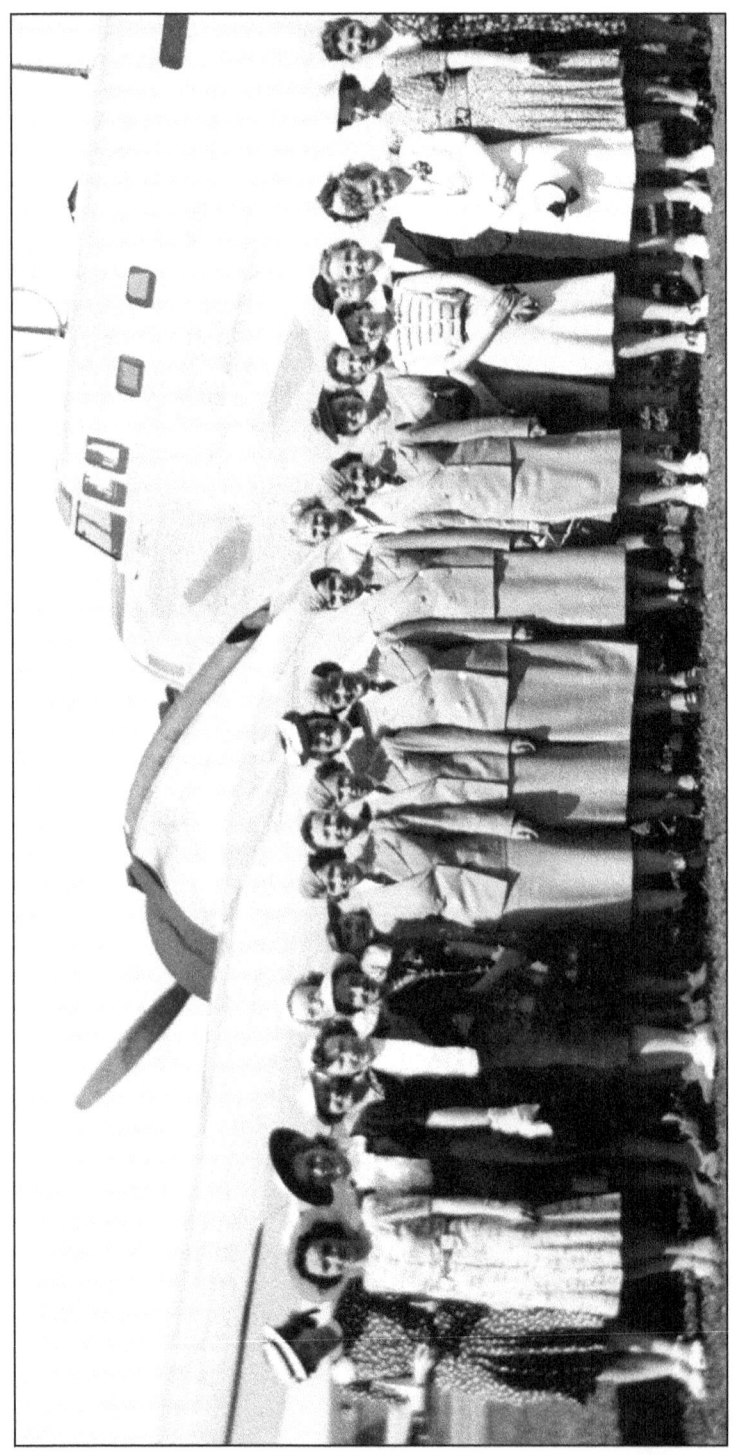

Figure 05.31. Company A-5 in front of a Douglas C-33 at Selfridge Field, U.S. Army Air Corps (now Selfridge Air National Guard Base), in Michigan. Leora Stroup is in the front row, seventh from right, 4 June 1939. MMM Collection.

Companies

The airplanes the group inspected during the tour:

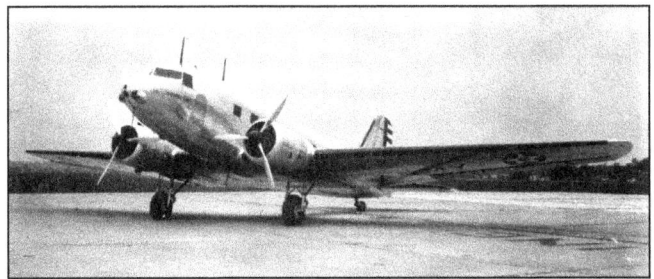

Figure 05.32. Douglas Cargo C-33

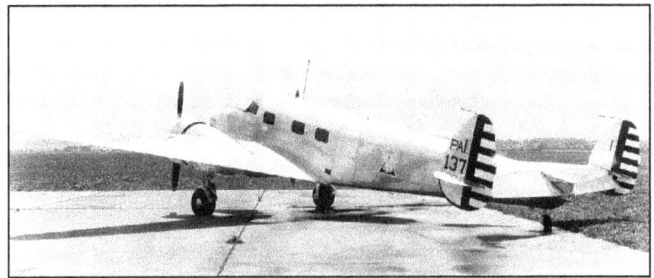

Figure 05.33. Lockheed Cargo C-40A

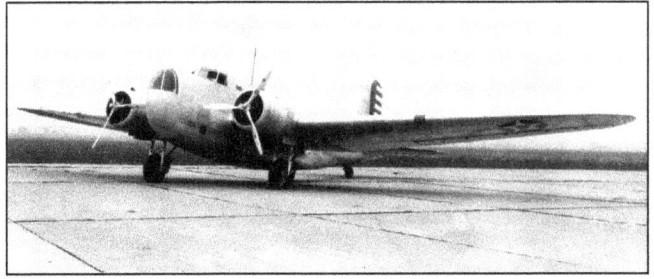

Figure 05.34. Douglas Bomber B-18

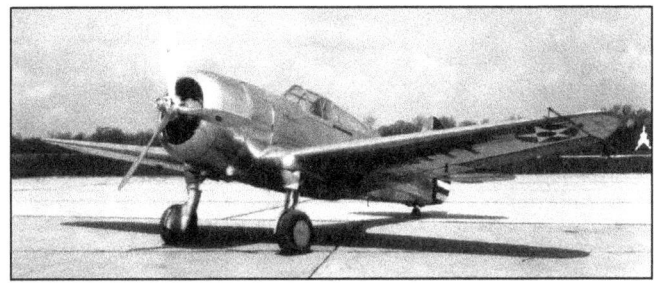

Figure 05.35. Curtiss Pursuit P-36

Chapter Five

Company B-5, Cleveland, Ohio

B-5 began on 5 August 1938

Company B-5 Officers

- Company Commanders: Florence Boswell, RN; Janice Porter, RN
- No emblems or mottos were located

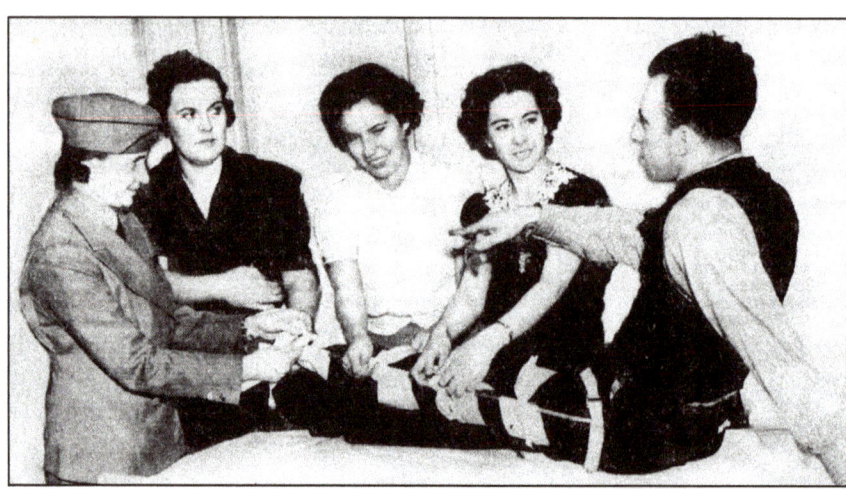

Figure 05.36. Company B-5 in a first aid demonstration, 1940. Janice Porter, Elinor Keeler, Katherine King, Ruth Esserman, with Verne Chapins. MMM.

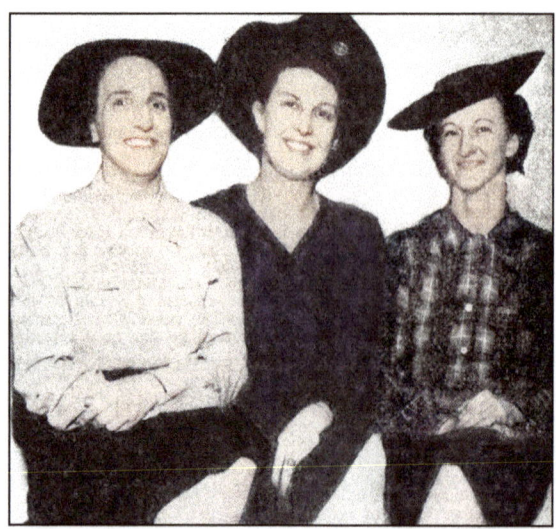

Figure 05.37. Elizabeth Mettie, Marjorie Patten, Mary Lawrence, and hats.

Company C-5, Dayton, Ohio

C-5 began on 24 June 1938

Company C-5 Officers

- Company Commanders: Merle McGriff, RN; Suzanne Finke, RN
- Adjutant: Erma Dobbertein, RN
- Quartermaster: Muriel Sinnott, RN
- Public Relations: Audrey Clingman, RN, Alma Krueger, RN
- Radio Department: Elsie Niehus, RN
- Recruiting: Laura Anderson, RN
- Photographic: Opal Downs, RN
- Athletic: Jeanette Rocky, RN

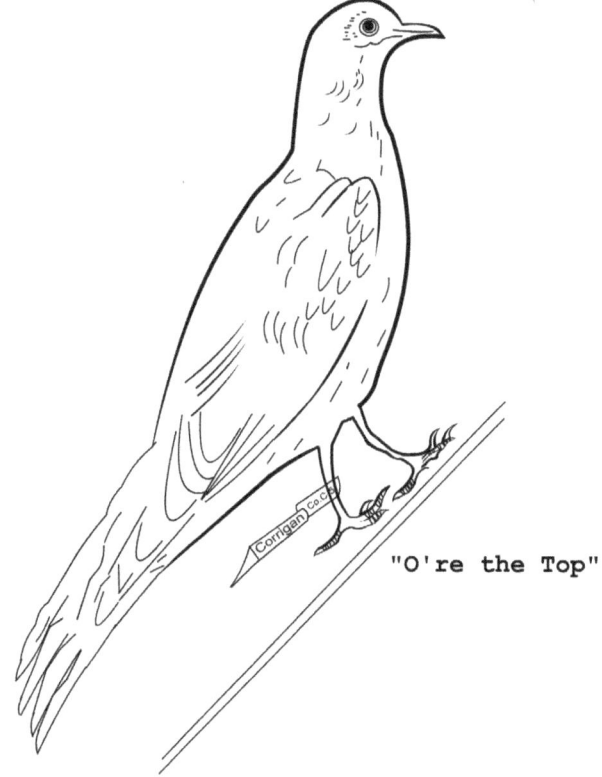

Figure 05.38. Corrigon the Pigeon, the C-5 Mascot, and Logo. Re-created from a *Flashes* sketch.

- Company Mascot: A pigeon named Corrigan
- Company Motto: "O're the Top"

Chapter Five

Company C Pep Song

Air-mates fly to-gether
We'll go o're the top
Fair or stor-my weather,
Friends and pals for-ev-er
Cap-tain to cadet
Aerial Nurses, Dayton Unit
Carry on, we dare not give up,
O're the top we go.

Although Merle McGriff had only joined the ANCOA on 24 June 1938, on 16 July, she led nine nurses to staff a first aid tent at the second annual Dayton Air Show. That first year they also staffed first aid tables at the Biltmore Hotel; at Patterson Field, during the Aero-Medical Association meeting; and at the 1938 National Air Races in Cleveland.

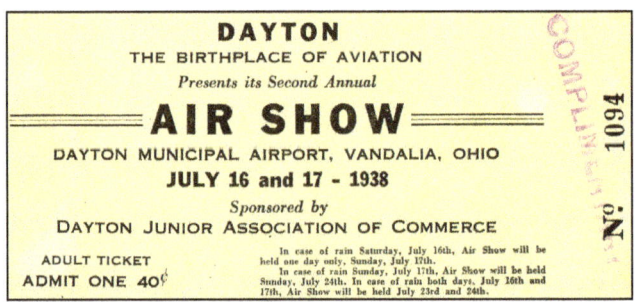

Figure 05.39. Ticket to the 1938 Dayton Air Show, C-5's first staffed event.

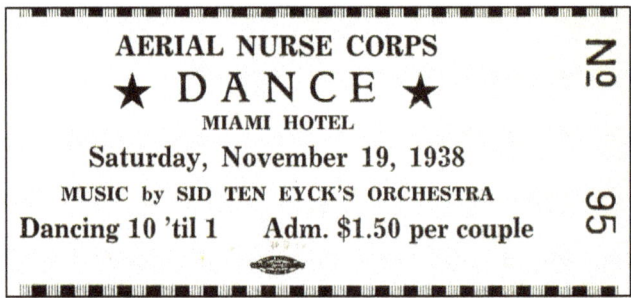

05.40. Ticket to the first fundraiser for Dayton Company C-5.

Company C-5 attended aviation classes at Miami Valley Hospital in Dayton. T.K. Kirk of the Reserve Officers Corps served as drillmaster and taught them military-style drills.[10] They held company fundraisers, including their first dance at the Miami Hotel with Sid Ten Eyck's Orchestra.

Companies

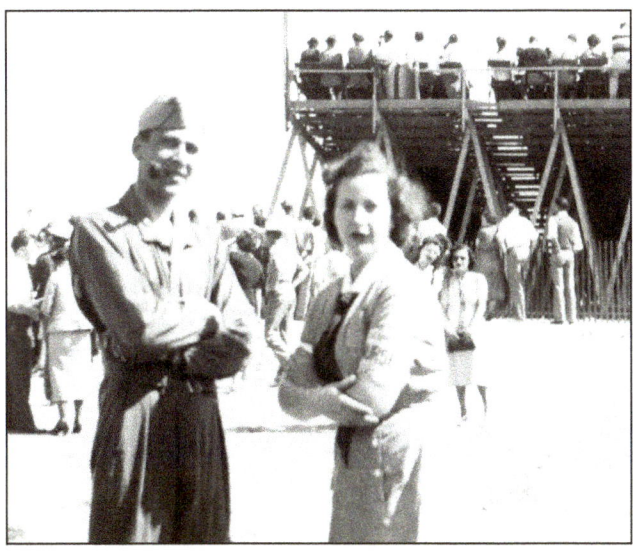

05.41. A pilot and Bessie Patrick, RN, at the 1938 National Air Races.

McGriff and Patrick represented the Dayton ANCOA at the 1938 National Air Races in Cleveland. The two nurses were busy—they applied first aid for 275 cases that ranged from support of simple fainters to more complicated treatments for injured parachute jumpers. [11]

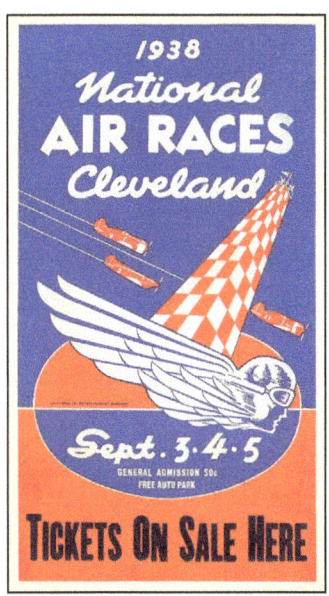

Figure 05.42. The 1938 Cleveland National Air Races poster. MMM.

Chapter Five

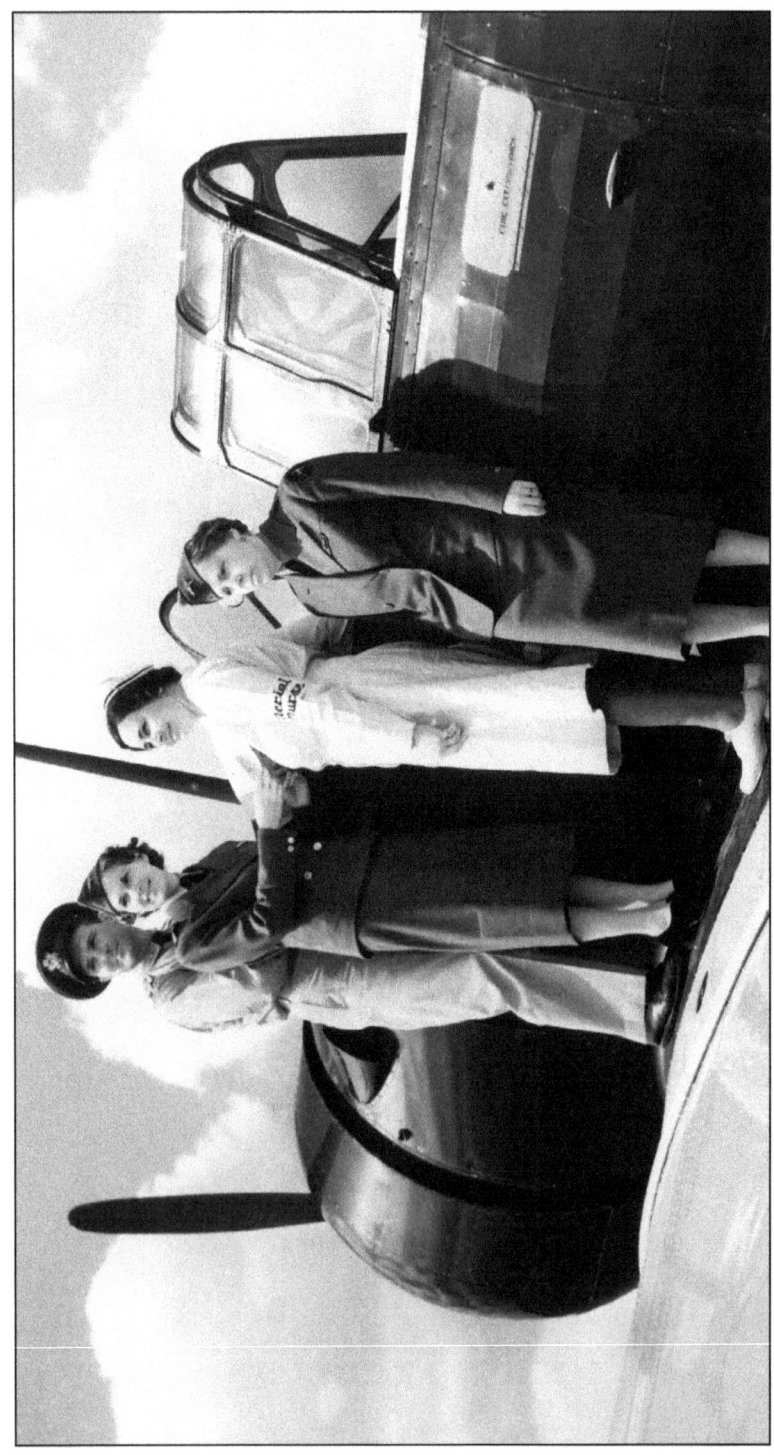

Figure 05.43. Captain Robert Morgan with Dayton ANCOA, left to right, Merle McGriff, Hilda Lackner, and Marie O'Brien at Wright Field, 1939. MMM Collection.

Companies

The Ohio ANCOA nurses trained with experts, such as Robert Morgan, at Wright Field. Captain Robert Morgan became famous during WWII for piloting the Boeing B-17 bomber, affectionately called the Memphis Belle. Morgan and his crew completed twenty-five bombing missions.

During one mission, they dropped bombs on a Nazi submarine base in the coastal city of Lorient while fighting a swarm of Luftwaffe fighters. Their aircraft's tail was shot to pieces and in flames. Morgan debated whether the crew should eject and become prisoners of war or continue before the tail ripped off. The tail did tear, but they survived the mission and seventeen missions after that.

The Memphis Belle became the first U.S. Army bomber to return to the U.S., despite the odds that German fighters with anti-aircraft fire downed eighty percent. Jeff Duford, museum curator, U.S. Air Force National Museum, Wright-Patterson Air Field, said, "In many ways, the Memphis Belle is the icon for the United States Air Force."[12] The military relocated the Memphis Belle to Wright-Patterson Air Force Museum in 2005, and after years of meticulous restoration, the museum placed it on public display in May 2018.

From 1930 until WWII began, airline companies required all stewardesses to be RNs. These companies must have noticed the ANCOA because United Airlines contracted with Schimmoler to review their new employee applications and train their stewardesses in 1938.[13] For whatever reason, perhaps just fashion, the uniforms styles looked similar. And just as it happened with the ANCOA, when WWII started, nurses left the private airline companies because the Army greatly needed them. Airlines adjusted their requirements and non-nurse stewardesses replaced the nurses.

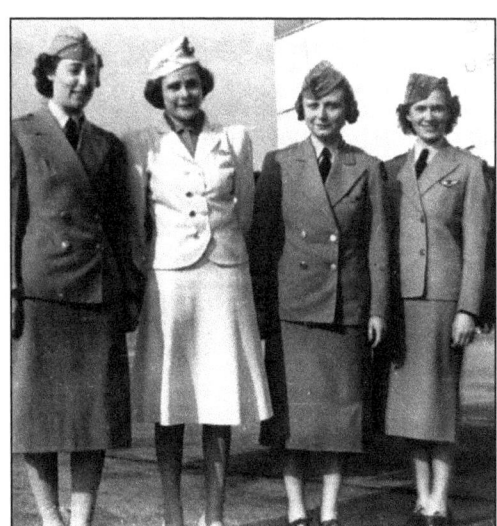

Figure 05.44. Dayton, Ohio ANCOA with a stewardess, 1938. Note the similarity in the design of uniforms. Jean McCallen, Mrs. Nelson (the stewardess), Rosella Herring, and Merle McGriff, left to right. MMM Collection.

Chapter Five

Company C-5 learned more about airplanes by touring and training at airports and manufacturing facilities. In July 1939, McGriff led six new nurses, who had yet to earn their official ANCOA uniforms, to Wright Field in Dayton to begin learning about air transport. McGriff somehow convinced the Army to allow the ANCOA to use an Army crash wagon ambulance and airplane for training purposes.

In 1922 the War Department had ordered flying fields in the U.S. to equip themselves with a new type of aero ambulance the engineering divisions at Wilbur Wright Field had recently developed—the most extensive aerial supply depot in the Army Air Service.

The Curtiss JN 68 with a Hispano motor of 180 horsepower, was the first medically-equipped airplane in the U.S. [14] But the ANCOA used a newer Waco model, recently built at the Troy Ohio Plant for the South American Government. [15] The Army called it "Snow White." Reporter Alexander McSurely, of *Aerial Age Weekly*, recounted the session:

> We went to watch the aerial nurse cadets go through their ambulance drill at Wright Field. It was one of those hot days when the sun beat down on the white concrete pavement of Wright Field flying line with unmerciful vigor. [16]
>
> Despite the white-hot day, nurse Elsie Niehus volunteered as the demonstration patient. They placed her on a stretcher in the crash wagon ambulance and wrapped her in heavy wool army blankets.
>
> Three men demonstrated the technique of moving the stretcher from the crash wagon in three counts: removing it from the wagon, lowering to the ground on the second count, and hoisting it through the airplane ambulance door on the third count. The gal was game and finally came out of her blanket shroud, perspiring but unharmed.
>
> Then the ANCOA girls tried, and aside from using three-girl power to a side of the litter, instead of one-man power, they handled the matter very satisfactorily. Actually, the nurses won't have to do much of the strong-arm work, except in special emergencies, but take it from us—they can if necessary. [17]

Wright Field allowed the nurses to attend to passengers aboard the plane. Riding onboard served a dual purpose: it calmed the patient's nerves and let the nurses satisfy their required air hours for certification.

The manager of the Springfield Airport, Harry Britton, promised he would make an aerial ambulance available as soon as the ANCOA qualified. This action would finally establish a private air ambulance service for the Dayton area. Wright Field was the only air ambulance transport in the region, but it was only available for military use. [18]

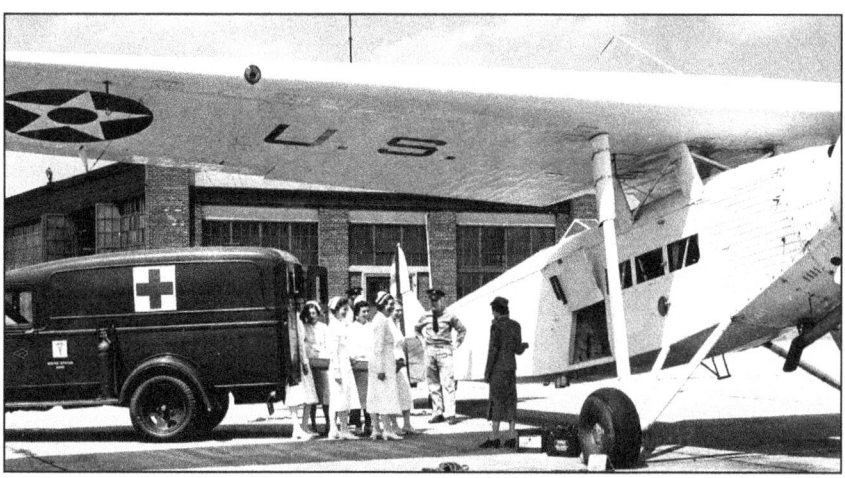

Figure 05.45. McGriff, far right, directing new ANCOA nurses, July 1939. They loaded patients from the crash wagon to the plane for their training exercises. The patient, on the stretcher, and the nurse had to squeeze through the small door of the cargo/passenger hold where they rode during the flight. The pilots called this plane "Snow White." MMM.

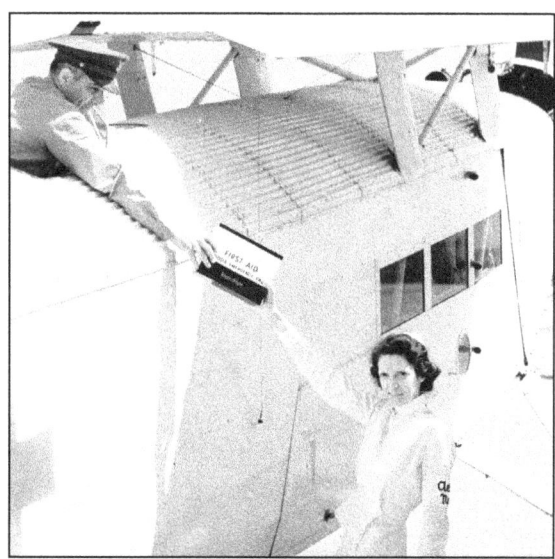

Figure 05.46. ANCOA nurse cadet-in-training Hazel Golly, RN, takes a first aid kit from the pilot, Captain C. W. O'Connor, July 1939. The pilot flew from the open cockpit area in the rear of the plane.

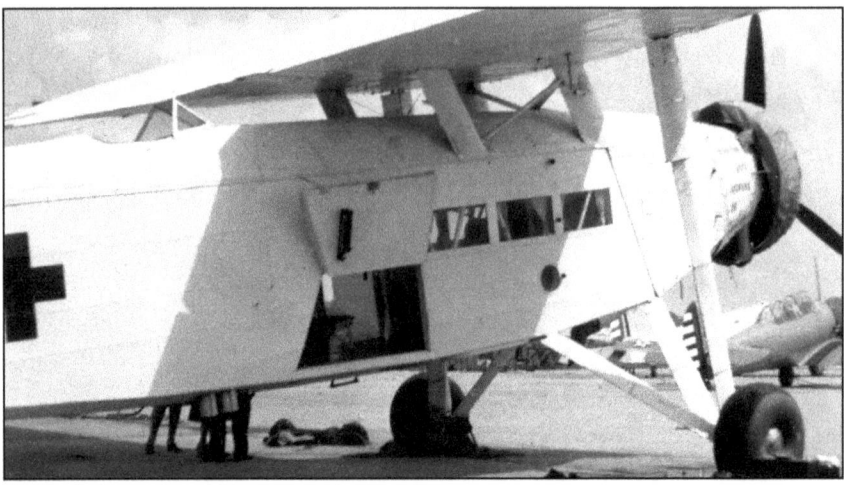

Figure 05.47. View to the open door of the small passenger area, 1939.

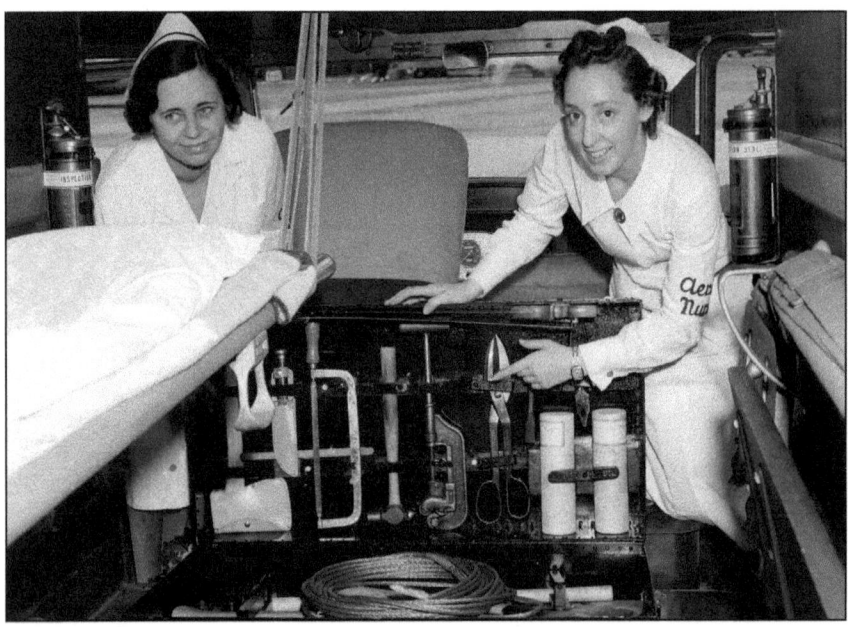

Figure 05.48. Hilda Lackner and Jean McCallen point out the lifesaving equipment in the crash wagon. Lackner was regularly stationed at Wright.

Airports equipped their crash wagons with fire extinguishers and various items to free victims from a plane crash. They carried an eighteen-foot-long steel rod with a large hook on the end. They used the hook to grab the pilot when the flames were too hot to permit a gentle rescue method.[19] In later years, fire engines with water tanks became crash wagons. Some airports still employed small trucks as first rescuers because they were able to reach the crash site quicker than a fire truck. [20]

McGriff's Dayton Company actively campaigned for members by placing flyers in hospitals. Local newspapers printed articles about their activities, bolstering interest and making area nurses aware of the organization. They established headquarters in the Fidelity Medical Building at 211 South Main Street in Dayton. The building housed doctor and dentist offices, a medical library, meeting rooms, X-rays technicians, and a pharmacy. [21]

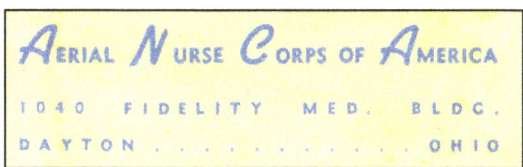

Figure 05.49. Company C-5 official stationary imprint. MMM Collection.

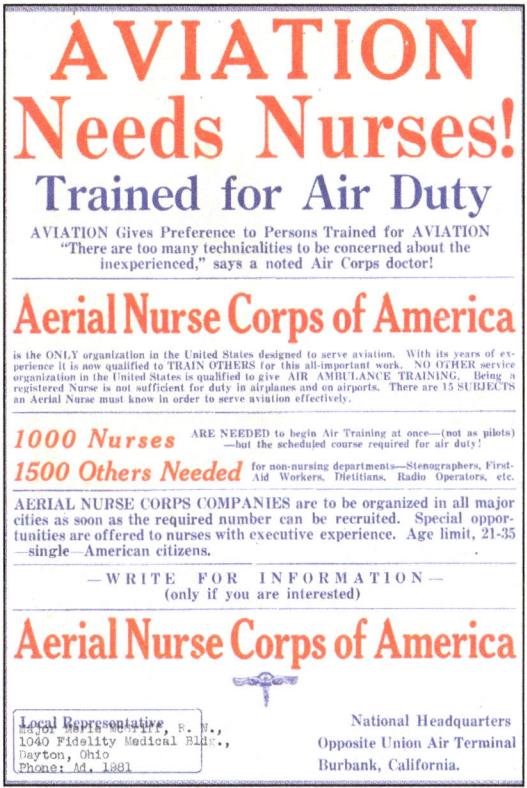

Figure 05.50. The flyer McGriff used to recruit nurses into the ANCOA.

Chapter Five

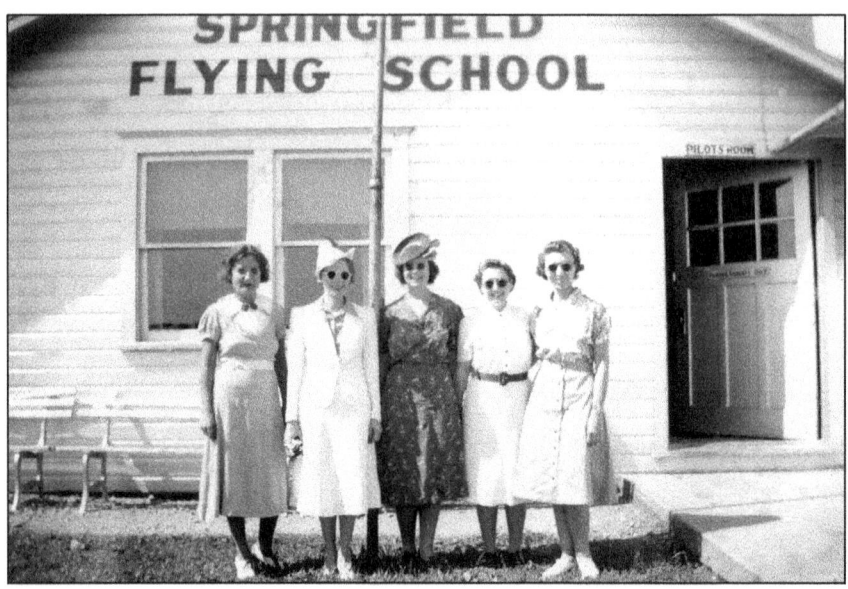

Figure 05.51. Flyers Audrey Clingman, Merle McGriff, Suzanne Finke, Alice Hendershot, and Jeanette Rockey of Dayton's Company C-5, in ground school training at Springfield Flying School, 1939. MMM.

Company C-5 created several pilots because of McGriff's influence; they learned to fly at the schools in Dayton and Springfield. In 2023, the Dayton area listed thirty flight schools—it still plays a vital role in flight training.

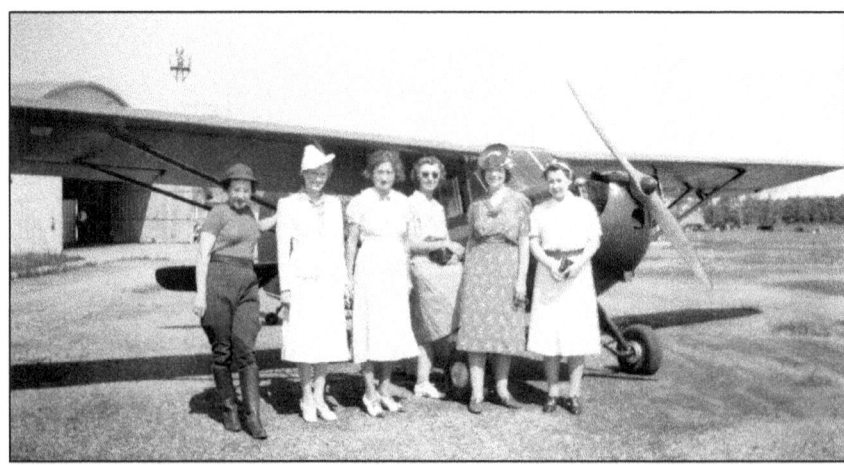

Figure 05.52. Audrey Clingman, Merle McGriff, Elsie Niehus, Suzanne Finke, Alice Hendershot, Jeanette Rockey, 1939. MMM Collection. This wasn't a ground school training day for these women—they were flying.

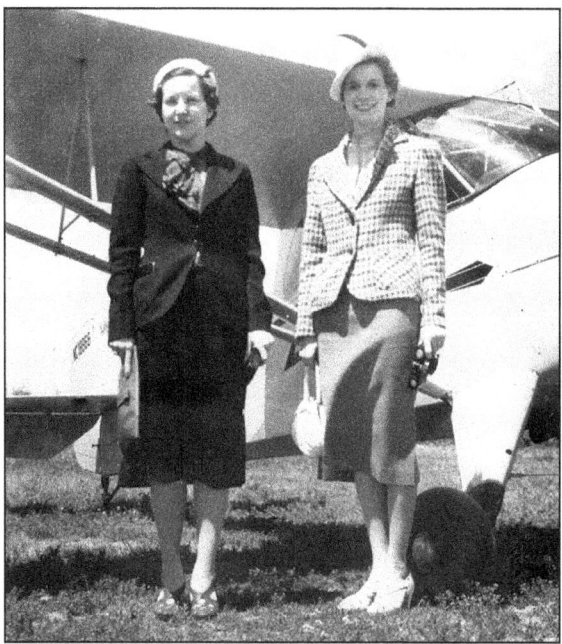

Figure 05.53. Audrey Clingman and Merle McGriff using Mr. Lee's Aeronca for their flying lessons, 1939.

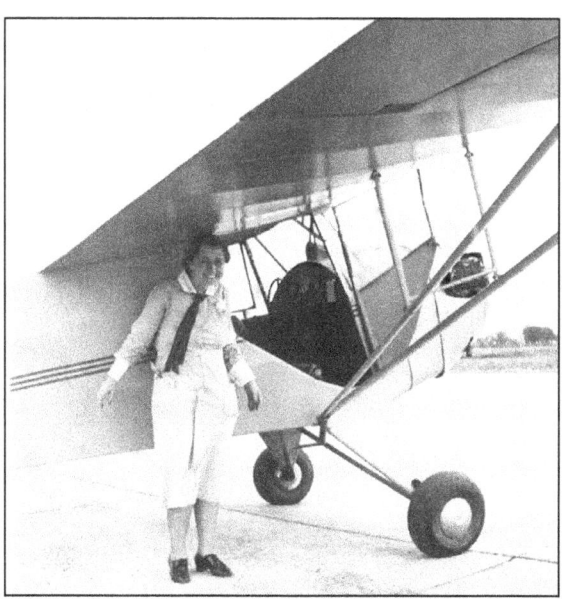

Figure 05.54. Alice Undershot learned to pilot, but this was the first time she ever flew as a passenger in an airplane, 1938. MMM Collection.

> **THE DAYTON NATIONAL AIR SHOW**
> Sponsored by Jr. Association of Commerce
> **MUNICIPAL AIRPORT, VANDALIS, SUN., JULY 23**
>
> Featuring...The Famous Aces Starred At The Mammoth Cleaveland National Air Races–America's Greatest Acrobatic Fliers Making Their First Dayton Appearance In A Thrill-Packed Program of Stunt Flying, Parachute Jumping, Test Pilot Demonstrations, Stunt Team Fling And Aerial Comedy Events...See These Thrilling Events:
>
> ************************************
>
> * HAROLD JOHNSON, AMERICA'S NO.1 STUNT PILOT, IN HIS SENSATIONAL STUNTING WITH A 6-TON TRIMOTOR TRANSPORT PLANE! A Giant Trimotor Performing Startling Tailspins, Barrel Rools and Whipstalls...Roaring Loops That Start and Finish only 15 feet Above the Ground...Hazardous One-Wheel Landings and Takeoffs!
>
> * A REAL "TEST PILOT" DEMONSTRATION! A Howling Pursuit Plane Diving Out of the Skies at 400 Miles and Hour... High-Speed Aerobatics and Gruelling Maneuvers Seen in Hollywood's Sky Productions!
>
> * CAPT. DICK GRANERE, WORLD-FAMOUS FLYING COMEDIAN OF THE NATIONAL AIR RACES!...The Hilarious Antics of Aviation's Noted Sky Clown in "How Not to Fly"!
>
> * A CHAMPIONSHIP AERIAL STUNT TEAM!...Brushing Wingtips with Dazzling Aerial Acrobatics in Close Formation!
>
> * DON WALTERS PRECISION STUNT ACT!...Breath-taking Upside Down Flights Only 30 Feet Above the Turf...Whirlwing Precision Acrobatics!
>
> * A 10,000-FOOT PLUNGE THROUGH SPACE BY BUDDY BATZEL, WORLD CHAMPION PARACHUTE JUMPER....A Two-Mile Plunge Through Space Before Opening His Parachute... Thrilling Test Jumps!
>
> * HUGH THOMASSON, RAPID-FIRE AVIATION COMMENTATOR AT THE MICROPHONE!
>
> MODEL AIRPLANE CONTEST AT 9:00 AM..SPOT LANDING CONTEST AT 1:00 PM-AND THE AIR SHOW AT 2:30 PM.
>
> SPECIAL ADVANCE SALE BOX SEAT:$10.00 FOR BOX OF 6 SEATS Includes General Admission and Free Parking
> RESERVED SEATS: $1.50, With Admission and Parking
> GENERAL ADMISSION: Adults 50¢ - Children 25¢

Figure 05.55. Ad for the 1939 Dayton National Air Show. Re-created.

Companies

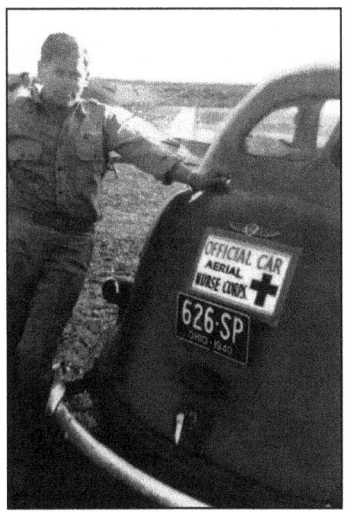 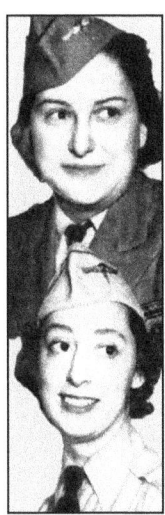

Figure 05.56. Official ANCOA car at the 1939 Dayton National Air Show.
Figure 05.57. Jean McCallen, RN, and Maxine McLaughlin, RN, nurses who attended to injuries sustained from the dangerous activities.

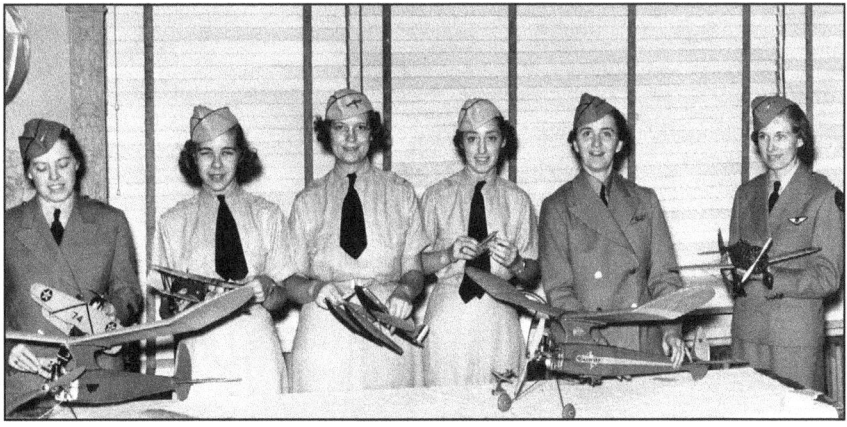

Figure 05.58. Dayton Company C-5 at the National Air Progress Week Air Meet, September 1939. Marie O'Brien, unidentified member, Suzanna Finke, Maxine McLaughlin, Janice Porter, and Merle McGriff. MMM.

Company C-5 staffed the first aide table during National Air Progress Week at Lansdowne Airport in Greenville, Ohio, on 24 September 1939. Participants staged test flights with gas and rubber-powered model planes. Aviators from Greenville, Dayton, Fort Wayne, and other cities exhibited stunt flying. Contestants competed in spot landings and navigation contests. Several thousand spectators attended. 22

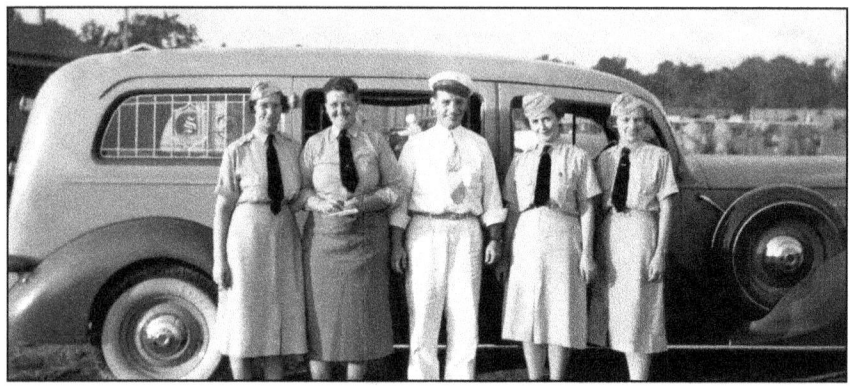

Figure 05.59. The 1939 Cleveland Air Show official ANCOA car. Suzanne Finke, Lauretta Schimmoler, Earl, Janice Porter, and Merle McGriff. MMM.

The Fifth Division, Companies A, B, and C, joined together again and staffed the 1939 Cleveland Air Show. Merle McGriff, RN, and Herbert Wright, MD, were in charge of the field hospital.

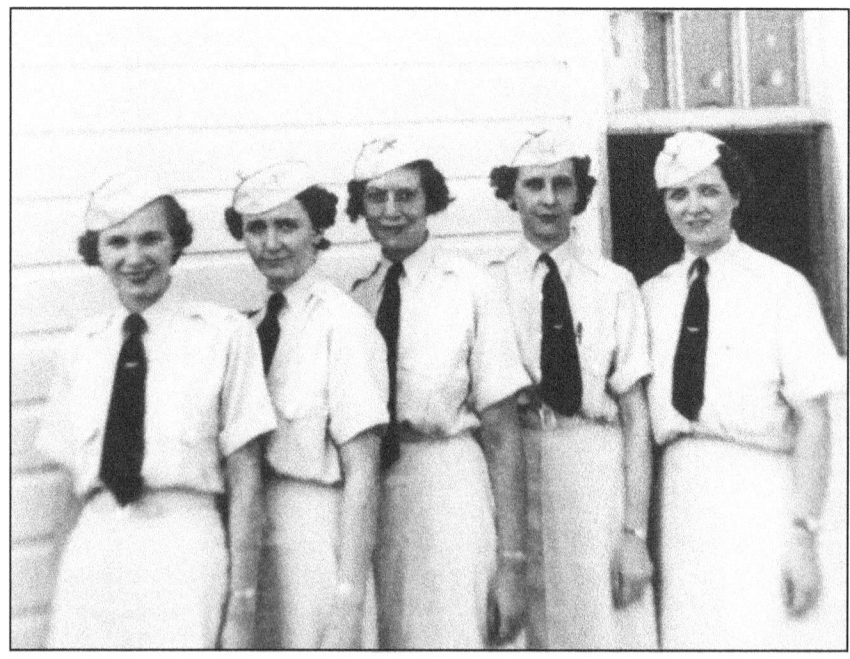

Figure 05.60. Members of the Fifth Division at the Cleveland Air Show field hospital, 1939. From left to right, Merle McGriff, Janice Porter, Suzanne Finke, Alice Newbeck, and Margaret Gudobba enjoying their cool summer uniforms. MMM Collection.

Companies

After the 1939 National Air Race concluded, McGriff received a stunning letter from the office of the Managing Director of the National Air Races, informing her that future races were suspended. Although the U.S. had not yet become involved in WWII, the letter indicated a growing concern:

> It is with profound regret that we bring to a close our active participation with the National Air Races project.
>
> This year, the 19th Anniversary of the National Air Race, will unquestionably stand out indelibly in the minds of the Air Race Committees and staff because of the unusual and uncontrollable elements...We refer, of course, to the devastating effect of yet another European war upon the American consciousness..."
>
> This note will covey, on behalf of the National Air Race Sponsoring Committee, along with our sincere personal gratitude, an appreciation for your effective participation as a member of the Aerial Nurse Corps of America, which constituted an important phase of this year's National Air Race project.

Officials suspended the National Air Races from 1940 until 1945.

The Dayton Tri-Flyers Club (Dayton ANCOA, Dayton Flying Club, and Wright Escadrille) sponsored the first Annual Aviation Ball at the Biltmore Hotel, 9 March 1940.

The Karl Taylor Orchestra, touted as Dayton's best band, played from 10 p.m. to 2 a.m. for 500 members and guests from the various flying clubs and local organizations around the Dayton area.

They used red, white, and blue as theme colors, with a parachute and an ancient propeller as a canopy for the dance floor. Leora Stroup and Margaret Gudobba from Detroit's ANCOA flew in for the festivities.

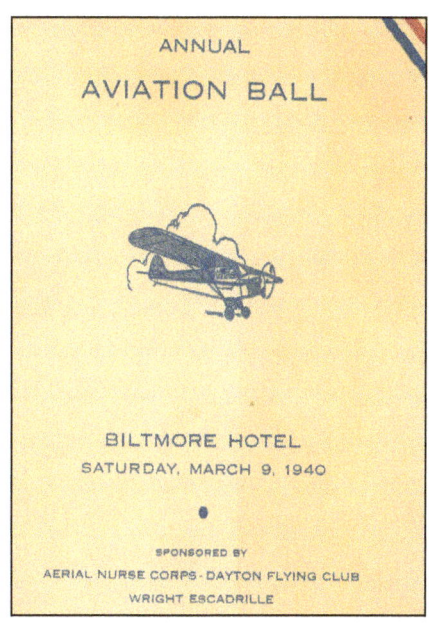

Figure 05.61. The Aviation Ball program doubled as an autograph book, 1940.

Chapter Five

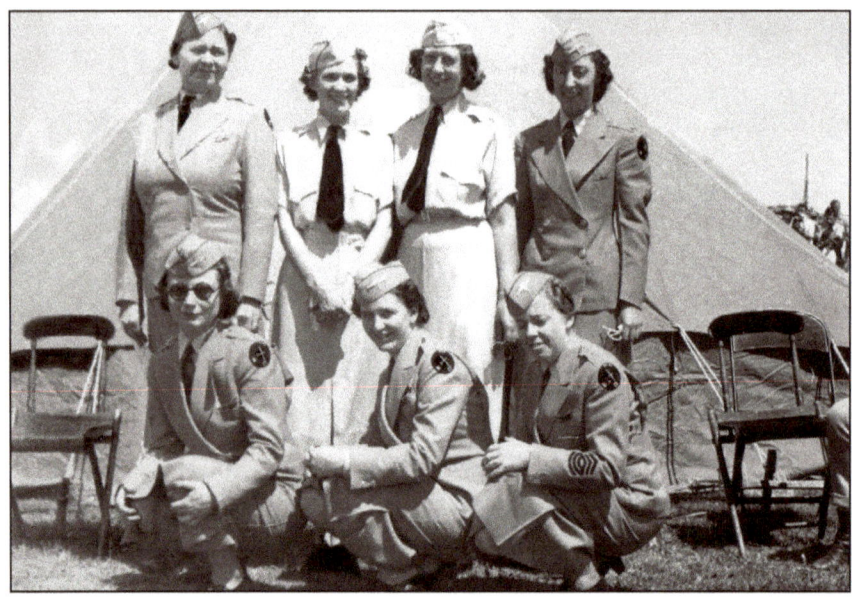

Figure 05.62. Company B-5 & C-5 at the 1940 Dayton Air Races. Rosella Herring, Janice Porter, Marie O'Brien in the front. Hilda Lackner, Merle McGriff, Florence Finke, Jean McCallen in the back. Despite war concerns, the Dayton Air Races continued—at least into 1940. MMM Collection.

McGriff remembered the year 1938: the world felt safer, the ANCOA was at its height, and they met the most respected aviator when Dayton officials summoned Company C-5 to serve at a special event.

The City of Dayton celebrated the 35th anniversary of the first successful flight. Henry Ford attended, as well as Orville Wright. The city laid a wreath on Wilbur's grave in Woodland Cemetery and set off 35 bombs at one-minute intervals.

At the meeting, they showed a movie on the progress of air flight from its earliest time. Dayton ANCOA members served as the ushers for the observance.[23]

Figure 05.63. Dayton's public celebration for the Wright Brothers and thirty-fifth anniversary of flight, 17 December 1938.

Ford to Dine With Wright

Public Will Join in Observance

Henry Ford, who is to join in Dayton's public celebration Saturday at 8 p. m. in the N. C. R. auditorium, honoring the thirty-fifth anniversary of the Wright brothers' first airplane flight, will arrive from Detroit by automobile between 5 and 6 p. m.

At 10 a. m. a wreath will be laid on the grave of Wilbur Wright in Woodland cemetery, and 35 bombs will be set off at minute intervals.

Mayor Charles J. Brennan is to preside at the meeting. A government-owned motion picture showing the progress of the airplane from the earliest days to the present will be shown. Members of the Dayton chapter of the Aerial Nurse corps are to serve as ushers.

230

Companies

Company D-5, Dayton, OH

Company D-5 Officers

- Company Commander: Alice Hendershot, RN; Dorothy Laska, RN
- Public Relations: Alma Krueger, RN, Elsie Niehus

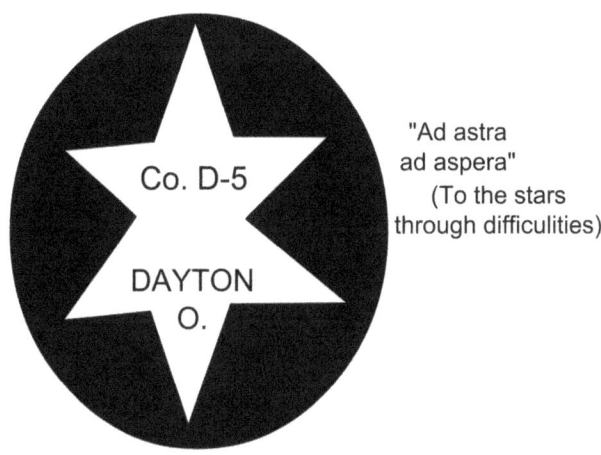

Figure 05.64. Company D-5's logo. Re-created from a sketch in *Flashes*. Lucius Annaeus Seneca coined the phrase, *per aspera ad astra*, c. 30 CE. Sustaining the trend, the show *Star Trek: Strange New Worlds* used it in 2023.

- Motto: "Ad astra ad aspera" (to the stars through difficulties)
- Song: "Star Dust." No lyrics were located

Company E-5, Toledo, Ohio
Company E-5 Officers: Company Commander Edna E. Sharritt, RN

Company F-5, Lancaster, Ohio
Company F-5 Officers: Not known

Company G-5, Cincinnati, Ohio
Company G-5 Officers: Not known

Company A-5, Louisville, Kentucky
Company A-5 Officers: Company Commander Euna Embry, RN

Louisville is listed as A-5 in *Flashes* August 1937 issue. Euna Embry, RN, its Commander, wrote articles in the first and second issues. In May 1938, A-5 moved to Detroit with Leora Stroup as commander. It might have moved due to a lack of members in Kentucky. Embry was only A-5 Kentucky member.

Chapter Five

2nd Wing

No 2nd Wing Commander is listed.

The 6th Division

Schimmoler initially slated the 6th Division Headquarters to start in Atlanta, Georgia. *Flashes* listed the start in November 1938 and its headquarters in West Palm Beach, Florida. No nurses are listed in West Palm Beach or Atlanta.

Division 6, Company A, started in Sarasota, Florida on 2 August 1940. The Sarasota roster included several members. Its headquarters likely changed to Sarasota because no members lived in West Palm Beach or Atlanta. [24]

Company A-6, Sarasota, Florida

Company Commander: Margaret Smith, RN. *Flashes* listed WWII CAP activities but no other officers for group A-6.

Company B-6, Fort Lauderdale, Florida

Company Commander: Fay McWorter, RN. McWorter was the only known member in B-6, *Flashes* listed no activities or other officers.

The 7th Division

Company A-7, Washington D.C.

Company Commander: listed as Mae Brickner, RN. Brickner transferred to D.C. from B-5 in Ohio. A7 probably did not form as no recruits are listed.

Company B-7, Johnstown, Pennsylvania

Company Commander: Josephine Cope, RN. *Flashes* listed no activities or other officers for group B-7.

The 8th Division

Company A-8, New York, New York

Company Commander: Matilde Grinevich, RN. *Flashes* listed no group activities or additional officers, but A-8 had at least sixteen members. Grinevich and Julian Sabat participated in the infamous event with Relief Wings. Grinevich collected ANCOA ephemera, but her files were lost.

Flashes published a quote about the start of A-8. The editor said the formation of the company became a reality because of the lonely Cadet in New York. The lonely Cadet's name wasn't noted but she said:

> During the recent hurricanes in the New England states, airlines and commercial operators were transporting the people who had been left homeless, and rescuing others that were stranded. It was doing its usual renewing of homes, bodies, spirits, and anything that was needed, and trying their best to keep up with temporary food supplies, and shelter, only to see another hurricane strike in nearly the same place. They kept on and saw it through working with what they had.
>
> In such tragedy, and loss of human lives, and suffering, ANCOA will soon give aid to those of similar circumstances in the future, like a guardian angel. I hope the future is near when our Wings will cover the whole United States of America and our unequaled example will make us the training ground and inspiration to others. [25]

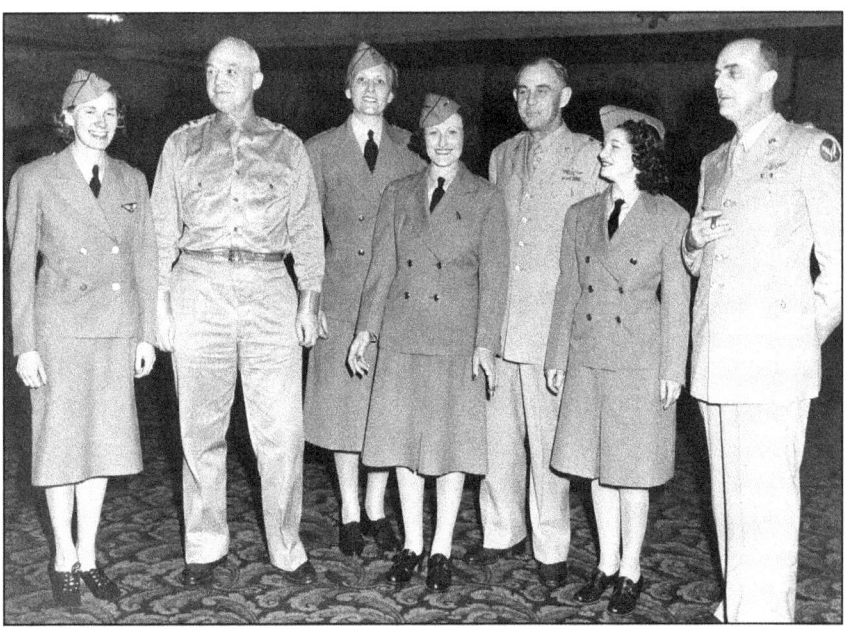

Figure 05.65. Merle McGriff, General Hap Arnold, and Irene Anderson, with two other high-ranking members of the Air Force and two unnamed AEC members. Schimmoler might never have met the infamous General Hap, but Merle McGriff did. And she had the photo to prove it.

Chapter Six

Commanders, Nurse-Pilots, & Flight Nurses

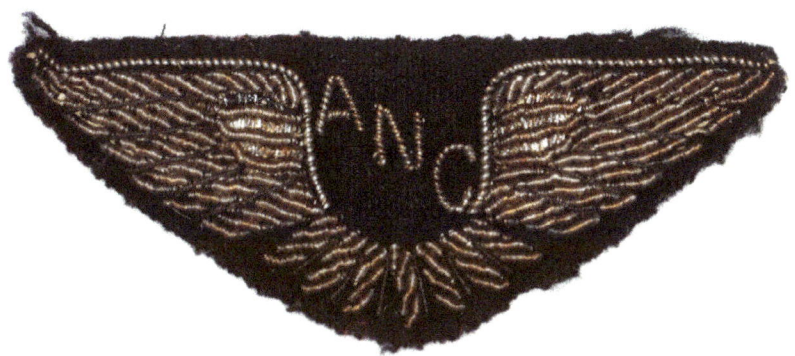

Figure 06.01. The ANCOA Commander patch, 1937.

Schimmoler chose most of the early commanders from the nurses who were also pilots, but that was neither a rule nor a requirement: not all pilots became commanders; not all the commanders were pilots.

Nurses entered the Corps with the rank of cadet. After six months, they took a written exam for the commission of Lieutenant. If they demonstrated an ability to organize and lead, Schimmoler might promote them to Captain or Cadet Captain.

A Captain advanced to Company Commander as the highest-ranking member of a regional company. A Division Commander, with the rank of Major, supported a division. A Lieutenant Colonel commanded a Wing. Only Schimmoler ranked as Colonel—the National Commander.

Commanders organized membership drives, approved new members, arranged basic training, and held drills. They sought out air meets and other first aid opportunities and set the details for the meets. Other group members assisted with the details as the companies grew.

The Company Commanders presented recommendations, to the General Headquarters, for appointments of senior members to various assignments within their company: Adjutant, Quartermaster, Public Relations, Athletic, Mess, Photographer, Recruiting, and Color Guard. The Chief of Staff or the Adjutant General approved and issued orders for the assignments.

AERIAL NURSE CORPS OF AMERICA
National Headquarters
Burbank, California

January 8, 1941

MEMORANDUM — Company Commanders

1. Chief of Staff:	Lt. Colonel Ruth G Mitchell, R.N. Oakland, Calif.
2. Adjutant General	Major Merle McGriff, R.N. Dayton, Ohio
3. Quartermaster General	Major Leora B. Stroup, R.N. Detroit, Mich.
4. Company A-1st	Captain Myrtle Martin, R.N. Santa Monica, Calif.
5. Co. D-1st	Cadet Captain Wanda Fill, R.N. San Diego, Calif.
6. Co. K-1st	Cadet Captain Alice Moyer, R.N. Seattle, Wash.
7. Co. B-4th Div.	Cadet Captain Florence Fintak, R.N Milwaukee, Wis.
8. Co. C 4th Div.	Captain Genevieve Waples, R.N. Decatur, Ill.
9. Co. A-5th Div.	Major Leora B. Stroup, R.N. Detroit, Mich.
10. Co. B-5th Div.	Cadet Captain Janice Porter, R.N. Cleveland, Ohio
11. C-5th Div.	Captain Suzanna Finke, R.N. Dayton, Ohio
12. D-5th Div.	Cadet Captain Dorothy Laska, R.N. Detroit, Mich.
13. Co. E-6th Div.	Cadet Captain Edna Sharritt, R.N. Toledo, Ohio
14. Co. A-6th Div.	Cadet Captain Margaret Smith, R.N. Sarasota, Fla.
15. Co. B-6th Div.	Cadet Captain Fay McWhorter, R.N. Ft. Lauderdale, Fla.
16. Co. A-7th Div.	Cadet Captain Mae Brickner, R.N. Washington, D. C.
17. Co. B-7th Div.	Cadet Capt. Josephine Cope, R.N. Johnstown, N.Y.
18. Co. A-8th Div.	Captain Mitilda Grinevich, R.N. New York City, N.Y.

Figure 06.02. ANCOA Commander List, 1941. Re-created from the original.

Commanders
Major Merle McGriff McAfee, RN

Commander of Wing 3 & Division 5
Commander of Co. C-5, Dayton, OH
Adjutant General; Licensed Pilot

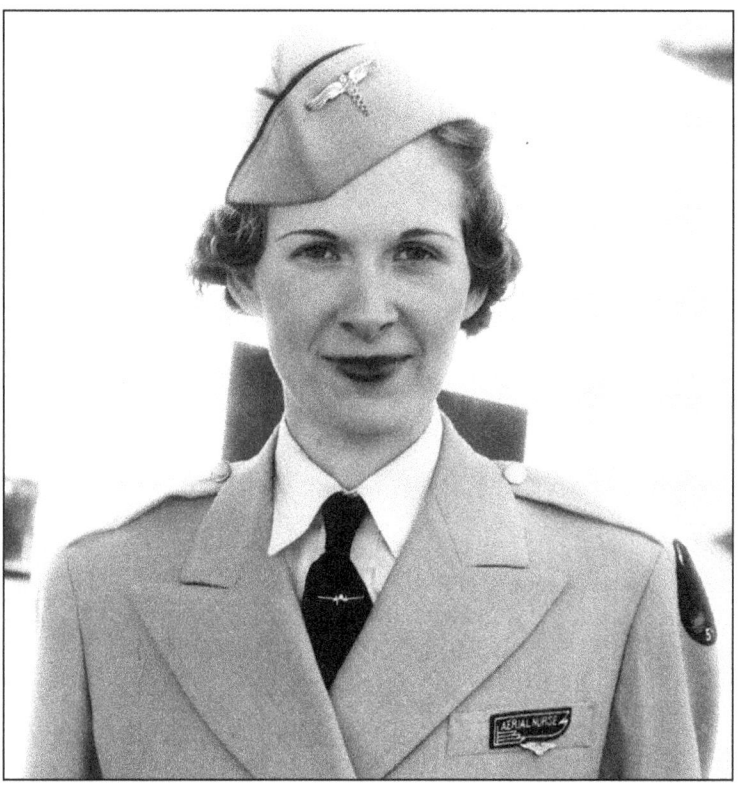

Figure 06.03. Merle McGriff, RN, in the ANCOA uniform, with the patches she wore prior to becoming the Division Five Commander, 1938. An Aerial Nurse pocket patch, a National Aeronautic Association pin below it, a 5th Division shoulder patch, an ANCOA nurse cap pin, and an unknown airplane emblem on her tie. MMM Collection.

Although petite in stature, McGriff was a powerhouse in action. She joined on 24 June 1938 as the 99th recruit and became one of ANCOA's most dynamic members. She quickly recruited others and started Division Five in Dayton, Ohio. By 16 July, only three weeks after she joined, her nine nurses staffed the first aid table at the second annual Dayton Air Show. She recruited thirty-one nurses in July alone. Without McGriff, the Ohio ANCOA would not have enjoyed its growth and success.

Chapter Six

Born on 18 June 1909, in Palestine, Ohio, to Perry McGriff and Pearl Sleeth, McGriff's father farmed; after five years, they moved to a farm near Arcanum and she attended the West Point county school. After Arcanum High School, she studied at Miami Jacobs Business College. She graduated from Miami Valley Hospital School of Nursing in 1931. She'd planned to attend medical school, but personal circumstances prevented it.

She studied a postgraduate course at Margaret Hague Maternity Hospital in New Jersey, then accepted an industrial nurse position in the Eye, Ear, Nose, and Throat department, Aero Products, General Motors Corp. in Dayton.[1] She became a charter member and the President of the Beta Mu Chapter of Beta Sigma Phi, a social and cultural service organization.[2]

Schimmoler must have felt delighted to find a nurse as devoted as McGriff, a nurse who could make the ANCOA succeed in Schimmoler's home state of Ohio. Naturally, she would have wanted Ohio to have an active ANCOA presence. Since Schimmoler could not be there, finding McGriff was a moment of great luck for her and the ANCOA.

McGriff arranged for Fifth Division members to staff the 1938 National Air Races in Cleveland, Ohio, on 2-4 September. She didn't just organize the Dayton crew, she also coordinated with ANCOA nurses from the Cleveland area and Leora Stoup in Detroit, Michigan. This made it the first all-Fifth Division event. No one owned regulation ANCOA uniforms yet, but they improvised and managed the field hospital.

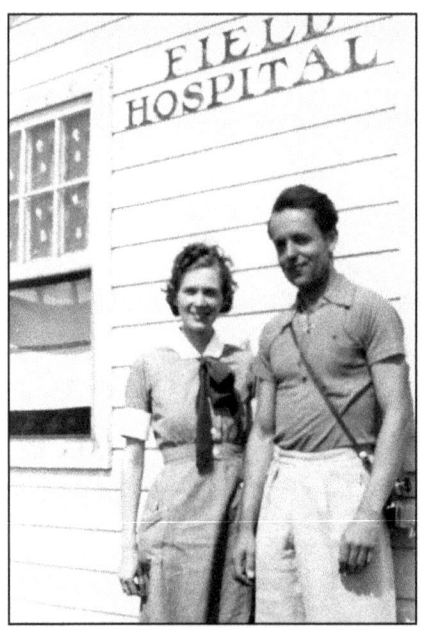

Figure 06.04. Dayton Commander Merle McGriff standing in front of the 1938 National Air Races Field Hospital with the infamous stunt pilot, Count Otto Heinrich von Hagenburg, of Germany. MMM.

Von Hagenburg—a master of the inverted flight—flew upside down, only mere inches from the ground, during air events.

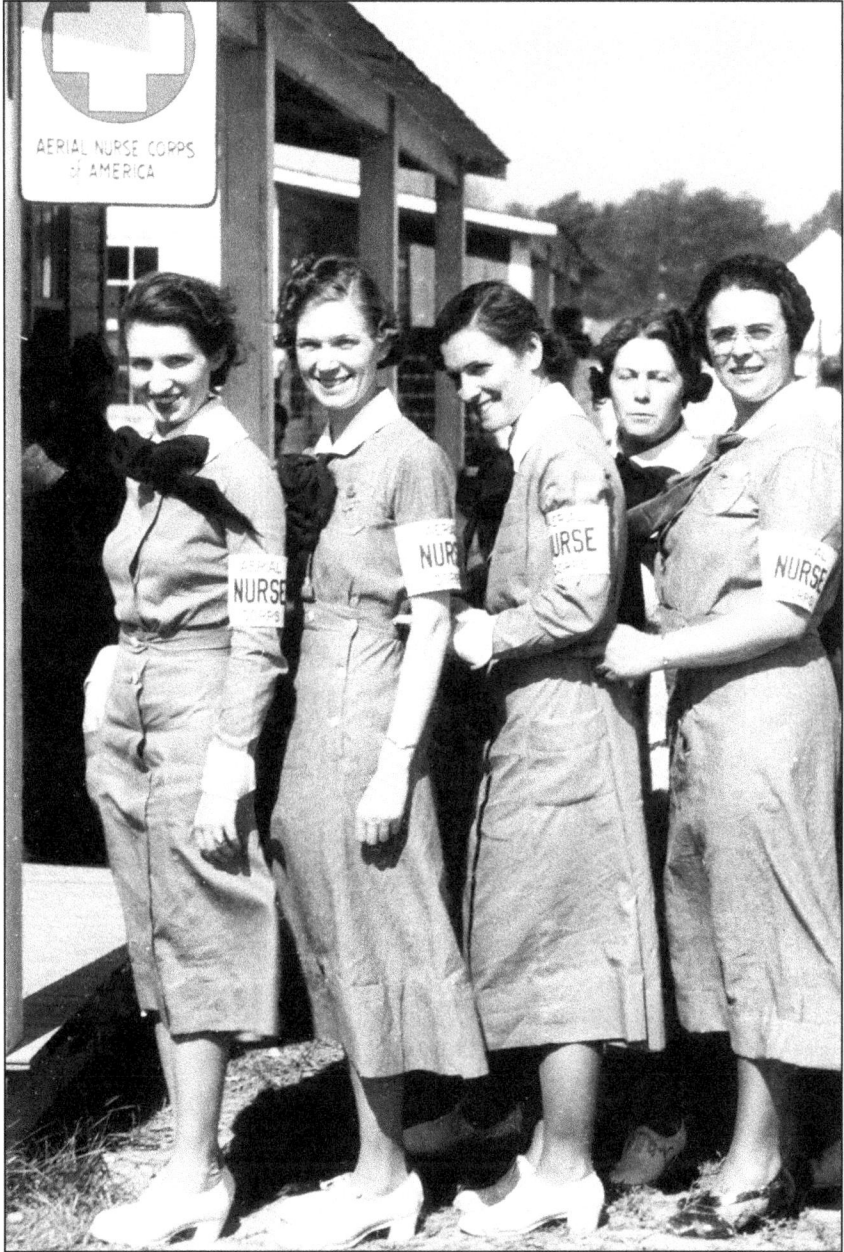

Figure 06.05. Nurse-pilots and soon-to-become ANCOA Commanders, are waiting in the wings to render first aid at the 1938 National Air Races in Cleveland: Merle McGriff, second; Florence Boswell, fourth; and Leora Stroup, fifth. New cadets Catherine Gerry, first, and Josephine Jones, third, are also pictured. Pre-official-uniform days. MMM Collection.

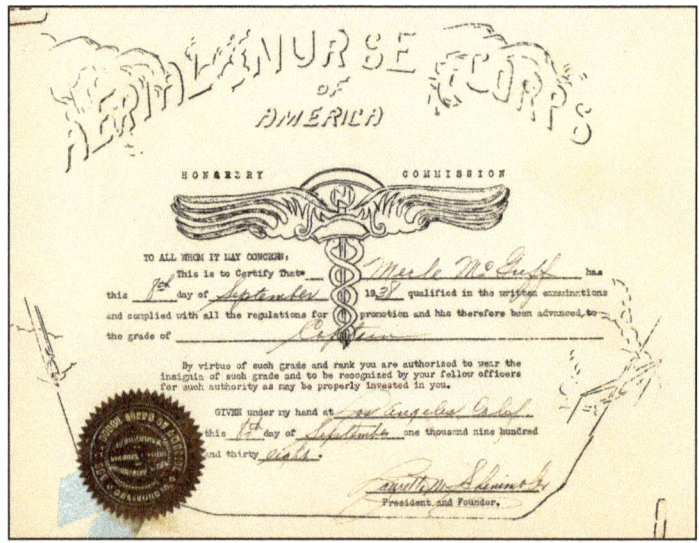

Figure 06.06. McGriff's ANCOA Certificate for advancement to Captain, 8 September 1938. MMM Collection.

Because of her efficiency and initiative, Schimmoler promoted McGriff to Captain, making her the first Commander of Company C-5. Schimmoler waived the three-month waiting period listed in the by-laws and advanced her rank immediately after the races. McGriff had undoubtedly earned it.

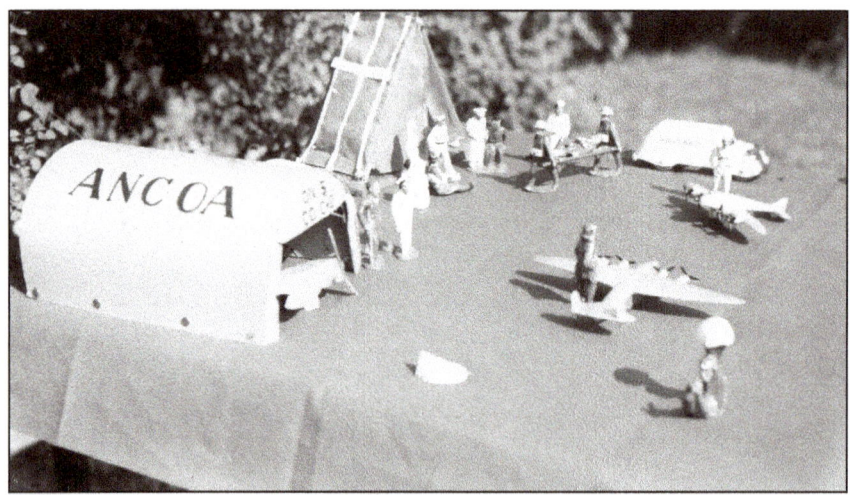

Figure 06.07. A miniature diorama depicting an ANCOA first aid tent at an air race, 1939. Created for the 1939 Michigan Air Races. Companies A-5, C-5, and D-5 staffed the first aid tent. MMM.

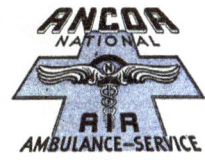

```
AERIAL NURSE CORPS OF AMERICA
2620  NORTH   HOLLYWOOD   WAY
OPP.   UNION   AIR  TERMINAL
BURBAND . . . . . . . CALIFORNIA        February 10, 1939

                                                THE SIGN OF SAFETY
                                                FOR THE . . PATIENT
        SUBJECT:  Appointment to Post of Division Commander.
                                                OFFICIAL . . NURSING
        TO    :   Captain Merle McGriff, R. N., 1040 Fidelity    ORGANIZATION . . FOR
                  Medical Building, Dayton, Ohio                 NATIONAL AERONAUTIC
                                                                 ASSOCIATION

        1.      In accordance with regulations Art. 206 and by virtue of
        your remarkable record and accomplishments during the past seven months
        you are this date appointed to the post of Division Commander of the
        5th Division of the Aerial Nurse Corps of America.

        2.      To accomplish all that you have in such a short period of time
        is indeed commendable and certainly not without much effort on your part.
        Success in any activity depends on the individual interest and you have
        manifested a sincere interest and have succeeded to a post that you are
        justly entitled to.

        3.      "Honor has Responsibility", and while this honor accorded you
        may increase your responsibility, every effort will be made to give you
        capable officers to assist you to carry on and we sincerely hope that your
        efforts will not wane but instead forge ahead to a higher post of
        recognition.

        4.      We wish to take this opportunity of expressing our very deep
        appreciation to you for your sincere efforts, your fine spirit of cooper-
        ation, and to tell you that it has been an unusual pleasure to work with
        one so capable and thorough as you.

        5.      With this added responsibility and new post of duty will come
        an added or new rank, namely that of Major, which will be conferred upon
        you within the near future.

        6.      We wish you every success in your new post and want you to
        know you can continue to count on us to stand by in all you do for the
        future growth and welfare of the Aerial Nurse Corps of America.

                                        Very sincerely,

                                        Lauretta M. Schimmoler
                                        Colonel, A. N. C. of A.,
                                        National Commander.
```

Figure 06.08. McGriff's letter of appointment from Schimmoler to Division Commander, 10 February 1939. MMM Collection.

Only seven months later, McGriff advanced again—this time to Commander of Division 5 and the rank of Major. She must have genuinely believed in the cause of aerial nursing and its importance for society; she worked tirelessly to advance the Corps.

Schimmoler could be rigid with rules—she liked to portray a military formality—but she also enjoyed displaying her flair to ANCOA members. She frequently sent letters with glowing words of appreciation and many certificates of achievements.

Chapter Six

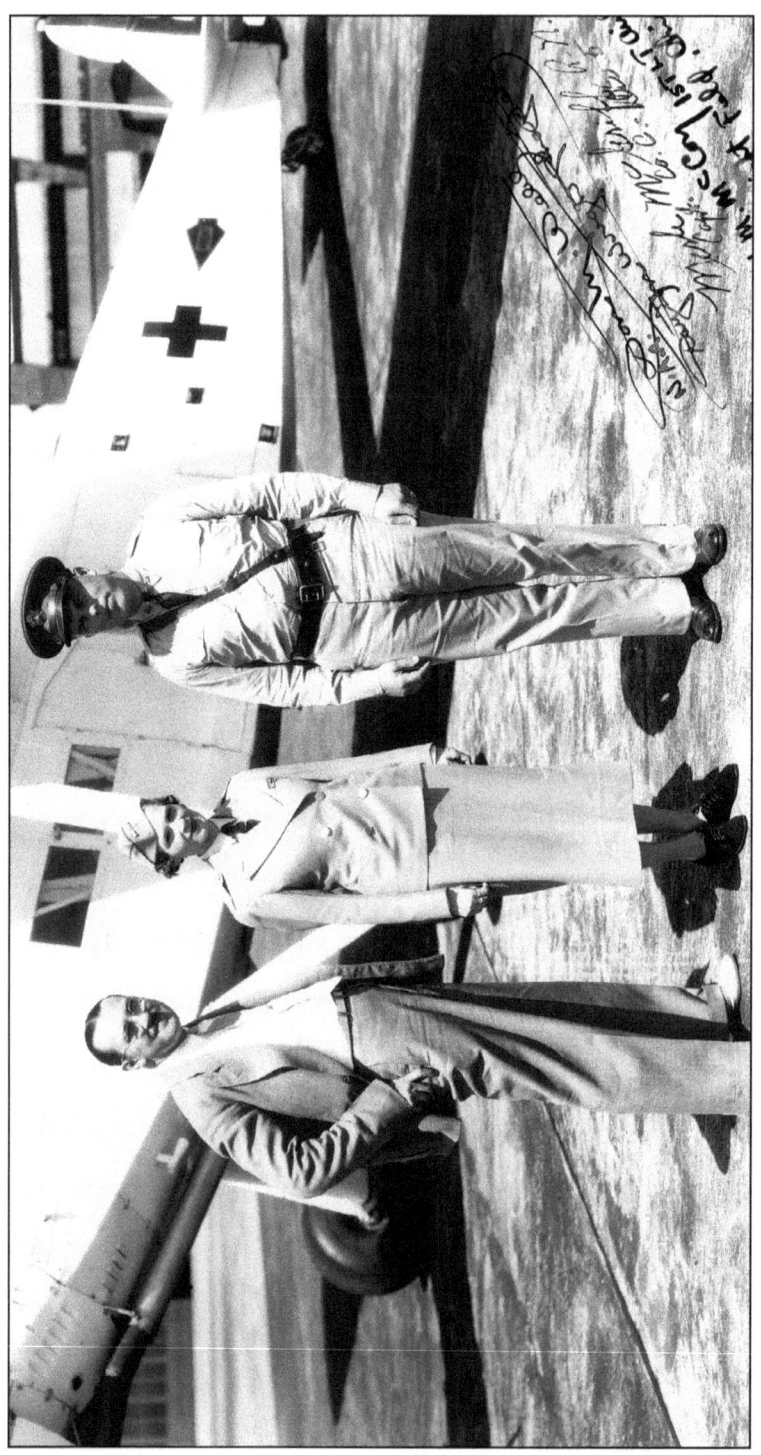

Figure 06.09. McGriff with Don M. of the NAA, 1st Lt. H.M. McCoy of the Air Corps, and the Snow White ambulance plane at Wright Field, July 1939. Courtesy of the International Women's Air & Space Museum, Cleveland, Ohio.

Schimmoler encouraged members to learn to fly. Several joined Dayton's Flying Club and attended ground school classes at the Gibbons Hotel. A local newspaper bragged, "The Flying Nurses are taking ground school and flight courses at Russ Moore's Flying School, Dayton Municipal Airport, and at the Air City Flying Service, East Dayton Airport. On Monday night, members of the newly formed pilot's club voted to let girl members in their club, thus allowing the Aerial Nurses to attend its meetings." 3

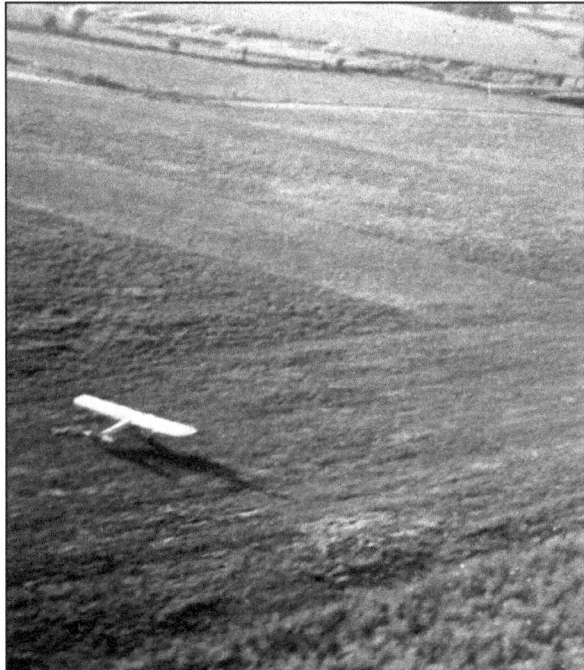

Aerial Nurses Given Flying Instructions

Members of the aerial nurse corps are learning to fly at various Dayton flying schools, according to Miss Merle McGriff, commander of the Fifth division ANCOA. The "Flying Nurses" are taking the flight courses both ground and air training at Russ Moore's flying school, Dayton Municipal Airport, and at the Air City Flying service, East Dayton airport.

Already several of the girls are attending the ground school classes of the Dayton Flying club held every Wednesday at the Gibbons hotel. And Monday night members of the newly formed Pilot's club voted to have girl members in their club, thus allowing the Aerial Nurses and other young women interested in aviation, to attend its meetings and benefit by its ground and air training courses.

More than 75 members attended the first meeting of the Pilot's club, but an error in the invitation kept away a good portion of the 200 expected. Meetings are to be held every Monday night.

The Pilot's club is the second flying club organized in this city. Plans are under way for making it a uniformed group such as the Dayton Flying club under Russ Moore.

Figure 06.10. McGriff landing a Cub Airplane on her first solo flight, East Dayton Airport, 10 August 1939. Figure 06.11. "Aerial Nurses Given Flying Instructions," unnamed newspaper clipping, 1939. MMM Collection.

McGriff chose the East Dayton Airport, across from Wright Field, and scheduled her lessons with the Air City Flying Service. They charged ten dollars for one-half hour. She finished ten lessons and then performed her solo. McGriff wrote a note about that day and told about a soloing tradition:

> When someone has their solo flight they have to treat all the people at the airport to Cokes. I treated several.

One day McGriff spotted a handsome pilot in khaki coveralls greasing an airplane that belonged to a Captain from Wright Field. Pilot met pilot and in 1941 she married him. She became Merle McGriff McAfee. 4

Chapter Six

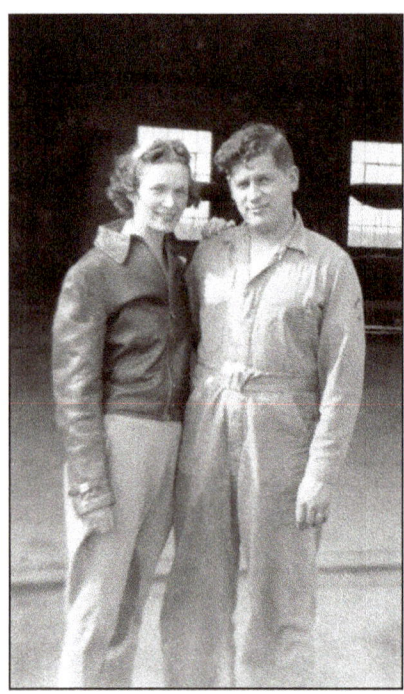 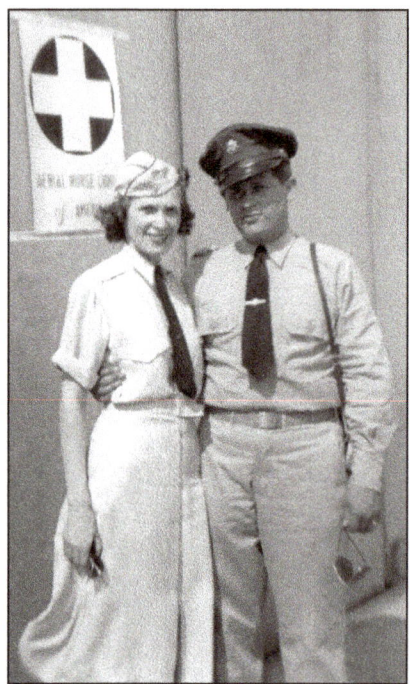

Figure 06.14. Merle McAfee and the Army Air Corps pilot who won her heart, Dean Robert McAfee, 1941. In WWII he achieved the rank of Major.

In 1954, the McAfee's moved to Orlando and then to St. Cloud, Florida. She worked in the newborn nursery and was appointed Director of Nurses at Wooster Community Hospital.[5] During her years in the ANCOA, she collected scrapbooks with photographs and ephemera. Her daughter, Judith Johnson, maintained them. Without Merle McGriff McAfee's scrapbooks (the MMM Collection) and the generosity of Johnson, we would know little about Dayton's activities.

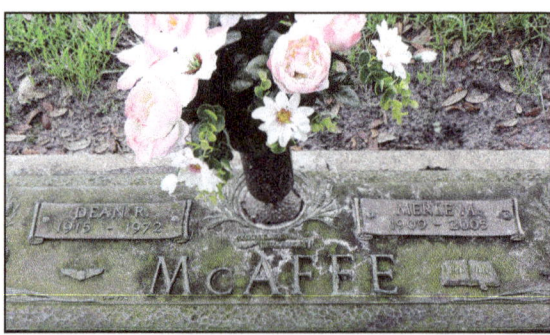

Figure 06.13. Merle McGriff McAfee's gravesite. She lived to the age of 96.

Commanders
Lieutenant Colonel Edith Corns Lloyd, RN

Chief of Staff, Commander of Wing 1
Commander of Division 1, Los Angeles, CA

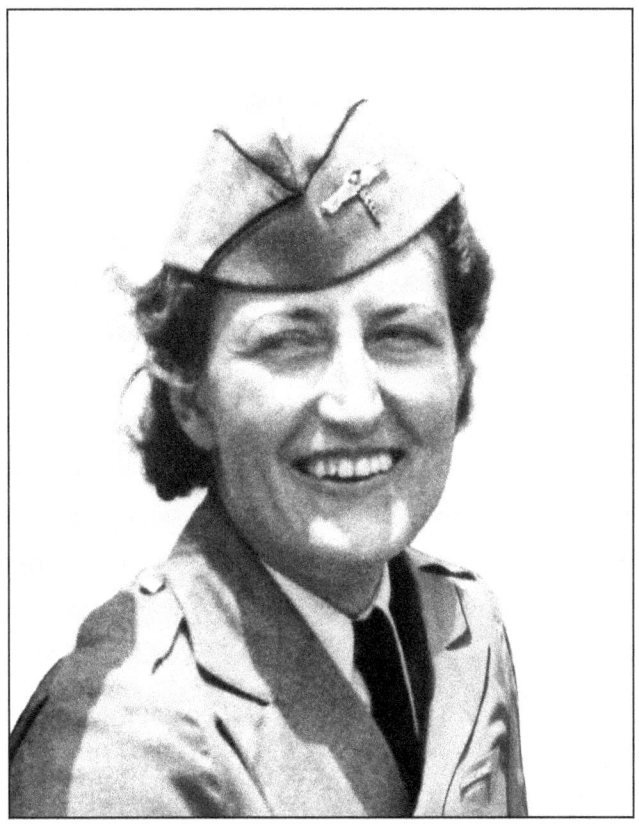

Figure 06.14. Edith Corns in her official ANCOA uniform with the cap pin and the first embroidered Aerial Nurse pin, 1937. Author's Collection.

Edith Mary Corns was born on 10 November 1913 in Ohio. James Corns, her father, must have died when she was young, and her family moved because in 1920, Corns' mother, Jennie Harris, is listed as a widow living with her mother in Los Angeles.[6] Corns graduated from the Los Angeles County General Hospital School of Nursing in 1935. The following year, on 15 September 1936, she joined the ANCOA as member #12—just one week after their inaugural post at the 1936 National Air Races.

She became the first Chief of Staff, the first member Schimmoler promoted to Lieutenant Colonel (April 1938), and the first Commander of Wing-1,

Chapter Six

Division-1, which included the California and Washington State companies. Initially, Schimmoler functioned as the only commander when just one company existed. But after ANCOA gained members, Schimmoler advanced herself to National Commander and promoted Corns to the Wing.[7] Corns remained active with ANCOA until WWII began.

Corns joined the Army Nurse Corps and was sent to the Philippines: a choice country with a tropical ambiance many nurses hoped to deploy to. But her enjoyment didn't last. The Japanese bombed the Philippines the same day they bombed Pearl Harbor. The military hurriedly moved Corns and 66 other Army nurses to Bataan—shortly before the Japanese capture of Manila.

Army Nurses set up two hospitals in the jungle of Bataan in outdoor tents. Hospital #2 stretched two and a half miles with more than seven thousand sick and wounded soldiers. The nurses worked 12-18 hour shifts as they tried to care for shrapnel injuries and tropical diseases with the few medical supplies they could scavenge.[8]

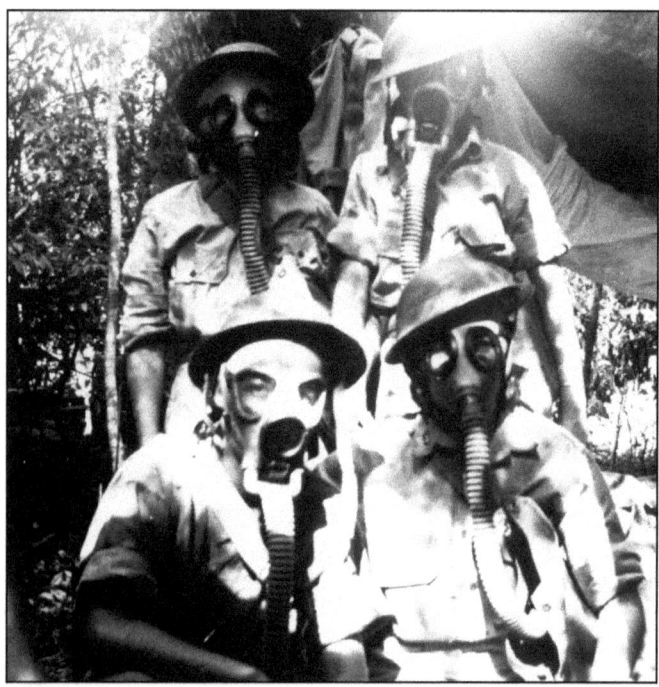

Figure 06.15. Army Nurses Edith Corns and Beth Veley, kneeling. Rose Rieper, and Mary Moultrie, standing, pose for a photograph in their helmets and gas masks in the nurses' quarters, General Hospital #2, Bataan, Philippines, 1942. Courtesy of the Army Nurse Corps Collection, Office of Medical History.

Just before the Japanese overtook Bataan, the nurses moved again—they transferred them to Corregidor, a huge hollowed-out rock with tunnels. More injured soldiers! Bombs continually shelled the island near "the Rock." Many died.

When the Japanese overtook the Philippines, 11 navy nurses, 66 army nurses, and one nurse-anesthetist were captured and interred as Prisoners of War (POWs). The nurses were separated from the military men and held with civilian POWs in Santo Tomas and Los Banos internment camps. Starvation, illnesses, injuries, and depression enveloped the camps, but the nurses continued to care for patients even as they became sick and lost weight. Corns lost 31 pounds.

After three years of imprisonment, the U.S. military liberated the nurses on 3 February 1945. Back home, citizens hailed them for their bravery. Carolyn See of *The Washington Post* said it best: "... they were plucky young girls on a mild adventure to authentic heroes."

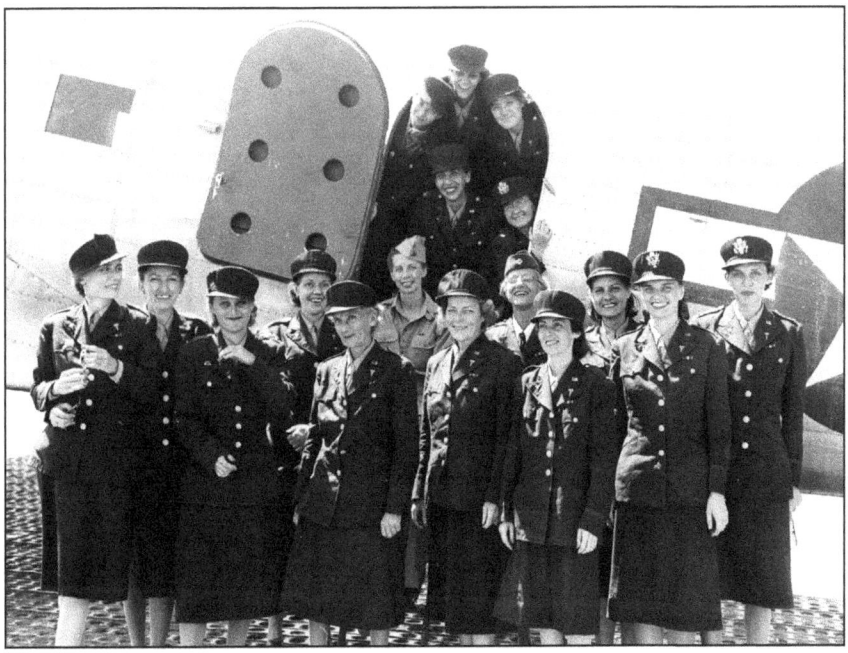

Figure 06.16. "The Angels of Bataan and Corregidor," in Leyte, 20 February 1945. Stroup flew to the Philippines to escort them to Hickam Field, Hawaii.

Once home, they were taken on war bond tours to raise money but told to keep quiet, not to tell their harrowing stories.[9] Many never would discuss it; eventually, some wrote books. Their stories are chilling.

Chapter Six

Before the nurses left for Hickam Field in Hawaii, they paused on Leyte Island to eat and rest. Chief Surgeon Brigadier General Denit awarded them two oak leaf clusters and one grade promotion.

With the many duties Corn performed for the ANCOA, and her infamous years as a POW Army Nurse, we should know more about her life, but she never told her story. She married Howard P. Lloyd in 1947 and died in 1988 at age 75. [10]

The Corregidor Foundation, Inc. erected and dedicated a historical marker on 6 May 2000, on Corregidor Island, to honor "The Angeles of Bataan and Corregidor," a name the public coined for the POW nurses. [11]

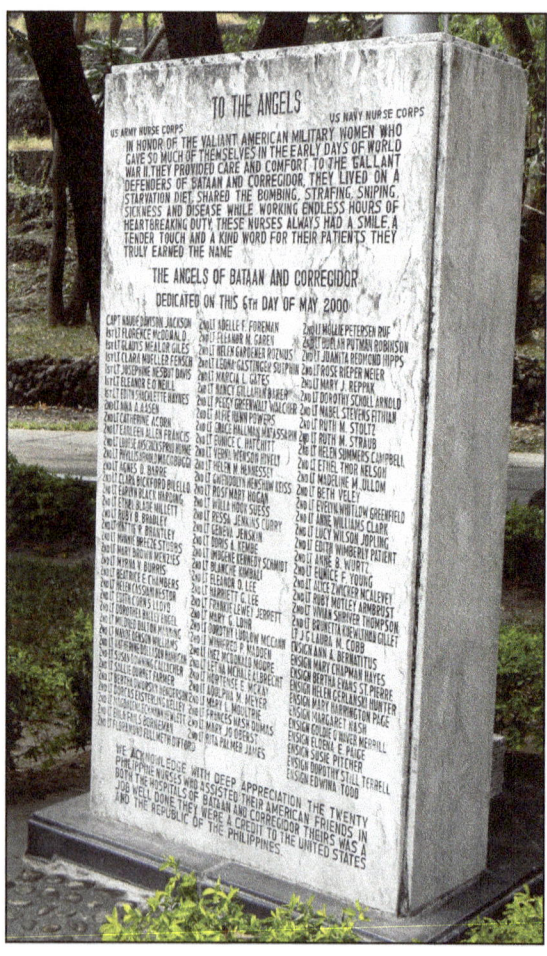

Figure 06.17. The marker, "To the Angeles," on Corregidor Island, Cavite, in the Philippines. Photo by Richard E. Miller, 2013. Courtesy of hmdb.org.

Commanders
Lieutenant Colonel Ruth G. Mitchell, RN

Chief of Staff
Vice President

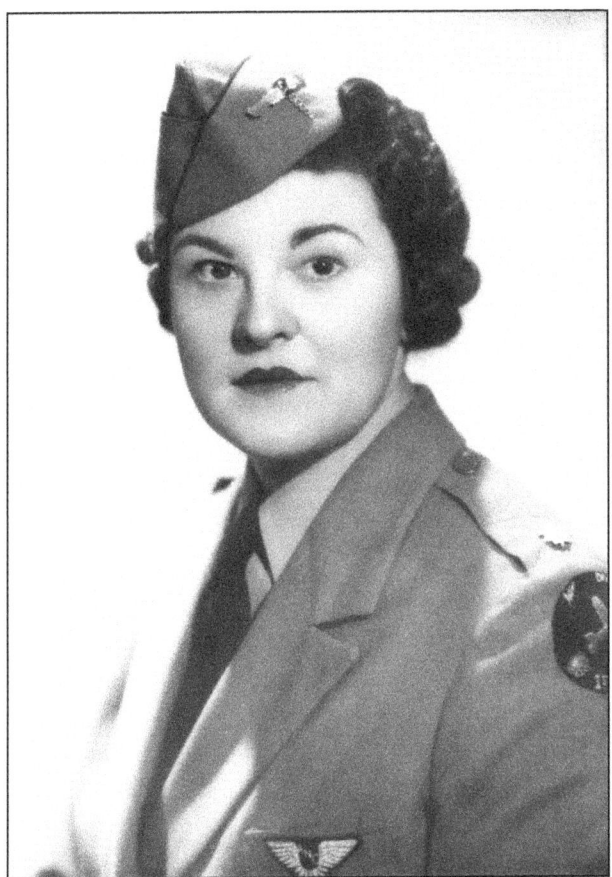

Figure 06.18. Ruth Mitchell's ANCOA photograph. She wears an eight-pointed oak leaf pin on her shoulder. Schimmoler might have awarded it with her promotion to Lieutenant Colonel; no other commander wore one except Schimmoler in the first year. A commander patch is on her pocket, and the 1st Division patch on her arm, 1939. MMM Collection.

Ruth Mitchell, RN, joined the ANCOA in December 1938. In April 1939, Schimmoler promoted her to Major and the Chief of Staff in charge of nursing.[12] Initially, she lived in the San Francisco/Oakland area. Later, Schimmoler promoted her to Lieutenant Colonel and Vice President—the highest rank possible then, next to Schimmoler.

Mitchell was born in Bay City, Michigan, in 1895 but moved to different cities. She spent her early childhood in Spokane, Washington, and Portland, Oregon. Mitchell secured a teaching job as an adult and moved to the University of Notre Dame in Indiana. She also studied there and graduated from Notre Dame with a Bachelor of Arts in Education. Teaching must not have been her ultimate goal because she moved back to Portland to enter the Good Samaritan Hospital School of Nursing, graduating from that program in 1932.

After several years of private duty nursing, the Industrial Hospital for the Montgomery Ward Company in Portland hired Mitchell as the head nurse. Next, she accepted the Director of Education position at Columbus Hospital and moved to Great Falls, Montana. Still not content with the limits of her education, she moved to the University of California, Berkeley, for a Master of Public Health degree with a planned doctorate. She became a member of the Alpha Tau Delta—the first chapter and the first nursing fraternity in the U.S. She joined the ANCOA during this time. [13]

Eventually, she moved to Pasadena, California, where she re-joined the ANCOA in December 1941 (members were required to re-join every three years). Her work and life after that time has yet to be discovered.

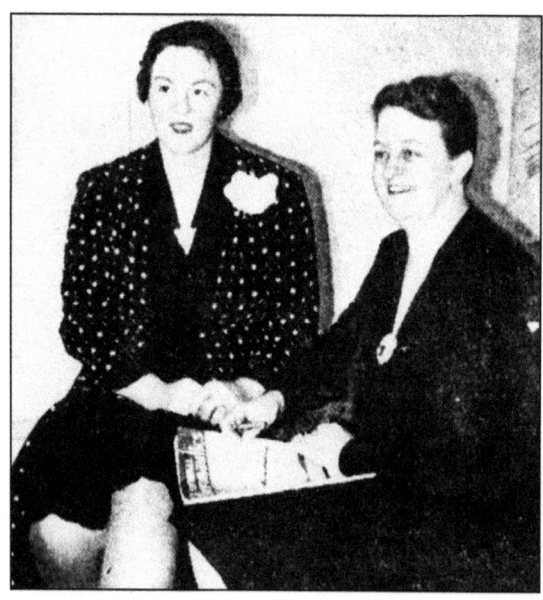

Figure 06.19. Ruth Mitchell and Lauretta Schimmoler attending the National Aeronautics Association Meeting, New Orleans, Louisiana, 1939. MMM. They hoped to recruit nurses and start a new company. No nurses lived in New Orleans, according to the roster. The plan must not have materialized.

Commanders

Captain Matilda D. Grinevich, RN

Commander of Co. A-8, New York, NY; Flight Nurse

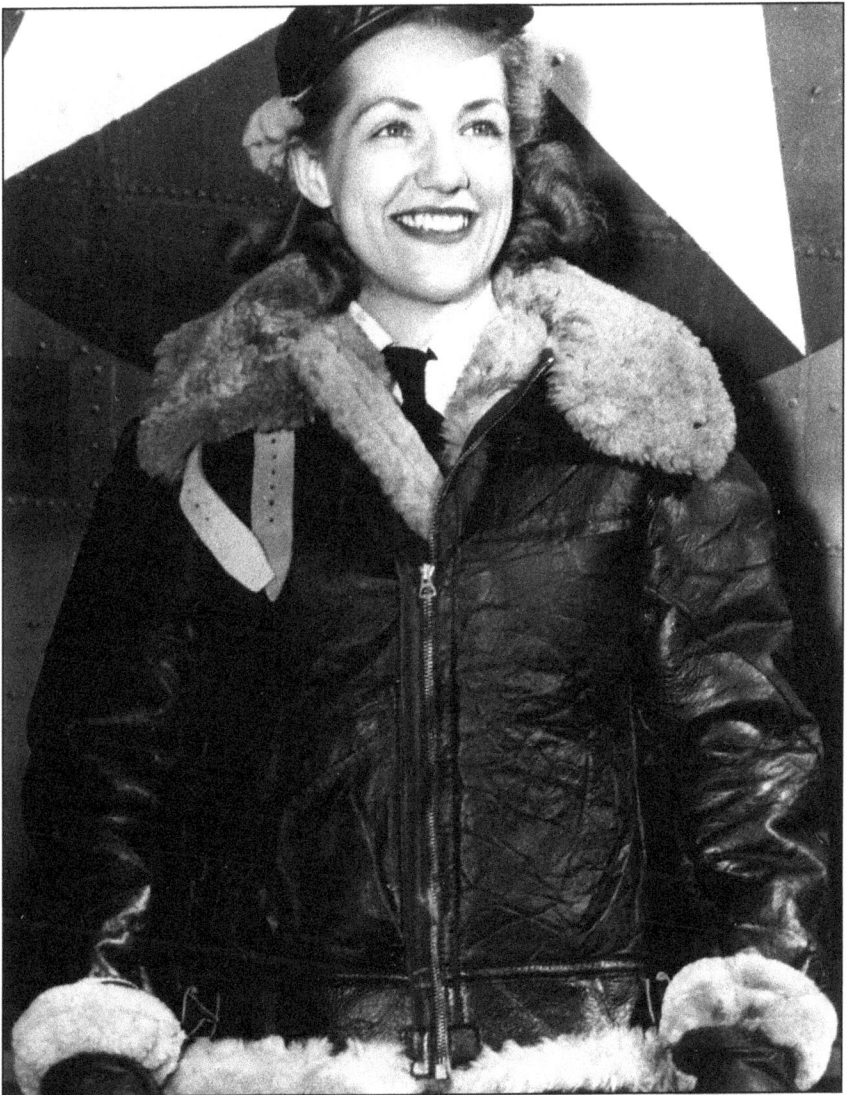

Figure 06.20. Matilda "Mickie" Grinevich in her WWII Flight Nurse jacket, in front of a military airplane, 1942. Courtesy of Adrienne Haddad.

A favorite Grinevich motto: "It's dull riding the end of a broomstick. I'd much rather be flying in the wild blue yonder." [14]

Chapter Six

Matilda D. Grinevich, Commander of ANCOA Company A-8, was born on 2 October 1915 in Mahanoy City, Pennsylvania, a region known for its anthracite coal production.

She graduated from Mahanoy City High School and began nurses' training at the University of Pennsylvania Training School for Nurses in Philadelphia. After she graduated in 1937, she moved to New York City to work as a private nurse. Celebrities of the era hired her. She often recounted stories about the celebrities who were in her care. [15]

Like many ANCOA nurses, when WWII began, Grinevich joined the Army. "My brother was in the war. I thought if he could go, I could go, too," she said. During her Army Nurse Corps training in Texas, she heard the Army had formed the Army Air Force Flight Nurse Corps. She volunteered. [16] No doubt, ANCOA developed her flying interest and helped her placement into the competitive field of the flight nurse trainee program.

We know little of her ANCOA activities except that she joined in the 1930s and was a lifelong friend of Schimmoler's. She knew a great deal about ANCOA's history; she directed Robert Skinner to historical information sources when he interviewed her for his 1984 ANCOA article. [17] She saved ANCOA photographs, but her family couldn't locate them.

Grinevich had four Flight Nurse careers:

- Aerial Nurse Corps of America
- Army Air Force, Flight Nurse Corps, in World War II
- Air Force in the Korean Conflict
- Air Force in the Vietnam War

She served on the 801st MAETS, the second group of flight nurses to leave overseas. Squadron 801 and 802 received different training than subsequent groups. History lists their training as haphazard: basic training, squadron administration, the use of the litter, and loading of air-evacuation aircraft. The military did not establish an improved didactic course until January 1943. Subsequent flight nurses graduated from the School of Air Evacuation; 801 and 802 did not. [18] Regardless, they had to care for injured soldiers inventing skills for those they had not learned during their experiences as civilian nurses. Grinevich said:

> Planes were not pressurized. They were not heated. You were so busy making continual rounds you didn't have time to think about being uncomfortable. Our hands got cold and we spent our time trying to keep patients warm with blankets to prevent hypothermia. We were flying in planes

designed for troop transport, not litter. The plane motors were loud, and the turbulence created issues when caring for patients. We had to stand on the litter below to reach the soldiers on the top, all while bouncing around from the turbulence. Some ideas, such as suctioning secretions, were new and proper equipment did not exist; we used primitive devices, such as a turkey baster, for a suction device. [19]

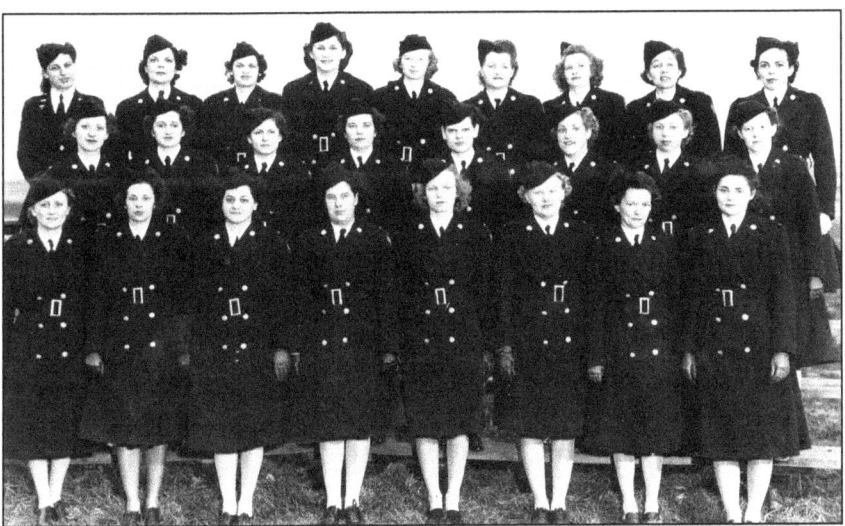

Figure 06.21. Grinevich, second row, third from right, with the 801 Medical Air Evacuation Transport Squadron, 1943. Leora Stroup Papers, AMEDD.

Figure 06.22. Grinevich receiving an Oak Leaf Cluster from General Henry Arnold for meritorious achievements in sustained aerial flights on evacuation transport missions, 10 August 1944. Bowman Field photo.

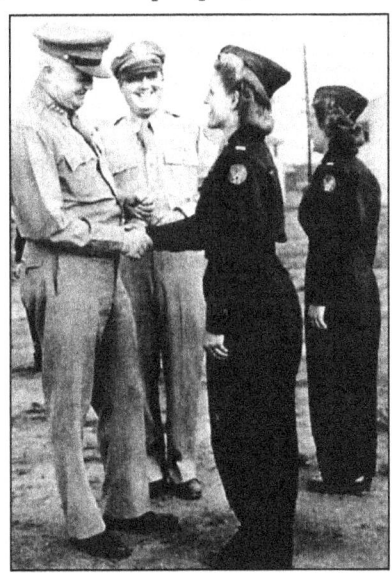

After WWII, she returned to civilian nursing as an industrial nurse at the *New York Daily News* and as a medical secretary at the National Biscuit Company in New York City. Around this time, the Air Force became an independent branch of the service. The potential rank might have tempted her because she re-joined the military as an Air Force Nurse in 1948.

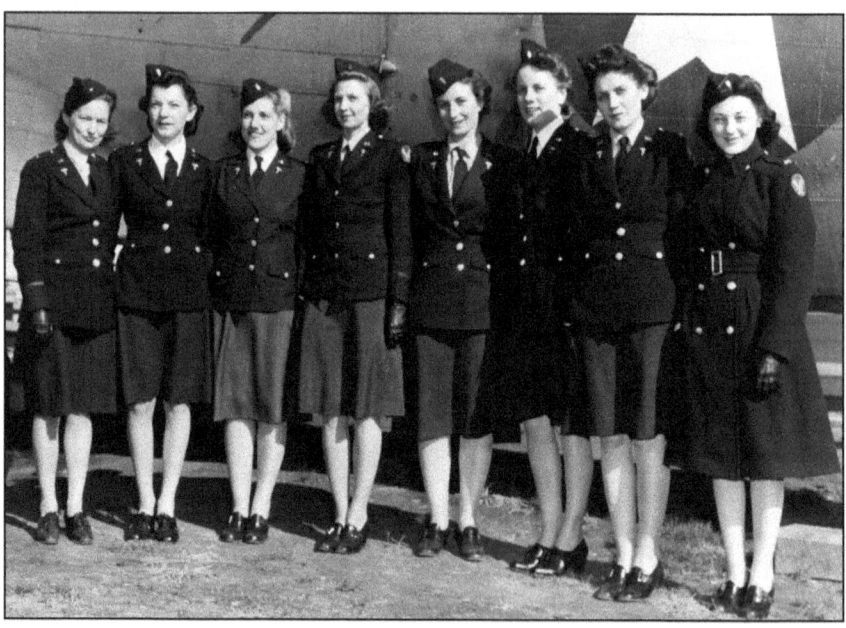

Figure 06.23. An unlabeled photo, either of the 1453rd MATS during the Korean Conflict or from WWII, Grinevich third from left. AMEDD.

During the Korean Conflict, the military assigned her to the 1453rd MATS at Hickam Field, Hawaii. She flew with patients to military hospitals in Hawaii and other Pacific islands. She and the nine other flight nurses of the 1453rd MATS helped to evacuate more than 45,000 sick and wounded personnel from the Korean Peninsula.

In 1959 the military assigned her to Pope Air Force Base in Fayetteville, N. Carolina. She earned her Bachelor of Science in Nursing at E. Carolina College, in Greenville, in 1963. After establishing her permanent residency in Southern Pines in 1967, the Air Force promoted her to Chief of Nursing Services at Pope Air Force Base.

During the Vietnam era, she served in several capacities:

- Chief Flight Nurse of the 1st Aero-Med Evac, Pope Air Force Base
- Chief Nurse, 811th Medical Group, Loring Air Force Base in Maine

- Chief Nurse, Langley Air Force Base in Virginia
- Chief Flight Nurse of the 1st Aeromedical Evacuation Group at Pope Air Force Base, where she taught air-evac to recruits—the same skill she had learned in World War II and which she now translated for modern warfare. [20]

Grinevich was the one who suggested that Flight Nurses should honor Schimmoler in a ceremony, organized the event in Las Vegas in 1966, and gave Schimmoler her flight wings.

While Grinevich never married, she did once fall in love with a pilot who asked her to marry him. Her mother forbade it because the man was not Catholic; she listened to her mother and ended the relationship. Her niece said, "Although it's a sad story, it wasn't an unusual sentiment for the time."

Grinevich received many awards: Victory Medal, Asiatic-Pacific Campaign Medal, Navy Unit Commendation, Air Medal with four Oak Leaf Clusters, Korean Service Medal, U.N. Service Medal, Army of Occupation Medal.

She logged 7,000 flight hours in C-47s, C-54s, C-97s, C-123s, C-124s, C-130s, helicopters, gliders, and "flying boats" called the PBYs. The PBYs were dangerous aircrafts used to rescue of aircrew downed over water. [21]

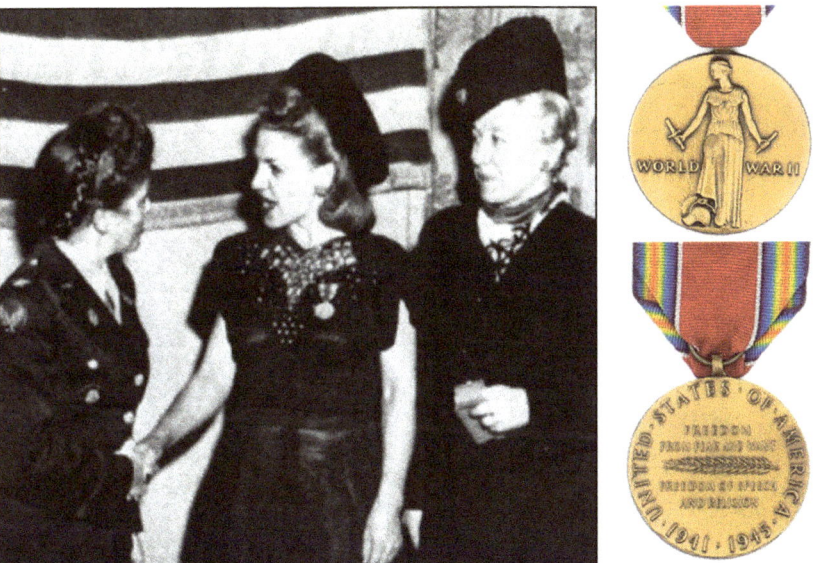

Figure 06.24. Grinevich receives the WWII Victory Medal from Colonel Mary Halleran, WACs Director. Mrs. Jimmie Doolittle looks on, 1944. Figure 06.25. The WWII Victory Medal. The medal's words: Freedom from War and Want. Freedom of Speech and Religion. USAF photos.

She retired from the Air Force in 1968 with the rank of Lieutenant Colonel, the highest afforded to women in the military then. Her registration was the first name entered into the Military Women's Memorial repository, at Arlington National Cemetery, on 6 April 1987.

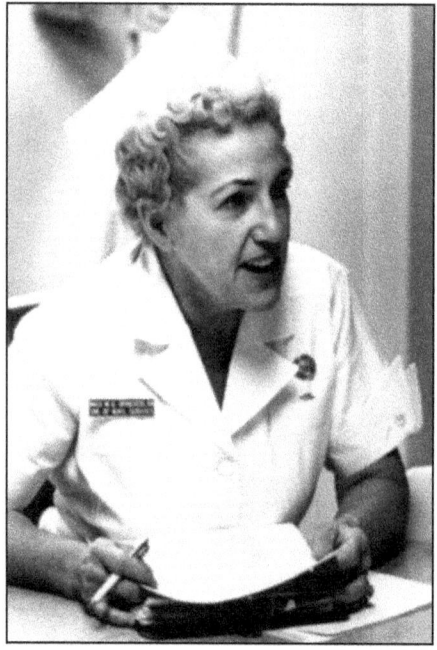

Figure 06.26. Grinevich, Director of Nursing Services at Cape Fear Valley Hospital in North Carolina. Courtesy of Adrienne Haddad.

After her military retirement, she accepted the Director of Nursing Services position at Cape Fear Valley Hospital, North Carolina. She directed a staff of 430 people. Then, after ten years, Grinevich retired from working life to enjoy the beauty of the Southern Pines area.

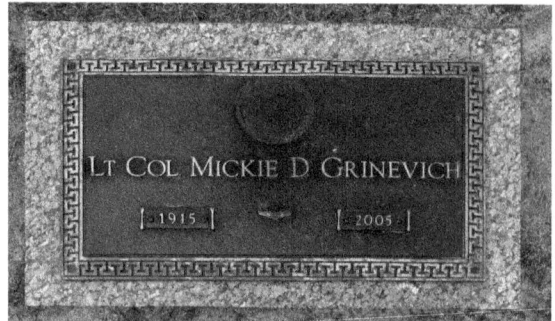

Figure 06.27. Lt. Colonel Mickie D. Grinevich was buried in Pinelawn Park, Pinehurst North Carolina. She lived to 89.

Shortly after she died, Sandhill Community College in Southern Pines established the Matilda D. Grinevich Endowed Nursing Scholarship with her estate gift, awarded to assist qualified nursing students.

Commanders
Captain Genevieve Waples Smith, RN

Commander of Co. C-4, Decatur, IL; Licensed Pilot

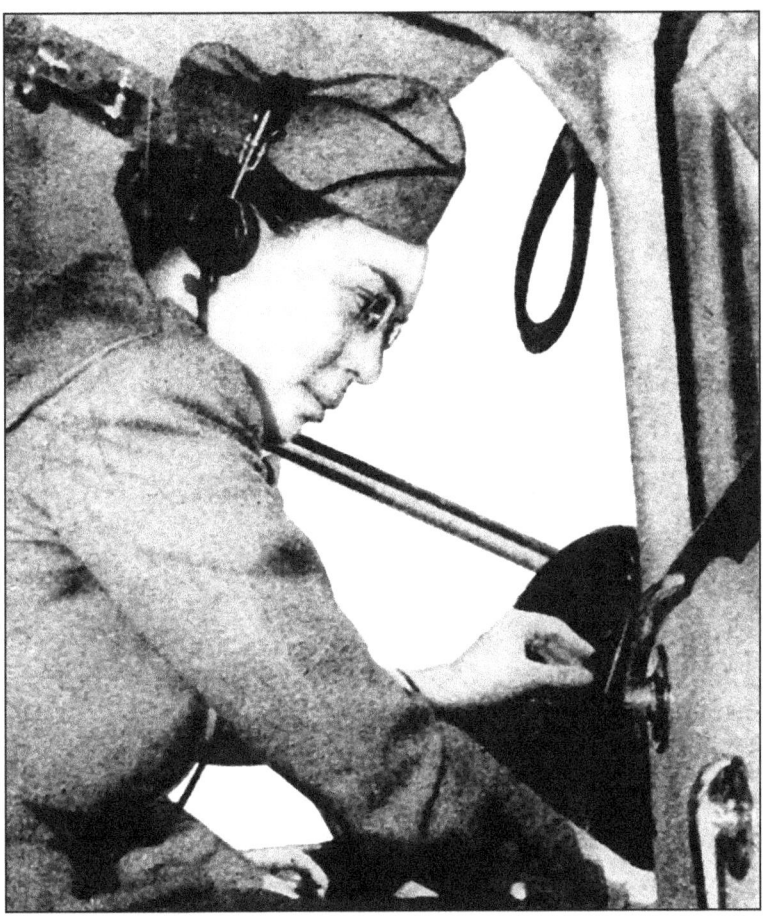

Figure 06.28. Waples at the controls of her Piper Cub, the "Zip n' Zephyr," and wearing the ANCOA uniform, 1940. MMM Collection.

Castana, Iowa's population was 360 when Genevieve Wilda Waples was born on 2 April 1913; her quaint town's growth has declined since then. She moved away from her parents, Jane Lawson and Eugene Waples, to the University of Iowa, where she earned a Bachelor of Science degree.

Her nursing degree from Iowa State University Hospital followed in 1935. After that graduation, St. Bonaventure Hospital in Boise employed her as Assistant Superintendent of Nurses for four years. [22]

Chapter Six

She earned her private pilot's license in 1937.[23] By the age of 27, she was a nursing instructor and an accomplished pilot—she had even won an award in a competition at the Illinois State Fair.[24] She must have developed a penchant to travel soon after she finished her education because a *Flashes* article in June 1939 said she stopped by the ANCOA General Headquarters before embarking on a boat to Australia.

Initially, she joined the ANCOA in Boise, Idaho, in 1937; two years later, in October 1940, she relocated to Decatur, Illinois, and formed the Fourth Division and Company C.[25]

She was not merely an occasional flyer. She did not settle in one area; local newspapers frequently listed the contests she entered in various states. In February 1940, she joined—as a founding member—the Idaho Chapter of the Ninety-Nines.[26]

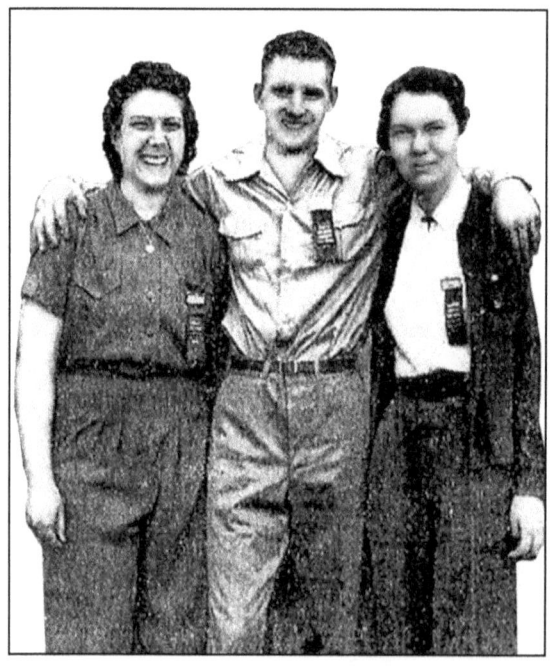

Figure 06.29. Adelade O'Brien, Humphrey Moody, and Genevieve Waples, L to R, wearing their ribbons after the 1940 Illinois Pilots Air Tour and Efficiency Competition. Courtesy of the Sangamon County Historical Society.

The local *Decatur Daily* reported Waples would represent Decatur in the 1940 Illinois Pilots Air Tour and Efficiency Competition. The contest traveled through eleven cities on the three-day flight and ended at the Illinois Fairgrounds.

She borrowed a plane, the "Miss Springfield," from the Aviation Hall of Fame flyers and brothers Humphrey and Hunter Moody, who had won the endurance flight in the exact plane one year earlier.[27]

The only other woman in the contest, Adelade O'Brien, became the first licensed female pilot in downstate Illinois at age 18. During WWII, O'Brien worked as a civilian ground flight instructor for the U.S. Army Air Corps and taught cadets.

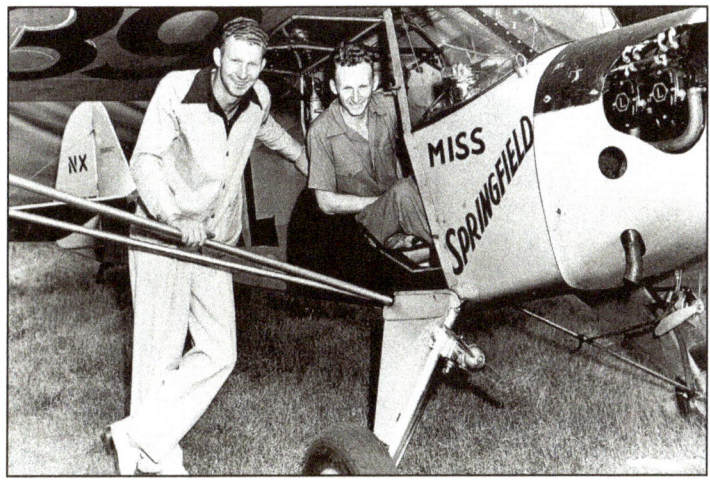

Figure 06.30. Humphrey and Hunter Moody, with Miss Springfield, 1939, the same plane Waples borrowed from them in 1940. Author's Collection.

In 1940 Waples finally bought a Piper Cub with fellow pilot and nursing instructor Alice Studer. They invited friends, threw a welcome party for the plane, christened it the "Zip n' Zephyr," and gave a prize to the woman who could demonstrate the quickest way to climb into a Cub. [28]

Waples had chosen a position as a science instructor at Decatur and Macon County Hospital School of Nursing in 1939. Studer was an instructor at the same school and an ANCOA Company C member. Local newspapers reported Studer and Waples flew together to events and conferences.

One newspaper ran their crack-up story. They had flown the "Zip n' Zephyr" to a nurse's convention. On the return, they had to make a forced landing. But they weren't dismayed; they calmly hunted for four-leaf-clovers until their rescuer finally arrived. [29]

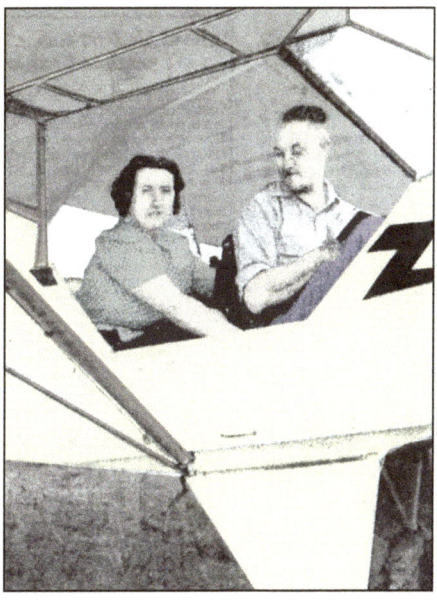

Figure 06.31. Alice Struder during a flying lesson in an unidentified open cockpit-style plane with instructor, Carl Lewis, 1940. Colorized clipping.

Meanwhile, Waples continued to move up the nursing hierarchy—in December 1942, Decatur and Macon County Hospital promoted her to Superintendent. [30] Like other ANCOA nurses, she traveled to various hospitals, clubs, and nursing conferences to present the topic of "Air Ambulance Nursing" and to promote joining. [31] But when WWII caused the demise of ANCOA, she started to teach home nursing classes with the Red Cross to help relieve the nursing shortages from wartime enlistments. Waples told the hospitalized patients:

> Half as many graduate nurses are available as there were during peacetime for hospital care. Make your arrangements. Be considerate. Leave the hospital when your time is up. [32]

Waples, as the Director of Nursing, met with St. Mary's Hospital members and a Red Cross nurse aide group to discuss the critical shortage of nurses. Hospital admissions were up from 145 to 175, and the graduate nurse staffing was down from 67 to 42. She said:

> People in Decatur Hospitals are accustomed to receiving luxurious nursing care; all they can expect now is necessary attention. They are lucky to receive the service they do. [33]

Perhaps this nurse shortage and patient need was the primary reason Waples chose not to join her fellow ANCOA nurses and enter the Army Flight Nurse program. She could have seen the world. Or, with her expert flying experience, she could've joined the Women Air Force Service Pilots. Unlike Schimmoler and Stroup, Waples was 30 when WWII started, well within the WASPs age limitation. Instead, she remained on duty at the hospital—a curious choice for a pilot who loved to fly and travel. For many nurses, it might have been the flip side of patriotism; some nurses needed to stay at home and care for U.S. patients.

Waples organized a Cadet Nurse Program. The government had passed the Bolton Bill in June 1943, which paid for women ages 18-35 to receive pay to study nursing and work in the hospital. They received $15 for the first nine months, $20 for the next 30 months, and $30 for the final six months. [34] The government gave scholarships for tuition, but students had to agree to work at their respective training hospitals through the duration of the war. Cadet Nurses stayed home; they were civilians and did not go to war overseas.

The Cadet Nurse Program was an excellent opportunity for women who wanted to study nursing but could not afford it. The government program, however, wasn't an easy sell. Women could obtain good-paying jobs by filling the factory positions men had abandoned when they went to war. Women could proceed straight from high school graduation to a lucrative

Commanders

paying factory job. Still, nursing had a future. The factory jobs did not. Women knew they would need to relinquish the factory jobs to the men when the men returned from war.³⁵

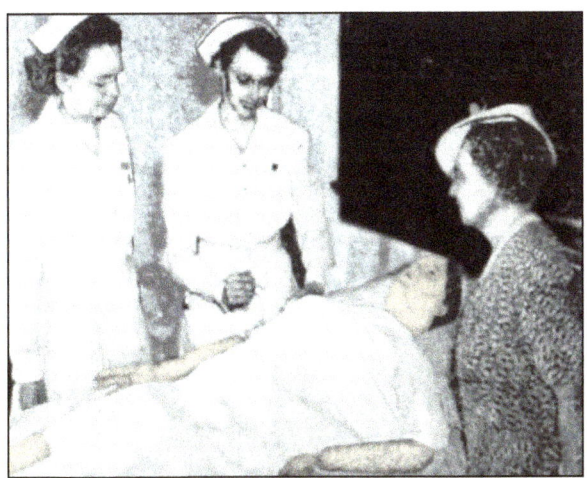

Figure 06.32. Waples, left, with the Permanent Patient donated to the school. Also in the photo are Margaret Faith, a clinical instructor, and Mrs. W. J. Grady, the mannequin donor, 1943. Colorized clipping, MMM.

A wealthy resident donated money for a healthcare mannequin they called the Permanent Patient, so students could gain confidence before caring for a live patient or administering injections.³⁶ Such expensive practice mannequins were a new idea and uncommon in nursing schools then; the Permanent Patient might have been one of the first medically simulated mannequins. Maybe Waples hoped it would attract more students by advertising it in the local newspaper.

Waples' Cadet program fell short of its desired enrollment; in January 1944, only 20 students began the class. She appealed to unemployed nurses to work at least four hours a week. She told a local reporter:

> It is worse than it ever has been. The nursing situation is critical. I have asked patients to share their private-duty nurses while in the hospital.³⁷

Six months later, the University of Oregon offered Waples a job teaching science and surgical nursing in their college program. She didn't hesitate. She resigned from Decatur and Macon County Hospital, moved to Portland, and never looked back. She immediately became an active member of the Oregon State Nurses Association (OSNA) and the Oregon Chapter of the Ninety-Nines, headquartered in Portland.

Chapter Six

The "University of Oregon Medical School Bulletin" shows she remained as a surgical nursing instructor at the university at least through 1948.[38] She completed her thesis, *Prediction of Student Deficiencies in Surgical Nursing with Methods for Correction,* and graduated with a Master of Arts in Nursing from Oregon State College.[39]

By 1947 the Oregon State Nurses Association had elected her as their field representative.[40] She organized a program with the Civil Air Patrol to train flight nurses in 1948. She said she started it "In order to have an efficient group ready in any local disaster of emergency. Oregon is the first state to undertake such a project."

This idea could have been straight from the ANCOA manual. They would conduct their training at the facilities of the Army Air Force. She asked nurses to volunteer; groups of twenty nurses from the Portland area started training on 1 July 1948.[41]

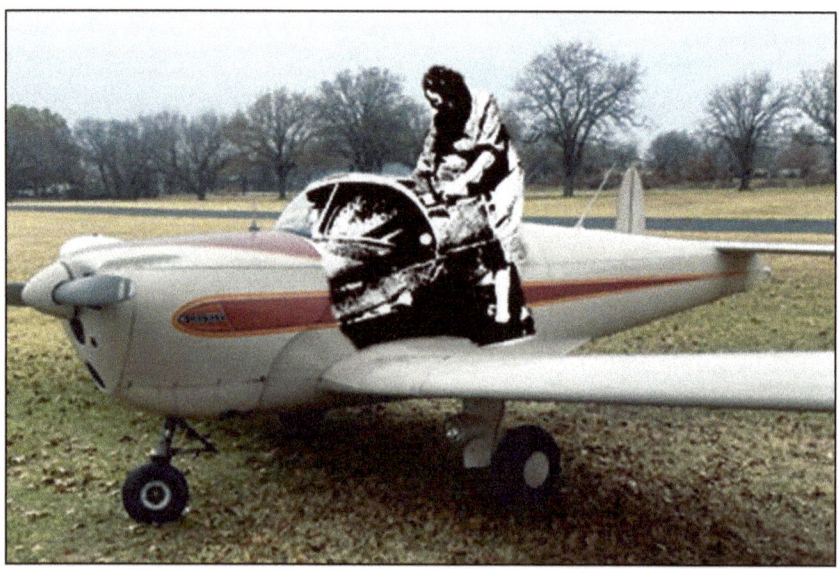

Figure 06.33. Waples prepares to take off from Vancouver Airpark in the Multnomah Flying Club's Ercoupe on a Flying Health Nurse visit, 1947. Created with a clipping of Waples standing on the type of Ercoupe she flew.

The State of Oregon hired Waples as their Flying Health Nurse to visit outlying Oregon districts—the only Oregon Ninety-Niner with a blanket permit that allowed her to fly any field at any time.[42] The *Sunday Oregonian* reported on her work; they called her the "flyingest nurse" of the Oregon flying nurses. As a member of the Multnomah Flying Club, she could use their Aeronca and Ercoupe planes for emergencies.

No articles mention if she took full ownership of the Piper Cub "Zip n' Zephyr," she'd purchased with her friend in Iowa. Probably not because she flew an Ercoupe plane in the "All-Girl Air Race" from Eugene to Hillsboro, Oregon. She won $150.00 for second place, close behind the winner. [43]

The Oregon Wing of the Civil Air Patrol featured this race as part of an Air Show at the Hillsboro Airport on 15 August 1948. Waples had become well known as an accomplished pilot.

She continued her world travel. By 1948 she had seen New Zealand, Hawaii, Australia, and the Fiji Islands—"lured by the warmth of island life." [44]

That same year the State Board of Aeronautics developed a plan to repaint the air markers of small airports. The board appointed Waples as committee chairman; they instructed her to choose co-workers from the Ninety-Nines and organize an immediate campaign. [45]

Congress had appropriated $100,000 in 1947 for states to repaint all the previously painted airmarkers they obliterated during WWII. But the money they gave was inadequate. The government encouraged the Ninety-Nines and other civic groups to paint the markers until they allotted more money. The government never reimbursed them; still, states continued the plan to repaint and install brand-new markers. [46]

Another major event occurred in her packed year of 1948: Waples married Gordon Smith from Corvallis. They moved to the beautiful seaside town of Arch Cape, population 200—even smaller than the farming community in Iowa where she grew up. [47]

Waples obtained a position as Administrator of nearby Seaside Hospital. She remained involved with the Oregon Chapter of the Ninety-Nines—she was vice chairman—and held meetings at her home to discuss preparations for the upcoming "All Girl Air Show." [48]

Next, they moved to the half-square-mile-sized community of Wheeler on the Nahalem River, twelve miles south of Arch Cape. She found a position as Superintendent of the Harvey Reinhart Memorial Hospital. Her husband had a stroke a few years later, and her life changed dramatically.

She needed to care for him at home without assistance. She felt frustrated with the lack of home care for patients in rural areas. While she'd had much hospital nursing experience, she had many questions about stroke care she couldn't answer. In the 1940s, schools had not yet included rehabilitative care of the post-stroke patient to the nursing curriculum; she had to learn by study, observation, and trial and error.

Chapter Six

Because of this experience, she published a book for families and nurses on home care and rehabilitation, *Care of the Patient with a Stroke,* in 1959. [49] She made her opinion clear that "home is the best place for such a patient." Her book contained simple explanations, dozens of drawings of exercises, and physical therapy suggestions to help patients walk and talk again. [50]

The book became a big seller and garnered reprints in 1967 and 1976. In the 1967 revised edition, she included book reviews from the rural hospital staff concerning the care of stroke patients. They said, "There is no longer that completely hopeless feeling when a loved one has a stroke." [51]

Her husband did not fully recover his physical functions: he needed a walker to ambulate, and his speech remained impaired. When she traveled to give author presentations, they often worked as a team to demonstrate to nurse groups the care of a patient with a stroke. Her husband told the patient's point of view. [52] Helping him recover from his illness must have curtailed her flying life as no further information exists on her membership in the Ninety-Nines, or her flying, after 1957.

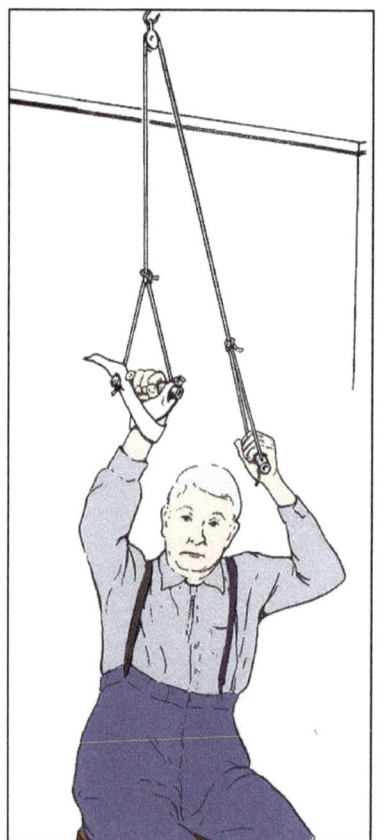

Figure 06.34. A re-created sketch of the Waples Smith pulley system she self-designed to rehabilitate stroke patients in the home in 1959.

Commanders
Cadet Captain Florence Frances Fintak, RN

Commander of Co. B-4, Milwaukee, WI
Licensed Pilot; Flight Nurse

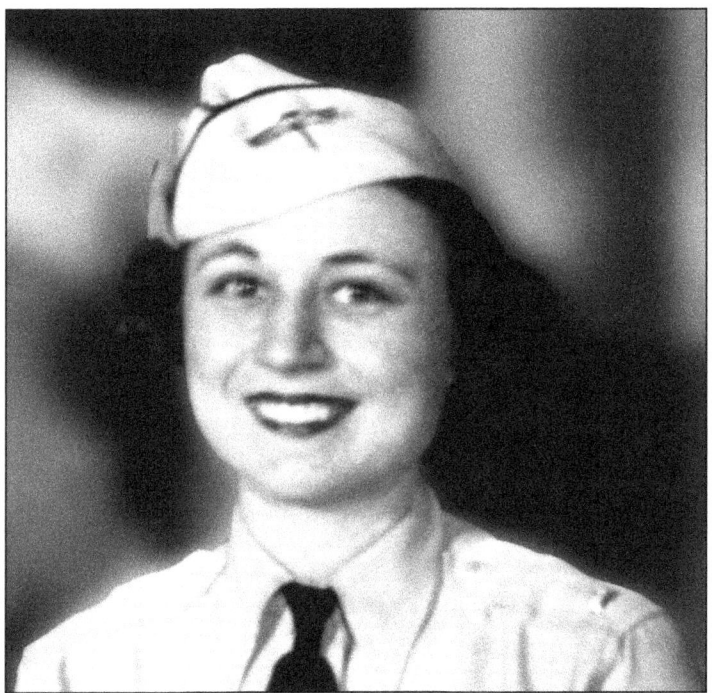

Figure 06. 35. Florence Fintak wearing the ANCOA summer uniform, before she became a Commander, 1939. MMM Collection.

Born in 1914 in Milwaukee, Wisconsin, Florence Frances Fintak graduated from New York's Misericordia Hospital School of Nursing in August 1936, then relocated to Chicago, where she worked for several years in Chicago's infamous Cook County Hospital.[53-54] She joined Chicago's ANCOA A-4, on 18 October 1938, as recruit #152. The details of when and where she learned to fly are unknown, but fly she did.

Moving back to Milwaukee in 1940, she started Company B-4, recruited the first ten nurses, and trained them in their new headquarters at 1410 N. Prospect Ave.[55] Schimmoler promoted her to Captain and Company Commander. Fintak organized twelve lectures on chemical irritants at Milwaukee Children's Hospital in April 1941.[56] Unbeknownst to them, she and other ANCOA nurses would use the knowledge they learned about chemical irritants when the U.S. entered WWII later that year.

Chapter Six

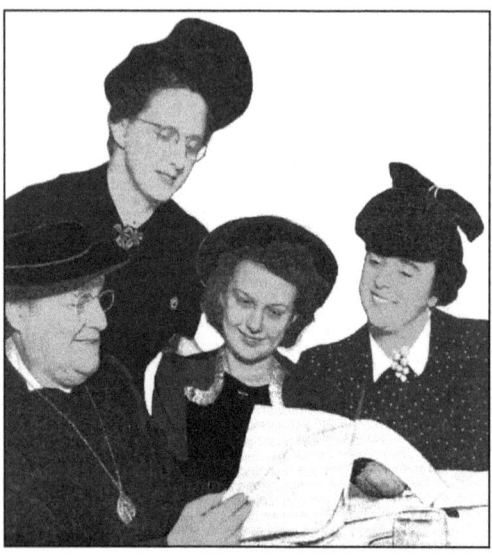

Harriet Fleming from the American Nurses Association paused in Los Angeles en route from the annual ANA Meeting in New York. 57

Later she would attend the theatre benefit the ANCOA conducted with an opening from the famed actor and singer Robert Taylor, titled "The Flight Command." Florence Fintak and Leora Stroup piloted-in to attend the big event.

Figure 06.36. Florence Fintak, center, Leora Stroup, right, and Mildred Mullikin, standing, met Harriet Fleming to discuss the ANCOA, 1941.

The war began; Fintak enlisted in the Army Nurse Corps, on 6 January 1942, with the rank of second lieutenant. She became a flight nurse in the Army Air Force, 814th Medical Air Evacuation Transport Squa`dron (MAETS). 58 Next, she transitioned to a Flight Nurse Instructor, where she taught courses in air evacuation, sea rescue, survival, and ditching classes.

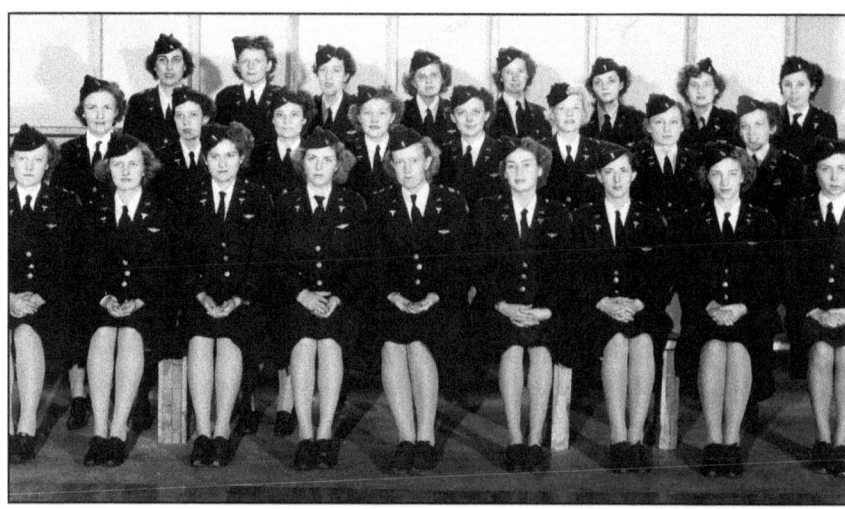

Figure 06.37. Fintak, second row, second from right, after graduation from Army Air Force Flight Nurse training, 1943. Leora Stroup Papers, AMEDD.

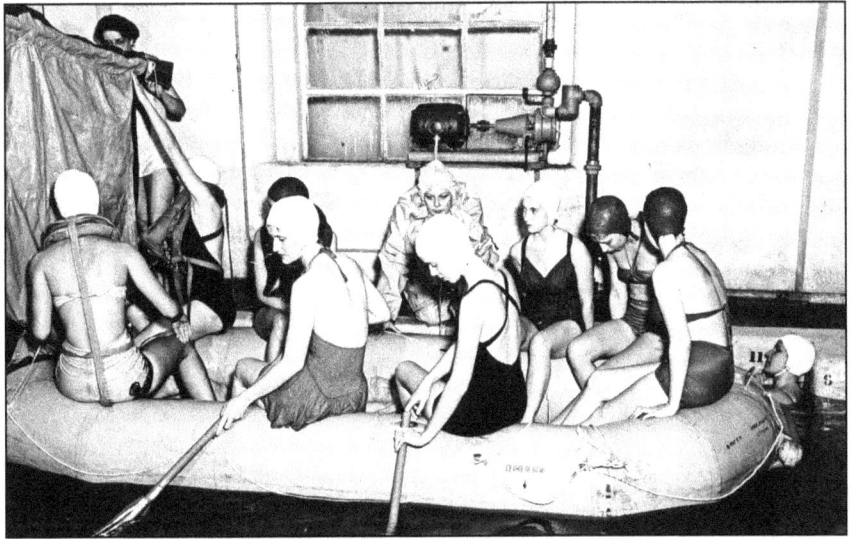

Figure 06.38. Fintak, center, dressed in a quick-donning, anti-exposure suit. She used the suit to demonstrate watermanship and ditching to the flight nursing students at Huntingdon College pool. U.S. Navy BUMED.

Fintak joined Jane Delano American Legion Post 408. The all-military nurse post in Milwaukee began in 1937 as the first post in the nation for women-only veterans. She held the Adjutant office in 1944. [59-60]

The military released her on 5 May 1946, but she continued her association with Post 408. She flew her plane from Racine to Billy Mitchell Field in Milwaukee to represent them in the 1947 American Legion Roundup. [61]

She helped form the Billy Mitchell Squadron (a Wisconsin CAP Wing) in 1948 and served as its first Treasurer and Secretary. But Fintak must have missed the military; she didn't remain a civilian for long.

She re-enlisted on 14 August 1948. By now, the Air Force had split off from the Army and was a separate branch; naturally, she joined the Air Force. She participated in the Korean Conflict and continued to use her flight nurse skills as a Military Air Transport Service (MATS) detachment member. The air evacuation group she served in also transported "mercy flights" for military families in emergencies. [62]

During her assignment in Alaska in 1954, she helped start the first chapter of the Ninety-Nines and became one of its eight charter members. She said the military hadn't stopped her flying; she could fly her plane after working hours "thanks to the midnight sun."

Chapter Six

After the Korean Conflict, one assignment included the flight evacuation demonstrations at General Mitchell Field in Milwaukee. During the open house events, she demonstrated some of the methods flight nurses used to arrange wounded soldiers and to care for them in the litters of the C-47 airplane. She said, "Participants enjoyed climbing inside transport planes to imagine the situation during the war." [63] Her assignments included:

- 1956, Flight Nurse Section, Gunter Air Force Base Hospital, AL
- 1959, Chief Nurse, Gunter Air Force Base Hospital, AL
- 1959, Chief Nurse, Eglin Air Force Base Hospital, FL
- 1962, Chief Nurse, 7272 Air Force Hospital, Libya
- 1964, Command Nurse, Langley Air Force Base, VA [64-66]

She remained in the military for twenty-five years; she retired as a Lieutenant Colonel—the highest rank for women then. They released her from duty on 30 September 1967. According to her separation record, she served in battle campaigns in Normandy, Northern France, Ardennes, and Rhineland.

She received many medals and awards: Air Medal, Meritorious Unit Badge, Air Transport Command, American Theatre Ribbon, European–African–Middle Eastern Theatre Ribbon, Four Bronze Battle Stars, Three Overseas Service Bars, and the Victory Medal.

After completing her Master's Degree in Nursing in 1968 from Marquette University, she became Director of Nursing Service at Trinity Memorial Hospital, Cudahy, Wisconsin. Fintak was President of the La Cross Flyers club in Wisconsin and still active in the Ninety-Nines in 1970. [67-69]

Fintak was the person who received Amelia Earhart's flight suit "from a friend" (most likely Schimmoler) when Post 678 disbanded. That's the infamous flight suit the Smithsonian now owns. [70]

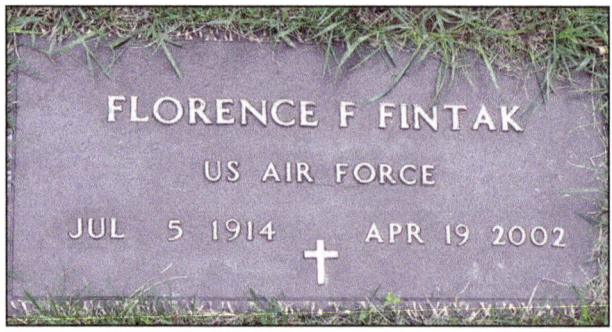

Figure 06.39. Florence Fintak's headstone in the Saint Adalbert Cemetery, Milwaukee, Wisconsin. She lived to 87.

Commanders

Captain Florence Haering Boswell, RN

Commander of Co. B-5, Cleveland, OH; Licensed Pilot

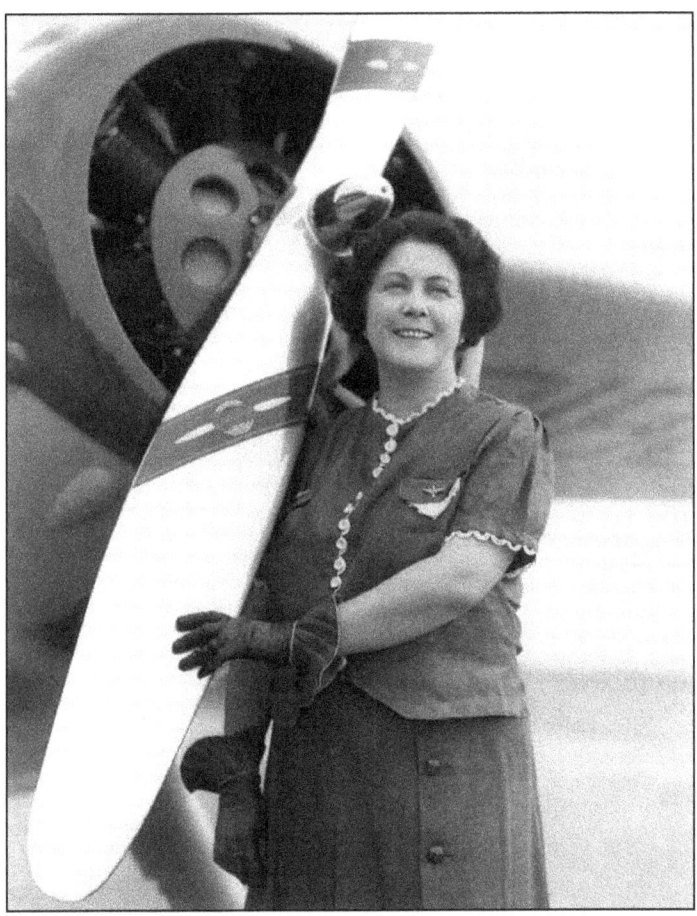

Figure 06.40. Florence Boswell with her Cessna C-37, 1937, a high-winged monoplane she named "Lady B." Courtesy of IWASM, Cleveland, Ohio.

> A matron steps out, stows away a pair of low-heeled flying pumps and radio earphones into her baggage compartment, shifts to high-heels, and arranges the purple plumes on her velvet hat. She immediately transforms into a pleasant-appearing housewife. [71]

Florence Boswell might have appeared a mere housewife on the surface, but that would be low on the list of her accomplishments.

Chapter Six

Florence Marguerite Haering was born in 1894, to 37-year-old Alfred Haering and 18-year-old Elizabeth DeLisle, in the Village of Bratenahl, Ohio, Cleveland's oldest suburb. Her father owned a professional wallpaper shop.[72] She finished eighth grade in 1909 at Bratenahl School—one of the first five students to graduate.[73] Later, she earned a teacher's degree in piano from Wolfram School of Music and professed a great love of music.[74]

Boswell graduated from St. Luke's Hospital School of Nursing in Cleveland and served as Alumnae Association President for three years. Next, she earned a degree from Colombia University with postgraduate work in six subjects.

She furthered her studies as a nurse anesthetist at University Hospital in Cleveland, and then married the well-known Cleveland surgeon, Louis Keith Boswell, on 25 June 1921. She lectured on child psychology, the nurse anesthetist profession, and the joys of flying.[75-77]

Boswell worked as an anesthetist, but the particulars of her anesthetist career aren't known. Since her husband was a surgeon, she might have assisted him. The National Association of Nurse Anesthetists began in 1931; Boswell became its first Executive Secretary (1933-1935) and President of the Nominating Committee.[78] She somehow had the time to lecture as a Professor of Speech. The student body of Purdue University said her talks were "invigorating and inspiring."[79]

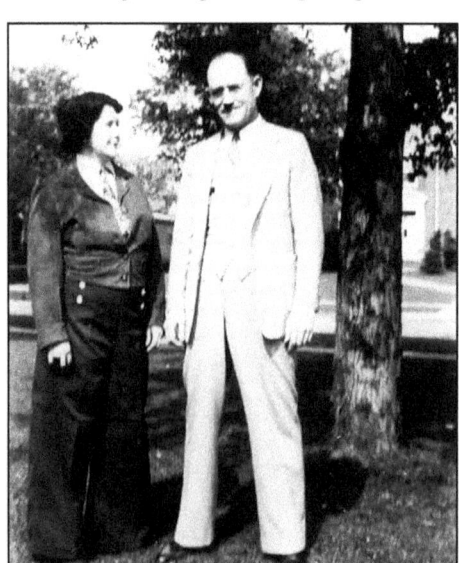

Figure 06.41. Florence Boswell with her husband, Louis Boswell.

Boswell joined the ANCOA on 20 May 1938 as the 95th member.[80-81] Schimmoler promoted her to Captain, then quickly to Commander when Boswell started Company B in Cleveland. She was friends with Schimmoler and Stroup and a respected pilot when she joined the ANCOA. Married women were prohibited from working as aerial nurses, but the ANCOA's enlistment board granted her a special waiver—she was too famous a pilot for them to reject her for most any cause.

Flashes news in August 1938 reported she formally presented the members of Company B to Mayor Burton; to the manager of the Cleveland Airport; to Dr. H. Wright, National Air Races Medical Director; and Clifford Henderson, the Director of the National Air Races. Four ANCOA nurses represented Company B at the August 25th presentation, although the member compliment was twelve. [82] Boswell resigned from the ANCOA on 20 October 1938—she only stayed active for five months.

She began her flying lessons at the non-tender age of 41, in a Stinson SM8A, NC220W, at Chagrin Harbor Airport Ground School. Charles Smith and Dewy Eldred taught her to fly. She first soloed on 7 December 1935 then tested and obtained her private pilot license on 4 May 1936—her 42nd birthday. She dashed to complete all three of her flying licenses in three months and a radio operator license within the year. At that stage, she became the only woman in Cleveland to hold an instructor rating. Her lists of aeronautical accomplishments were many:

- Limited Commercial License, 1 July 1936, tested by W.M. Robertson at Akron City Airport
- Transport Rating 17 August 1936—the only woman in Cleveland with a Transport Pilot's License
- Radio Operators License issued in Ohio—the third in the state
- The first woman in Ohio to receive an Instructor's Rating
- During the Ohio River Valley Flood in 1937, she flew typhoid serum to Pittsburgh and remained on duty to administer the vaccines

She obtained a Non-Scheduled Instrument Rating on 26 April 1937, the fourth female pilot in the world to earn the distinction. The first three women were already flying legends: [83]

- 1st Amelia Earhart
- 2nd Margaret Kimball
- 3rd Jacqueline Cochran
- 4th Florence Boswell

The Department of Commerce awarded the most coveted Non-Scheduled Instrument Rating (NSIR); it enabled pilots to fly when the weather was so severe it grounded all aviators who didn't hold this rating. To qualify, Boswell took the test in blind flying and radio-beam flying wearing a hood that prevented her from seeing anything but the plane's instruments.

Chapter Six

Male pilots said of Boswell's exceptional abilities, "There is none better. She gets through when others fail." [84]

Boswell first purchased a Cessna C-34, NC16455, and later a Cessna C-37 she called the "Lady B." Whether it's fact or not, she became known as "the first person to be struck by lightning when piloting a ship." Boswell told the story to Memphis friends:

> While flying through showers near Memphis one day, my plane was suddenly sucked into a tunnel cloud—the same type pilots dread. It was like heading into the Holland tunnel. When I saw the streak of lighting heading towards me, I tried to swerve, but the lighting hit directly on the speed ring within a quarter inch of a cylinder.
>
> My plane stalled. I was forced to dive. When I finally got control of the ship, I was obliged to scoot over to Kentucky to make a landing as the ceiling on the nearest emergency field was zero. The plane's spark plugs were charred and were unusable. My radio and most of my instruments were destroyed. My wristwatch was very damaged. It looked like a sheet of flame spreading over the wings. [85-86]

Being a pilot might sound unlikely for the wife of a prominent surgeon, particularly since she was raising three young children, but it worked for Boswell. Louise was born in 1923, then her sons Louis Jr. in 1924, and John Robert in 1925. She wasn't the type to stay at home, yet her practical mother-duties were initially responsible for her decision to fly.

Her two sons were in summer camp at Put-in-Bay on South Bass Island in Lake Erie. She needed to return them home to Cleveland for dinner on Sundays. A car ride, plus a boat trip, would be arduous to manage quickly. She decided to learn to fly and bought a Cessna.

Her instructor thought she'd be the last person who would want to fly. She didn't understand the reason he felt that way. She said:

> If a woman has use for a car, she buys one and learns to drive it. I bought an airplane and learned to fly it because I had a use for it. [87]

Eventually, she flew the camp counselors and other young boys to and from Camp Wa-Li-Ro on Put-in-Bay, South Bass Island. [88] She must have enjoyed transporting people in her Cessna because she decided to open an air taxi service, Florence H. Boswell's Flying Service, Inc.

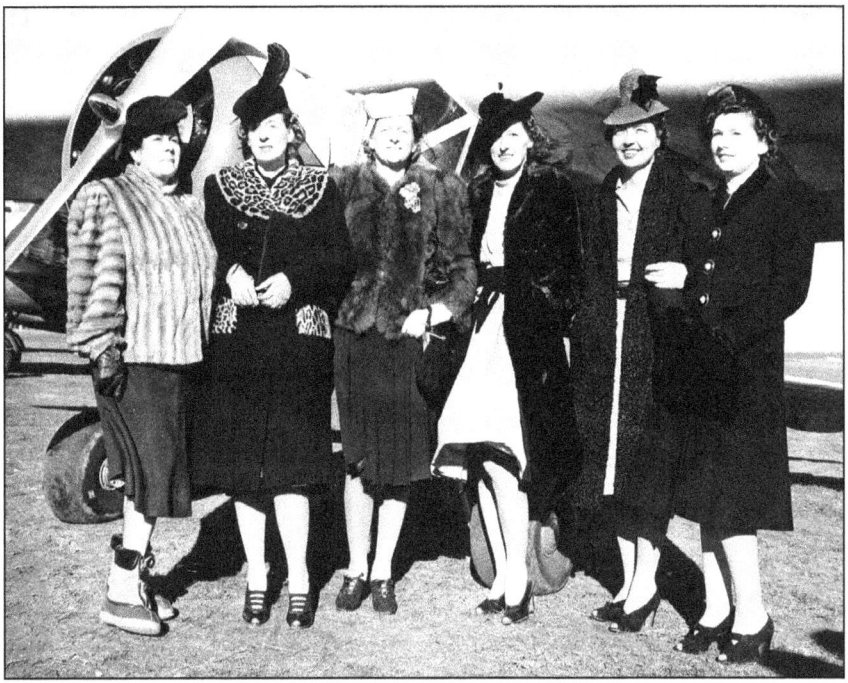

Figure 06.42. Florence Boswell, her Cessna, and fancy-dressed women in Dallas, TX, 2 February 1941. The passengers posing in front of this plane aren't known, but you can easily spot the pilot by her shoes and gloves. Florence Boswell, on the left. Courtesy of IWASM, Cleveland, Ohio.

Boswell knew Schimmoler years before she joined the ANCOA; they were members of the Ohio Ninety-Nines. Stroup and Boswell were also friends who flew around Ohio and Michigan together. It wasn't uncommon for Boswell to gather Ninety-Niner friends, like Schimmoler and Stoup, and fly them in her four-seater Cessna to a meeting of the National Aeronautics Association or a Ninety-Nine's convention. [89-90]

Her leadership and flying reputation garnered progressive club positions: Chairman of the All-Ohio Chapter, Secretary and Treasurer of the North Central Section, and Governor of the North Central Section. While in Texas, she organized the state's first chapter of the Ninety-Nines. [91]

She chaired the Ohio National Air Race Committee for two years, became President of the Cleveland Women's Chapter of the NAA, and served on the Cleveland Junior Chamber of Congress' Advisory and Aeronautical Committee. "I want to do all I can to help underprivileged pilots," she told fellow Ninety-Niner Ann Barille. She also told Barille her three children had become as air conscious as their mother. [92-94]

Chapter Six

Flashes documented only a few Boswell ANCOA activities. The reason she resigned after a mere five months isn't surprising; she involved herself in non-stop flying activities, volunteer groups, and was a wife and mother.

She occasionally held unusual jobs: Official Hostess at the Miami to Havana Air Cruise and as a judge for the radio air quiz *Wings Over Cleveland*. [95] She flew to air races in many states and Monterrey, Mexico, where she garnered her fair share of wins. [96] A few of her race wins:

- 1939, K.K. Culver Trophy, Free-For-All Handicap Race of 50 Miles, Miami, Florida [97]
- 1940, First Place in the National Sportsman's Pilot, Cruise Navigation
- 1940, Second Place, Sportsman Pilot Association Winter Cruise
- 1941, Fourth Place in the Culver trophy in Miami, Florida
- 1941, First Place, Western Wing, SPA, Winter Cruise to Mexico

In June 1941, she organized the Cleveland Unit of the American Women's Voluntary Services and became the State Chairman. The Cleveland Unit provided free preparedness instruction on topics from first aid to mass evacuation and communal feeding. Boswell told a reporter:

> This is an important and crucial moment in the lives of all American women…driving trucks, aeronautics, evacuation, mass feeding, first aid, communication, and agriculture are essential tasks that women can learn to do. [98] Whether a country is preparing for an emergency or digging itself out of a bomb crater, women have shown what they can do. American women now realize they, too, can help fortify democracy's defense by training for service. [99]

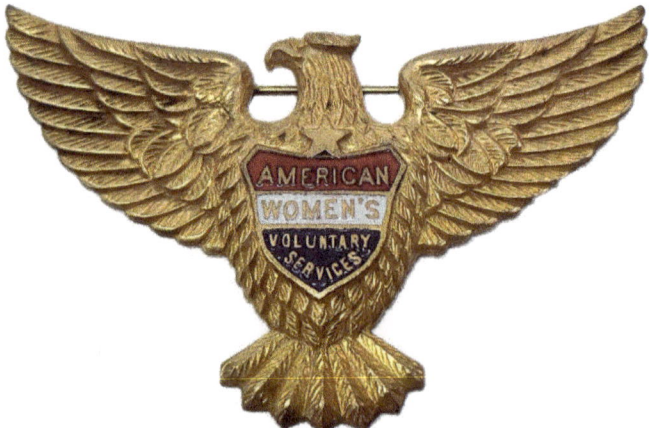

Figure 06.43. American Women's Voluntary Services pin, 1942. Author's photo.

Commanders

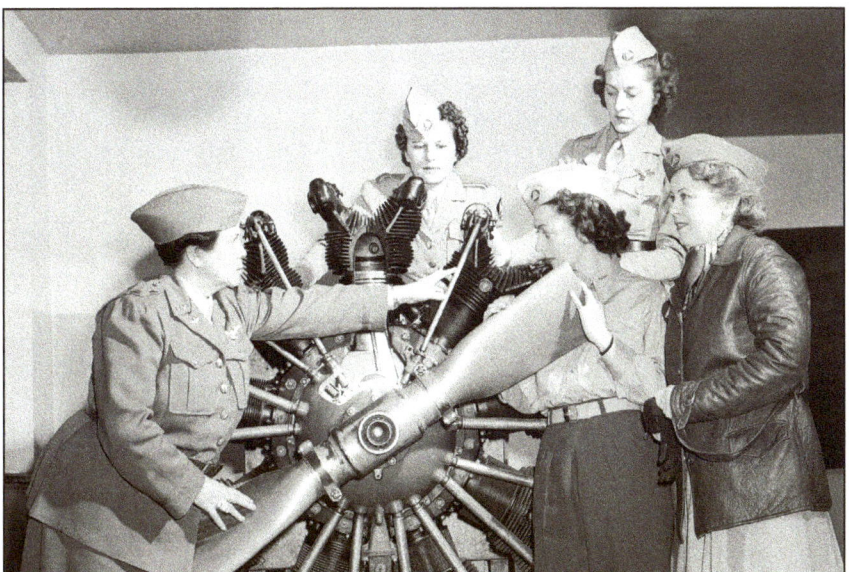

Figure 06.44. Lt. Florence Boswell explains a push-rod function to CAP members, 1942. Boswell, front left, Lt. Ardelle LaBrake, and Lt. Arlene Davis. Private Hazel Gristock and Flight Officer Annabelle Kekic in the back. An expert flyer, Kekic piloted for the historical Women's Air Force Service Pilots (WASP).[100] Photo courtesy of AP.

The women pilots are wearing various CAP uniforms: an indoor style with a skirt and an indoor one with pants. Boswell is wearing a formal uniform with a skirt. Several pins are visible: a Civil Air Patrol Pilot's Pin, the CAP device, the CAP lapel pin, and a U.S. Air Force Pilot's Pin.

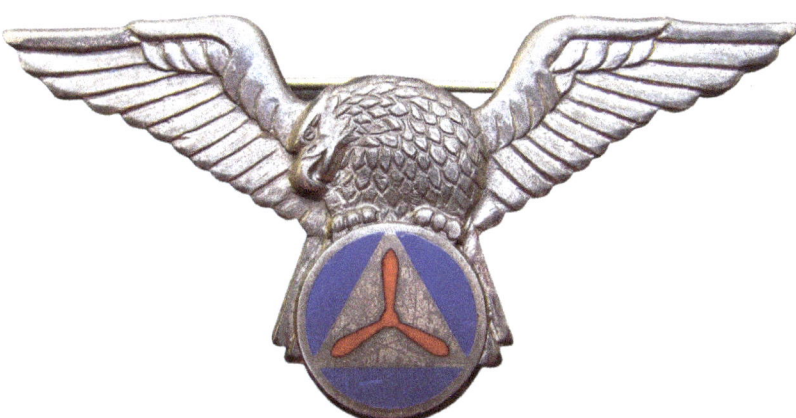

Figure 06.45. Civil Air Patrol Pilot's Pin, 1942. Cliff Presley Collection.

275

Chapter Six

When the Japanese attacked Pearl Harbor, Florence sold her Cessna to the government to aid in the airplane shortage. World War II cut short the adventures of many pilots during those years anyway. While the rules had curtailed her flying activities, she joined the Civil Air Patrol as a pilot and remained committed to various civilian war readiness activities:

- She became a Lieutenant in one of the first all-female squadrons of the Civil Air Patrol, Squadron 1. [101]
- She instructed Civil Air Patrol members in navigation problems and preparatory flight plans for their training missions in Cleveland.
- She served as one of four nurses assigned to the medical unit of CAP.
- She attended the War Department Civilian Protection School in Amherst, Massachusetts; she returned to Ohio to teach Air Raid Protection, as an instructor, in the Office of Civilian Defense and the Chairman of the Women's Defense League.
- Ohio selected her to direct the state's Aeronautics Training Course and courses in auxiliary nursing, first aid, communications, in motor transport, emergency services, photography, and others.
- She formulated plans for volunteers in Omaha, Nebraska, Denver, and Colorado. She taught map reading and motor transport. [102]

Nothing is available about her flying life after WWII. Perhaps she didn't purchase another airplane after the war, like many aging pilots. Indeed, a woman as dynamic as Boswell did not stop her activities, but when the war was over, many stories ceased to be printed.

Boswell held multiple leadership appointments and memberships throughout her life:

- First Executive Secretary, National Association of Nurse Anesthetists (NANA) 1933-1935
- President, St Luke's Hospital Nursing School Alumnae Association, for three years
- President of the Nominating Committee, NANA, 1933-1935
- Governor, North Central Section of the Ninety-Nines, 1938-1939
- National Membership Chairman of the Ninety-Nines, 1940-1941
- President, Cleveland Women's Chapter of the NAA, 1940-1941
- Chairman, Vitamin Committee for Allied Children
- State Chairman, American Women's Voluntary Services, 1941-1942
- Civil Air Patrol, 2nd Lieutenant, 24 August 1942
- Member, Cleveland Shaker University Heights Women's Club
- Captain, ANCOA, 5th Division, Company B, 1938
- Member, Florida Alligator Club
- Sportsman Pilots Association—First Woman Awarded Membership
- Secretary/Treasurer, N. Central Section, Ninety-Nines, 1938-1939

- Chairman, All-Ohio Chapter, Ninety-Nines, 1942
- Member, National League of American Pen Women
- Member, American Nurses Association

In 1947 the National Board of Directors of the National Aeronautics Association elected her for membership—the first woman elected. She served on the Board of NAA for several years and attended the National NAA conventions as a delegate. [103]

Boswell's grave is near where she was born, raised, and died, in the famous Lake View Cemetery, in Cleveland, Ohio. [104] Her accomplishments were too many to adorn a single headstone. Hers is simply marked, Mother.

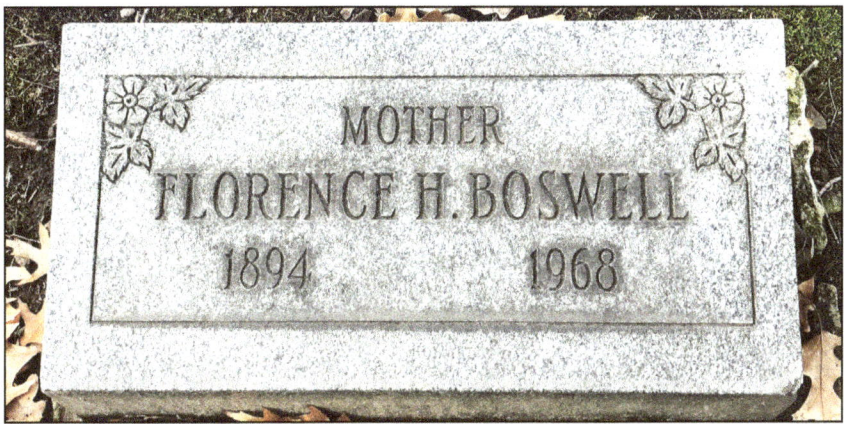

Figure 06.46. Florence Boswell's headstone. Photo by Robin Slater Boyd.

Chapter Six
Cadet Captain Fay M. McWhorter Mayes, RN

Commander of Co. B-6, Fort Lauderdale, FL; Licensed Pilot

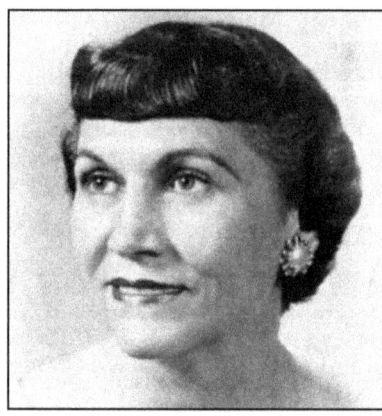

Figure 06.47. Fay McWhorter during her flower years, 1976. *Florida Gardener.*

Fay McWhorter joined the ANCOA on 10 October 1940 as recruit #319 in Fort Lauderdale, Florida. By January 1941, she was listed as Commander of Company B-6. Like many other commanders, she became a pilot.

McWhorter received her pilot's license in August 1941, ten months after she joined the ANCOA. [105] She was a charter member of the Fort Lauderdale Cloud Chasers and held several leadership positions within the Ninety-Nines, including Chairman. In 1942, she married Army Major Robert Mayes. After the war, they started Mayes Chevrolet—one of the first car sales agencies in Pompano Beach. [106-108]

She taught parliamentary law and was the President of Florida's Association of Parliamentarians. She was active in the popular post-WWII Blue Star Memorial, a project named for the blue star that homes and businesses hung in their windows to honor service men and women. [109-110]

McWhorter Mayes affiliated with multiple garden clubs: she edited *The Florida Gardener* magazine and was a Master Flower Show Judge. In 1958 she wrote *Program Patterns for Gardeners*; in 1963, she authored the book *Public Relations and Publicity Pointers*. [111]

She established the Weskiva Youth Camp Fund, a camp whose purpose was to instill love and respect through nature study, conservation, and protection of the environment. Friends said she was "Blessed with joy in her heart and a dynamic, sparkling personality. She lived a rich, full life."

Commanders
Captain Wanda Irene Fill, RN

Commander of Co. D-1, San Diego, CA; Flight Nurse

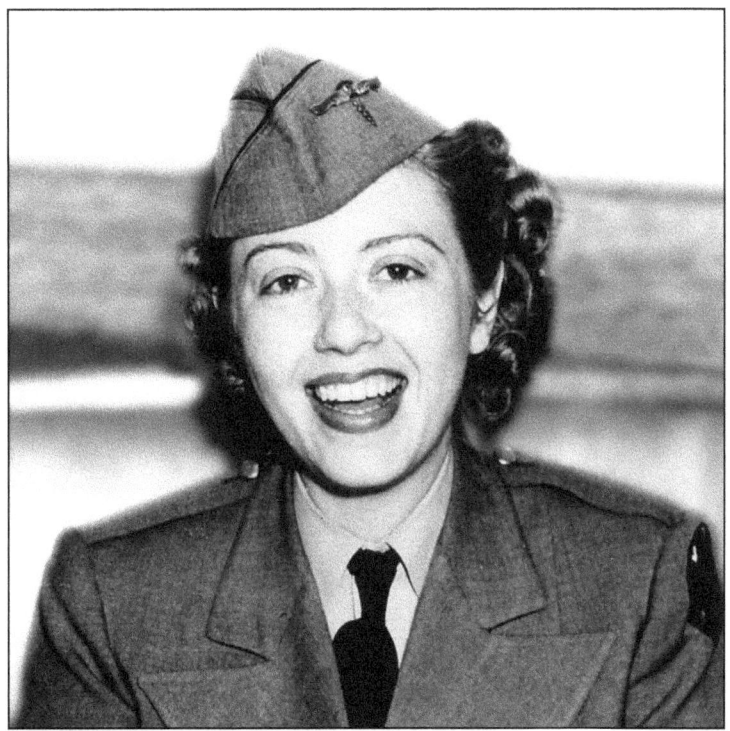

Figure 06.48. Wanda I. Fill in her ANCOA uniform, 1941.

Wanda Fill started life in 1914 in the often-chilly city of Greenville, Michigan. After graduating from the Harper Hospital School of Nursing, she stayed in Detroit and joined Stroup's Company A-5, on 3 May 1939, as recruit #215. [112] *Flashes* reported she visited San Diego Company D-1, in June, during a month-long vacation traveling in the western states. [113]

Perhaps the California portion of her vacation had an ulterior motive: four months later, she left her visiting nurse position and moved to San Diego to become a school nurse at the Memorial Junior High School. [114] Margaret Gudobba, Editor of *Flashes Great Lakes Breeze's* page wrote, "Our loss is San Diego's gain," and they threw a going away party for her. Significant changes awaited Fill in 1939.

After her move, she became the commander of Company D-1. She spent the next two years at the beach in San Diego on the picturesque Strand Way.

Then, like many ANCOA nurses, she answered the "call to the colors." She entered the Army Nurse Corps in September 1941, shortly before Pearl Harbor happened, and a few months too early to train as a flight nurse for WWII. The details of her Army Nurse Corps service are yet to be known.

She joined the Air Force in 1947 and served as a Flight Nurse in Korea. Next, the military assigned her the role of Chief Nurse at the brand-new Air Force Hospital in Colorado in 1959. Her service date ended on 30 September 1967. By then, she had achieved the rank of Lieutenant Colonel and had participated in three wars: WWII, Korea, and Vietnam.

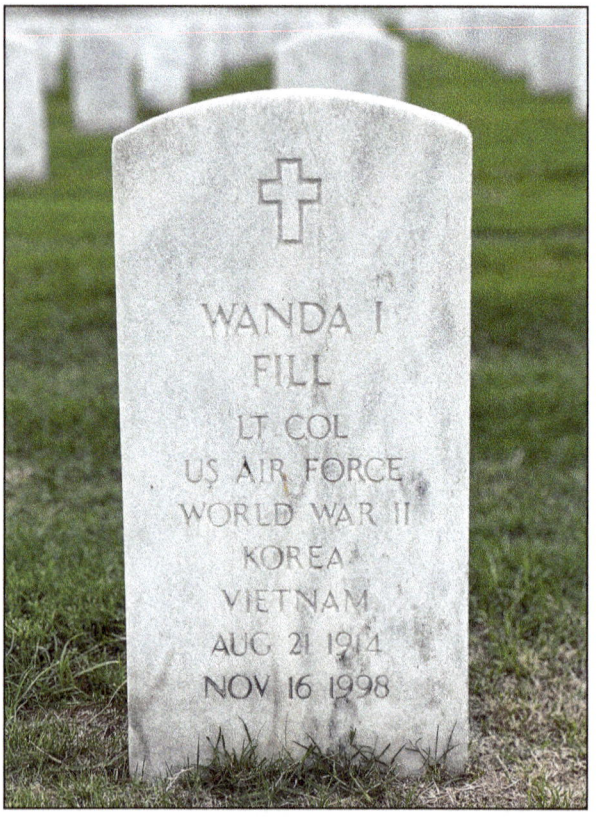

Figure 06.49. Wanda Fill's beautiful headstone, Fort Sam Houston National Cemetery in San Antonio, Texas. She lived to age 84. Author photographed.

Captain Carol Landis

Commander, Aviation Emergency Corps

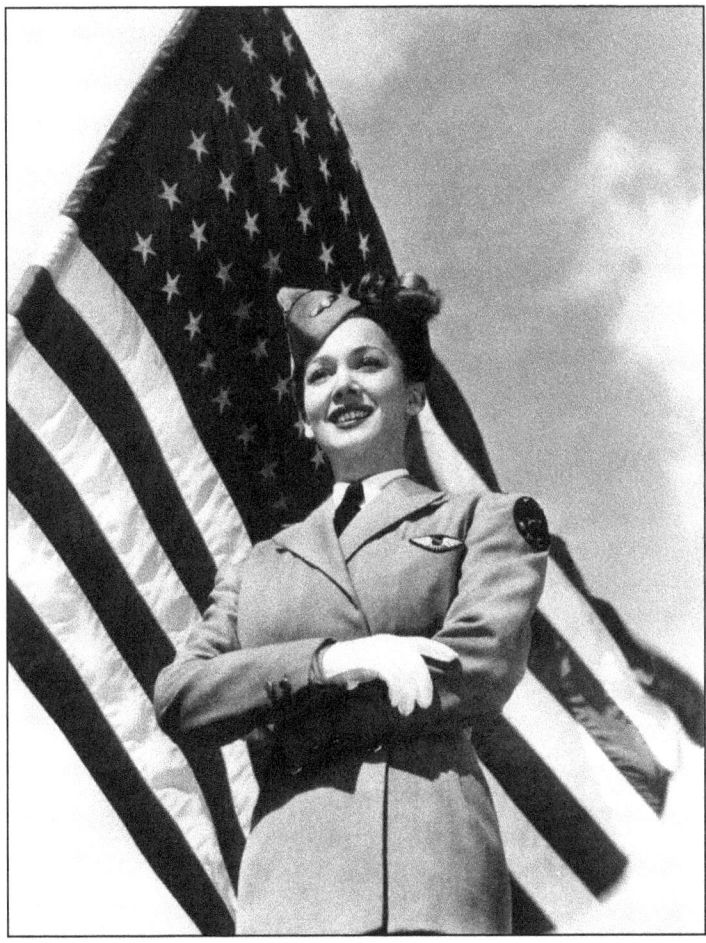

Figure 06.50. Carol Landis wearing her Aviation Emergency Corps uniform with the commander pocket patch, 1942. BHS Collection.

Frances Lillian Mary Ridste was born in Fairchild, Wisconsin, on 2 January 1919, to Clara Agnes Bernice and Alfred Leonard Ridste.[115] In 1922, her family moved to San Bernardino, California.[116] She changed her name to Carol Landis in 1942—a better stage name. She debuted as a film star in 1937 and posed as a pin-up model. Landis sang and acted: the studio didn't need to dub her singing voice, as they did for other stars, because she knew how to sing.

Chapter Six

Like many celebrities, when WWII began she joined volunteer para-military organizations. Although the ANCOA roster doesn't list her name or a date, the 1942 *Tampa Bay Times* article stated she joined on 12 December 1941—just five days after the Pearl Harbor attack. [117]

The article stated she was a commander in the Aerial Nurse Corps of America, First Division. [118] They should have said the Aviation Emergency Corps because only RNs were commanders in the ANCOA. The newly formed AEC auxiliary, however, wasn't a familiar name like the ANCOA, so they probably used it for easy recognition. Only four months for the extremely busy celebrity volunteer to become a commander? Schimmoler might have quickly promoted her for publicity.

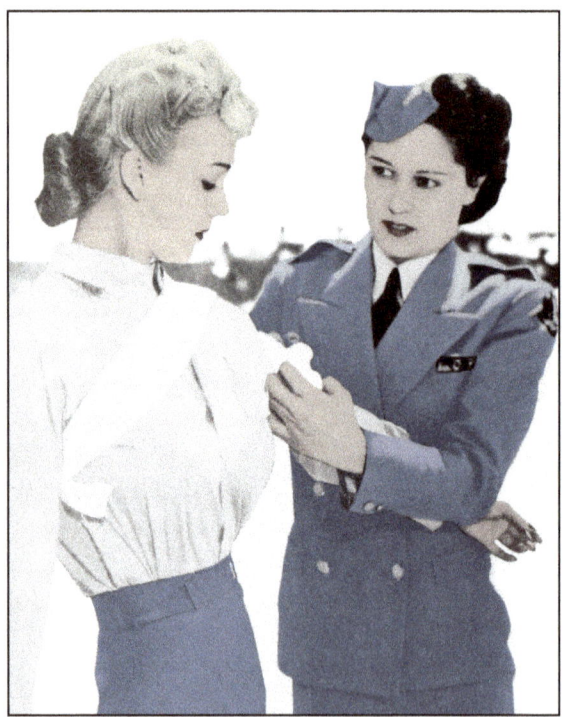

Figure 06.51. Sergeant Genevieve Dow of the AEC, demonstrates bandaging on Carole Landis, 1942. Colorized clipping, BHS Collection.

Pages in Schimmoler's archive, dated May 1942, report Landis spent her Sundays training for first-aid work, clerical duties, and communications. [119] A Missouri newspaper photo shows her teaching a class in first aid and says she helped fingerprint the workers in airplane factories. [120] Fingerprinting was the first job the Los Angeles Sheriff's Civil Division assigned to the ANCOA/AEC.

Commanders

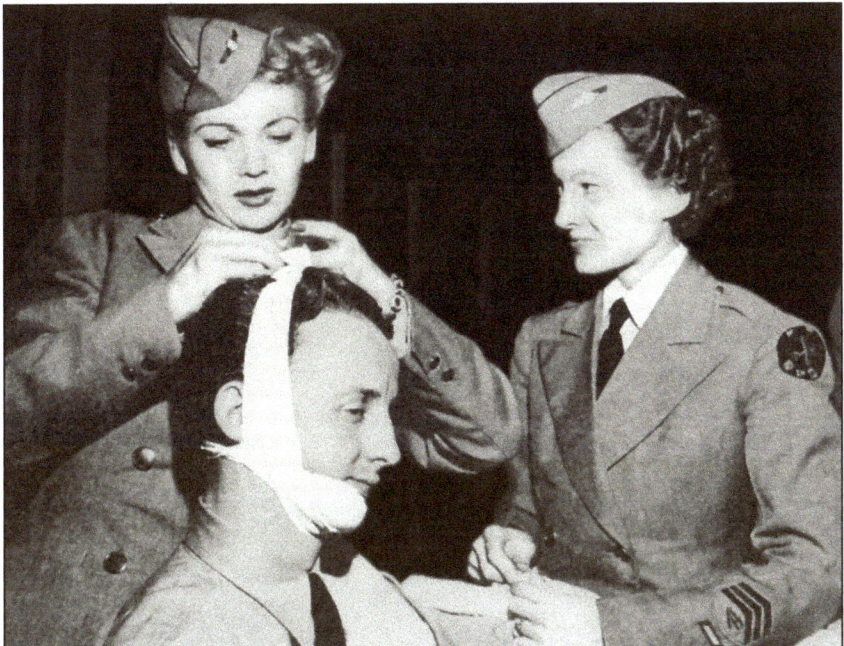

Figure 06.52. Carole Landis practices bandaging as an AEC member assists, 1942. BHS Collection.

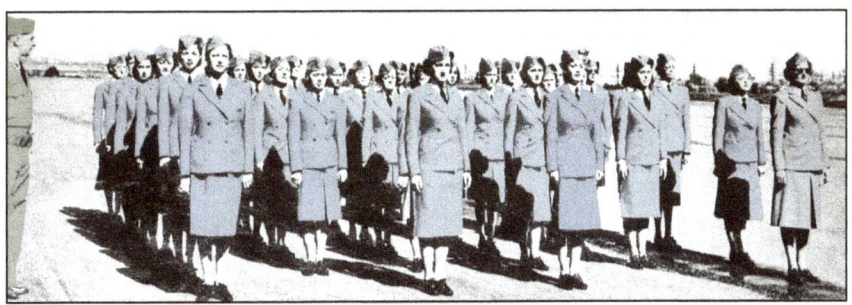

Figure 06.53. The AEC practice drills, 1942. Landis stands in the front row, third from the left. Colorized clipping. BHS.

The AEC wasn't the only wartime group Landis joined. She also volunteered as a Storekeeper, 3rd Class, with Bundles for Bluejackets, a charity collecting personal items and knitting clothing for service members. [121-122]

Figure 06.54. A Bundle for Blue Jackets pin used for fundraising. Author photographed.

Chapter Six

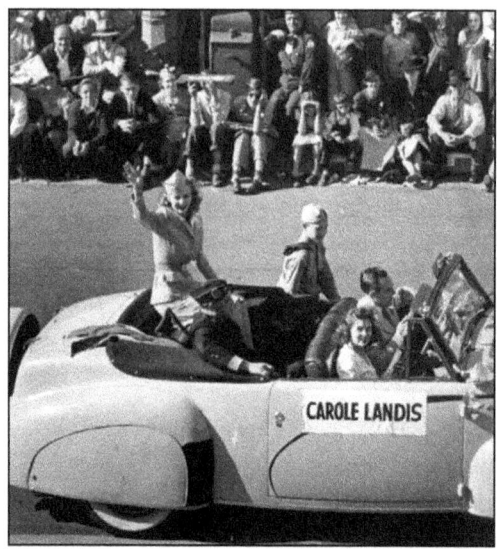

Figure 06.55. Carole Landis waving in American Legion's National Convention Parade, in October 1941. Milwaukee Public Library.

The Hollywood Post 43 of the American Legion, commissioned her as an honorary colonel in March 1942. She had ridden in the American Legion Parade the prior year at their National Convention in Milwaukee. [123-24]

Still, not enough for Landis, she volunteered as a Santa Monica Air Raid Warden. When air raids siren sounded, Air Raid Wardens walked the neighborhood to ensure people turned off their house lights. At night, she patrolled Santa Monica Beach with her Great Dane named Donner. [125]

In September 1942, she began a five-month tour for the USO (United Service Organization) with fellow actors Kay Francis, Martha Raye, and Mitzi Mayfair. The women traveled to England, Bermuda, Africa, and Ireland—more than 50,000 miles by plane, truck, and Army Jeep, giving 150 personal appearances and 125 shows.

Landis published several magazine articles about her experiences during wartime. She wrote a foreword for Victor Herman's popular cartoon book, *Winnie the WAC*. Random House contracted her to write a book about traveling and performing for the soldiers: she wrote *Four Jills in a Jeep*. In the book, she said of her experience:

> We had a wonderful time overseas, but it was hard. For five months, we never gave less than five shows a day. It was too cold to sleep and there wasn't enough water to take a bath. We bathed and shampooed in cold water—there was no hot. I had to do my own washing. And I ate more sand and fog than food. [126]

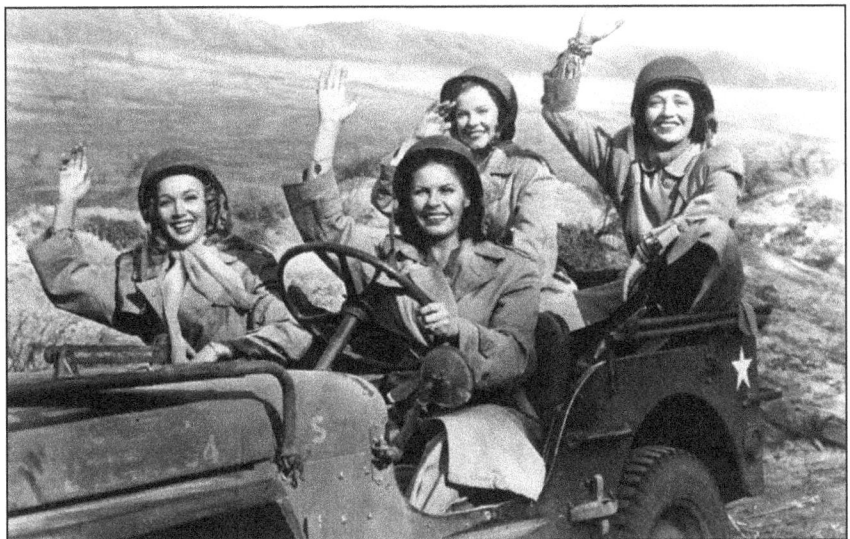

Figure 05.56. A lobby Card from *Four Jills in a Jeep*. Carole Landis, Kay Francis, Martha Raye, and Mitzi Mayfair, 1944. Author's collection.

Twentieth Century Fox Studio turned her book into a movie, *Four Jills in a Jeep*—the (mostly) true story of the four-girl USO team, entertaining American troops overseas. Francis, Raye, Landis, and Mayfair played themselves while re-creating their tour of Europe and North Africa. [127]

Landis met U.S. Air Force Captain Thomas Wallace while traveling with the show. On 5 January 1943, they married in London, England—her third of four husbands. Wallace was a twenty-five-year-old pilot in the Royal Air Force's American Eagle Squadron. They divorced two years later. [128]

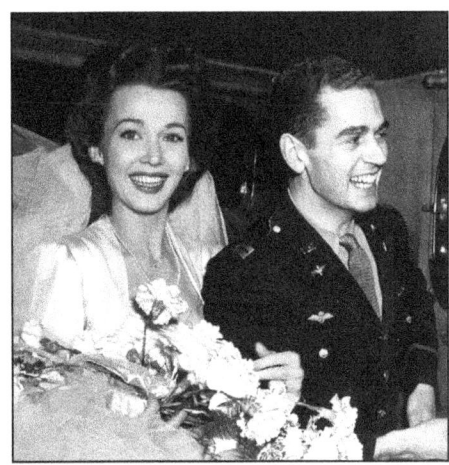

Figure 05.57. The beautiful couple Carol Landis and Thomas Wallace on their wedding day in 1943.

She had a relationship with a studio executive during her contract days with Twentieth Century Fox Studio. She'd acted in more than fifty-three movies between 1937 and 1948, but her film career declined to B movie status when she ended their relationship. [129]

After her fourth divorce, she began an affair with a famous married actor Rex Harrison. She became despondent when he refused to leave his wife for her. Landis died at home in Pacific Palisades at 29 from an overdose of Seconal. A note to her mother said: "I'm really, really, sorry to put you through this but there is no way to avoid it." [130-131]

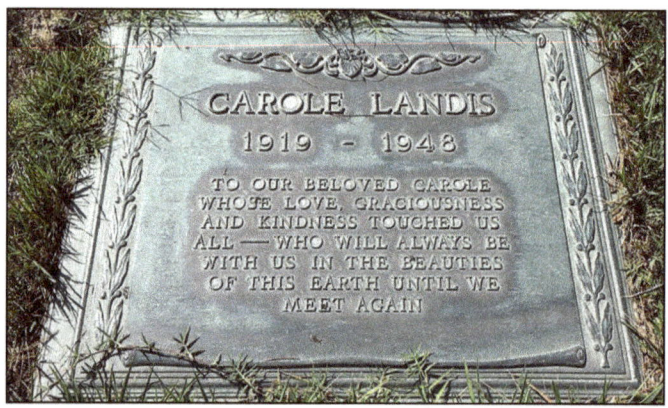

Figure 06.58. Headstone of Carole Landis, Forest Lawn Memorial Park, in plot 814, of the "Everlasting Love" section. Arthur Dark, Wikimedia.

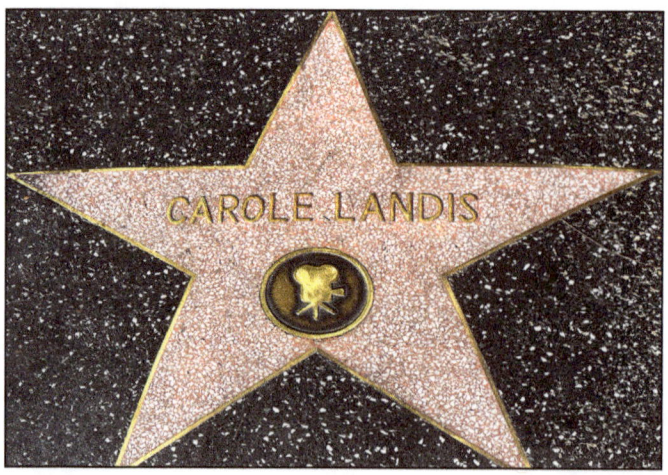

Figure 06.59. Carol Landis' movie category star on the Hollywood Walk of Fame, 1765 Vine Street, Hollywood. Her fans dedicated the star on 8 February 1960, twelve years after she died. [132] Author photographed.

Commanders
Ellen Church Marshall, RN

Adjutant of Co. B-4, Milwaukee, WI; Pilot; Flight Nurse

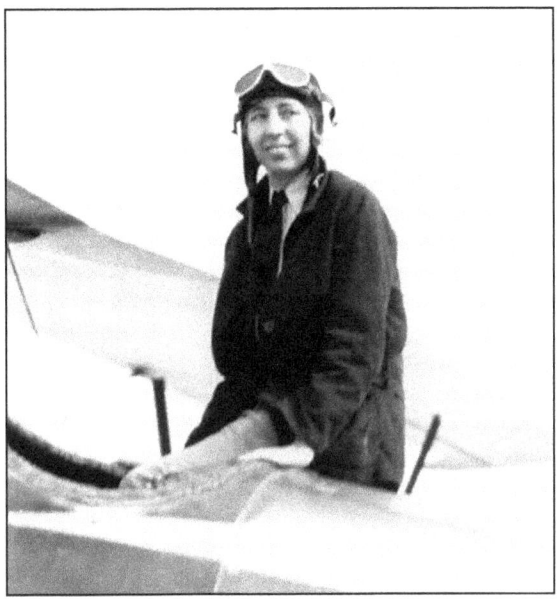

Figure 06.60. Ellen Church in the pilot's seat ready to fly, c. 1930. UAHF.

Ellen Church might be the most written-about ANCOA nurse. Although she accomplished much in her life, the one fact most people remember about her is her novel idea to hire nurses as the first airline stewardesses.

Her interest in airplanes began as a young girl when she watched Ruth Law perform stunts in a pusher plane at the Decorah County Fair—the first time she saw anyone fly. Then the neighborhood boys took lessons to prepare for WWI; they flew over and landed near her family's farm in Cresco, Iowa. She took her first flight in 1924 at the county fair: $7.50 for five minutes. Her subsequent flight happened during nursing school when the pilot-husband of an appreciative patient took her up in an Army plane in St. Paul, Minnesota. He performed stunts: barrels, falling leaves, dives, and the loop-the-loop. "Very exciting," Church said. [133]

After graduating from the University of Minnesota School of Nursing in 1926, Church started her first job at Munsing Hospital in Michigan; she soon moved to the University of Chicago for her Master's Degree in Nursing Administration. The French Hospital, in San Francisco, offered her the Director of Nurses position in 1929 and her life veered toward a change.

Chapter Six

She began flying lessons in a field in San Francisco and completed 13 hours of solo flights. She said, "One time, I forgot to fasten my seat belt and almost fell out of the plane. It scared me to death." But she never obtained her pilot's license because she started working with Boeing and moved to Wyoming.[134]

During lunch breaks at the French Hospital, she'd walk by the Boeing Air Transport office. Boeing had begun commercial flights with twelve to eighteen passengers. Once when Church stopped in to ask about airfares, she told the manager, Steve Stimpson, she was learning to fly. She continued to stop and chat with him. She wanted a job combining nursing and aviation. He didn't encourage her—airlines wouldn't hire women.

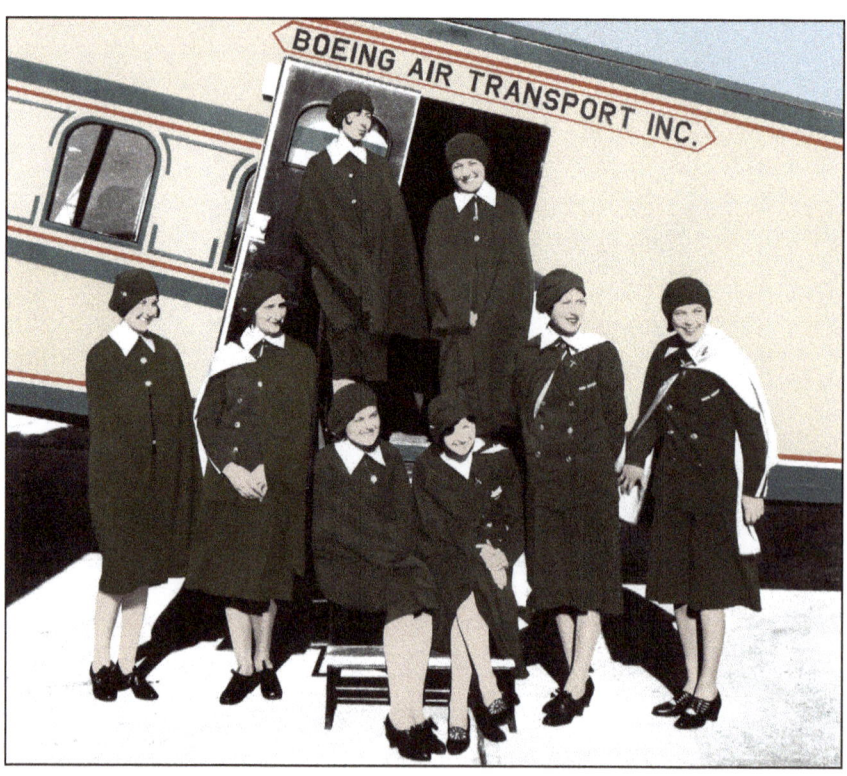

Figure 06.61. The original eight air hostesses, Ellen Church at the top left, on the only day all eight appeared together, 1930. From Ethel Pattison, UAL.

Stimpson said he planned to hire young Filipino men as cabin stewards. She thought nurses could calm passengers better than young men and said, "…what man could say he was afraid to fly if a woman was doing it?" Stimpson agreed. At first, Boeing officials resisted; ultimately, they gave Church a three-month trial. Her parents initially said, "No." Church must have had excellent convincing skills because her parents eventually agreed.[135]

Stimpson charged her to find seven nurses 5'4" and 115 pounds or less (planes were small).[136] Nursing organizations opposed her idea. She couldn't understand that as many nurses were unemployed due to the Depression.

On 15 May 1930, Church rode the first flight from Cheyenne, Wyoming, to Oakland, California: 20 hours, 13 stops, and 14 passengers.[137] The nurses worked hard to prove themselves: they took tickets, served lunch, cleaned the plane, assisted airsick passengers, and even tightened seat bolts. The experiment became a great success—the flying public loved it, so other companies adopted the idea. The airlines used RNs exclusively as their stewardess Sky Girls until WWII began, and the war needed nurses.[138]

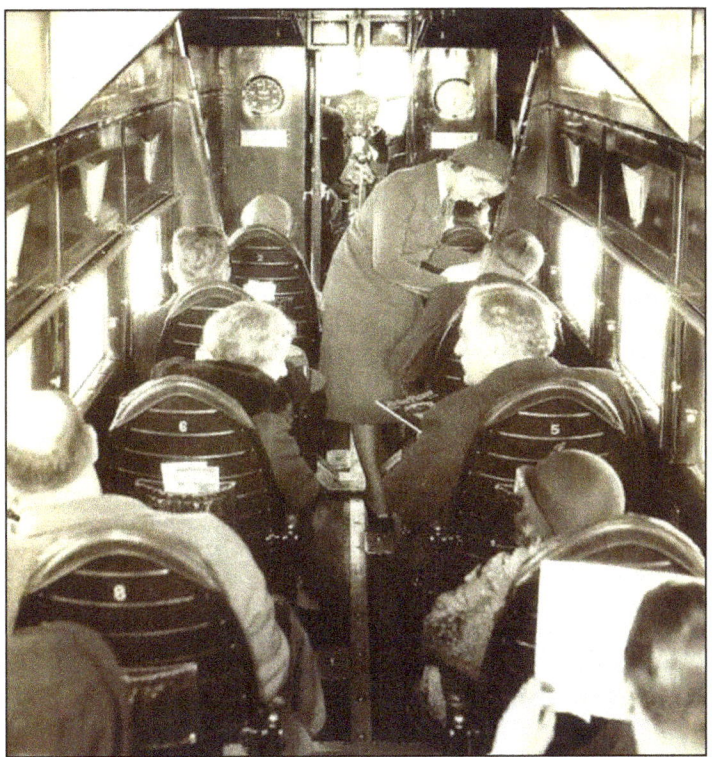

Figure 06.62. Church assisting passengers aboard a Boeing 80A. Courtesy of Vicy Young, UAL.

Unfortunately, Church fractured her ankle in a car accident, forcing her to leave Boeing after 18 months. She accepted a job in Wisconsin as the Superintendent and Faculty of the Milwaukee County Hospital. She joined ANCOA on 9 August 1940, as recruit #293, Company B-4, in Milwaukee. With her experience, National Headquarters quickly promoted her to the Adjutant. They already had a Commander.[139]

Chapter Six

Always a woman on the move, Church soon transferred to Louisville, Kentucky, in 1941, as the Director of Nurses at Children's Free Hospital. There is no record of any ANCOA members in Kentucky in 1941. She must have continued to believe in their mission, however, because that year, she told a Kentucky reporter about the ANCOA:

> It's quite possible the nurses could be of use now with the Air Corps, just as Army and Navy have their nurses. With times as serious as they are, we can't start figuring out all the angles too soon. [140]

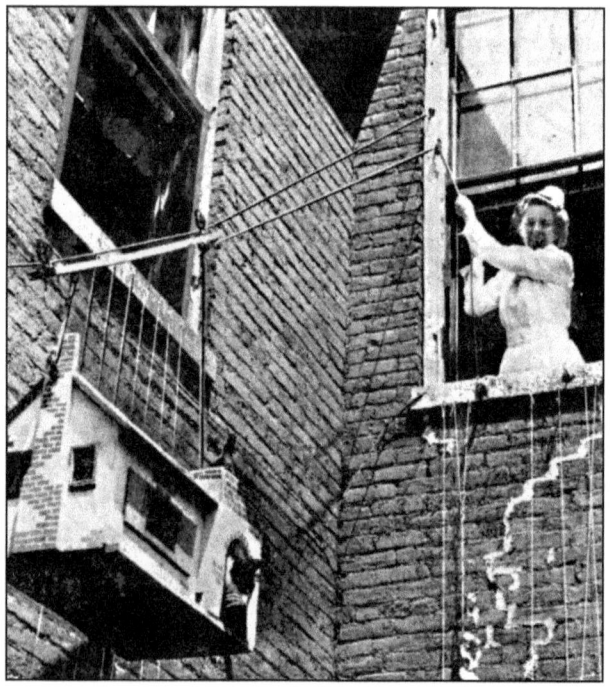

Figure 06.63. Church and her cat elevator. ©Davis–USA Today Network

Another reporter revealed her inventive side. Church lived on the second floor of the nurses' home at Children's Free Hospital—inconvenient for cats.

She owned brother and sister cats, Cap and Mittens, who she said, "would persist in waking me at dawn demanding their release." She devised a cat elevator: she painted a doll house and hung cables and pulleys outside her window. The door swung both directions so her cats could push it open. A button on the bottom automatically opened the door when it touched the ground. The cats didn't initially appreciate the elevator but quickly accepted it when they realized the device would grant them early morning exits. [141]

Kentucky didn't last; WWII beckoned. Since she was a former pilot, air hostess, and ANCOA member, she joined the Evac Nurses. She served in the 802nd MAETS. Church and Josephene Sansone, another ANCOA nurse, deployed with the first group. The Army transferred Church and Sansone to England to coordinate the air evac.[142]

During a rest from duty in 1945, she told an Air Transport Association reporter she was ready to return. "I'm trying to get sent back overseas. When I'm done, no plans to retire again (as a stewardess)...I'd like to fly from one end of the country to the other."[143]

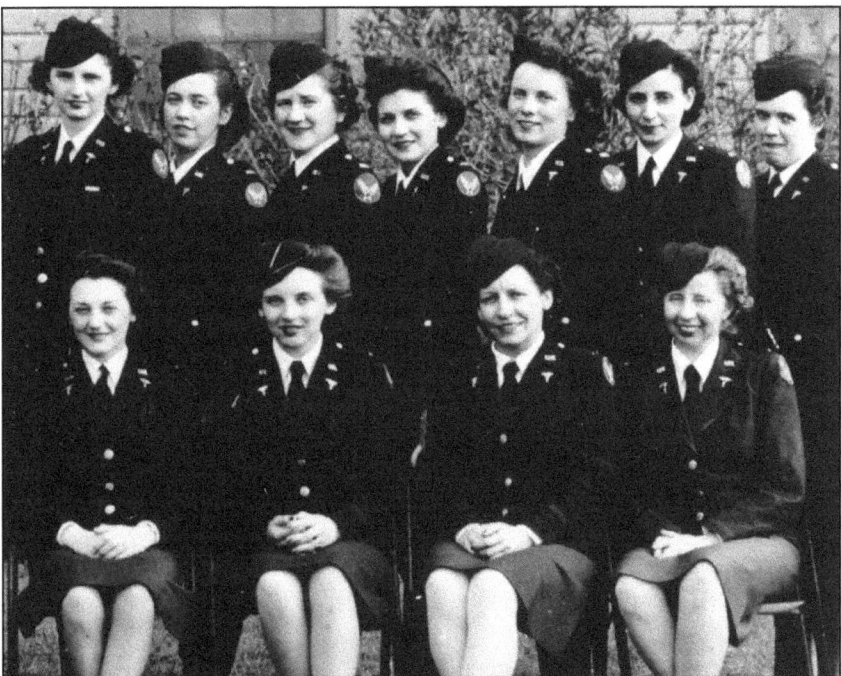

Figure. 06.64. Church, sitting right, and Josephene Sansone, standing second from right, in the 802nd MAETS (half of the squadron), 1943. AMEDD.

When asked about her experience, she told Air Transport:

> Compare it with a rolling hospital ship, the jolting of an ambulance, or even a hospital train. The pilots and nurses team up to give their passengers a good ride. We've learned to handle out-of-ordinary situations, and that helps. If we have lung cases, we try to stay under 10,000 feet. We put more serious cases in forward litters, the steadiest part of the plane. And the pilots go out of the way to fly at levels

where smooth air prevails. The fears proved groundless that brain or abdominal or certain unusual cases would be poor sky-borne risks.

She said the passengers asked many questions:

> They want to know how fast and how high we're flying. And food. That seems to be the major interest. I think they're almost more interested in 'when do we eat' than how soon they're going to get home. And finally, they start showing me pictures of their wives, sweethearts, and youngsters.

Her in-country flights usually started 10-12 miles behind the front lines, landing on rugged airstrips. They often had to dive into foxholes during enemy raids. After loading the patients, they'd fly back to hospitals 200-500 miles from the front. She logged about 90,000 miles in two years. [144]

Before she retired, she obtained the rank of Lieutenant. She received the Air Medal, the European-African-Middle Eastern Campaign Medal with seven campaign stars, and the World War II Victory Medal. The military released her from service on 18 June 1946.

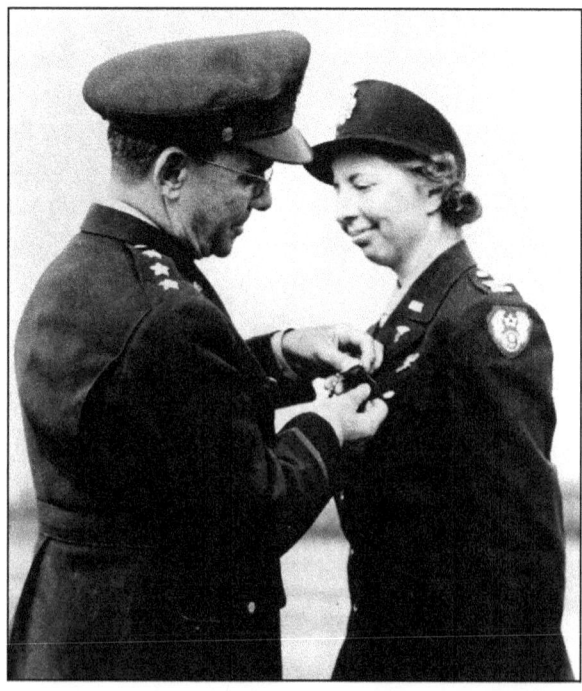

Figure 06.65. Church receiving a WWII medal. ANC photo.

In 1952, she became the Administrator of Union Hospital in Terra Haute, Indiana; she improved working conditions and added a modern psychiatric ward. In early 1965, she married Leonard Marshall, President of the Terra Haute First National Bank.

Church sustained a head injury while riding a horse on 27 August 1965. An ambulance immediately transported her to Union Hospital, but she died six hours later.[145]

Several agencies have sought to preserve her memory and achievements:

- The United Airlines Stewardess Management Center, at Chicago's O'Hare Airport, was dedicated to Church, and a statue erected.
- United Airlines (previously Boeing Airlines) contributed $25,000 to Union Hospital in her memory.[146]
- In 1966 United Airlines commissioned the noted South African sculptor, Rene Shapshak, to create copper bas-relief plaques about Church's life as a humanitarian, a war heroine, and an aviation pioneer. United Airlines placed the plaques in their headquarters in Chicago, in other airline training centers around the world, at Union Hospital, and in various organizations.
- She received a posthumous Aviation First award.[147]
- Iowa's Aviation Museum inducted Church into their Hall of Fame in 2004.[148]
- Cresco renamed their airport the Ellen Church Field. The public airport sits on 125 acres, about one-mile southwest of Cresco, in Howard County, Iowa.[149]

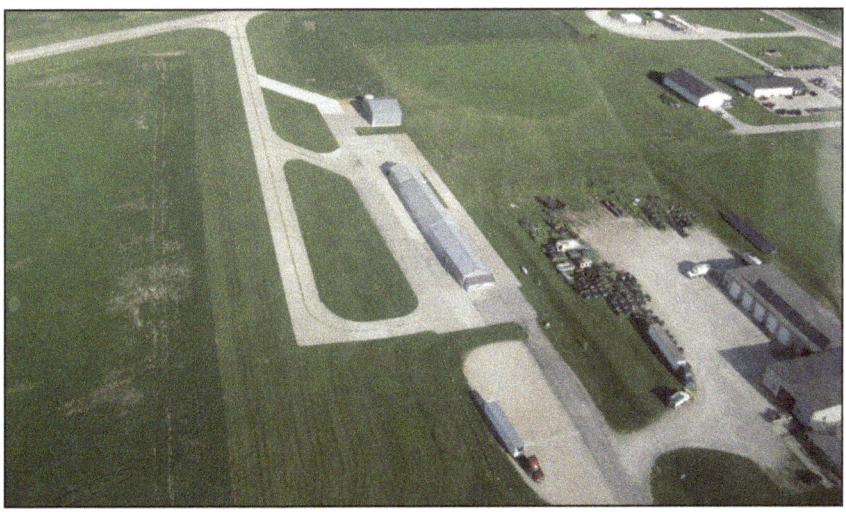

Figure 06.66. Ellen Church Field, Cresco, Iowa. Photo by Clair Pecinovsky.

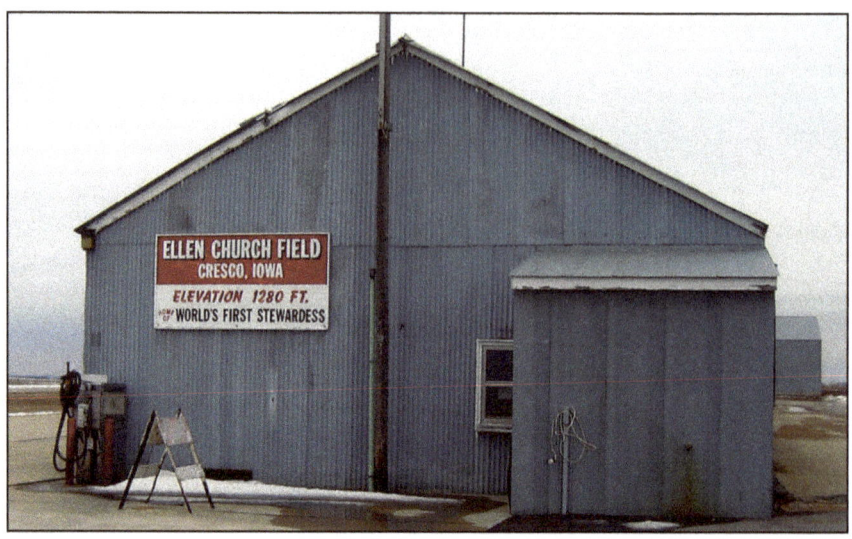

Figure 06.67. An original building at Ellen Church Field, Cresco, Iowa. They have since modernized the facilities. The Church Memorial plaque is at the side door of the airport where pilots enter. Photo by Tyler Vachta.

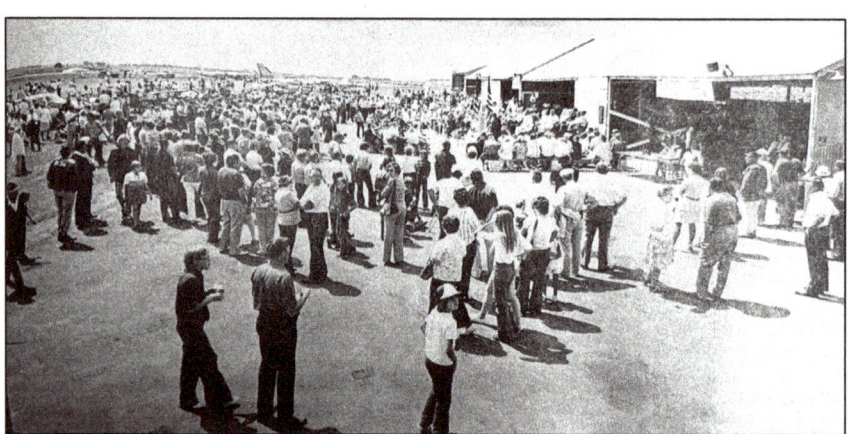

Figure 06.68. Attendees at Ellen Church Field dedication day, 13 July 1975.

On 13 July 1975, Cresco (Church's birthplace) dedicated and re-named the airport as the Ellen Church Field. More than 3,000 people and 200 planes attended, including a two-seater, experimental Pietenpol Air Camper Plane powered by a 60 horsepower Corvair car engine. [150]

Iowa Department of Transportation Official and Ninety-Nine club member, Ann Pelegreno, paid tribute to Church and presented the dedication. Cresco unveiled a new airport sign for the building, which they still use today.

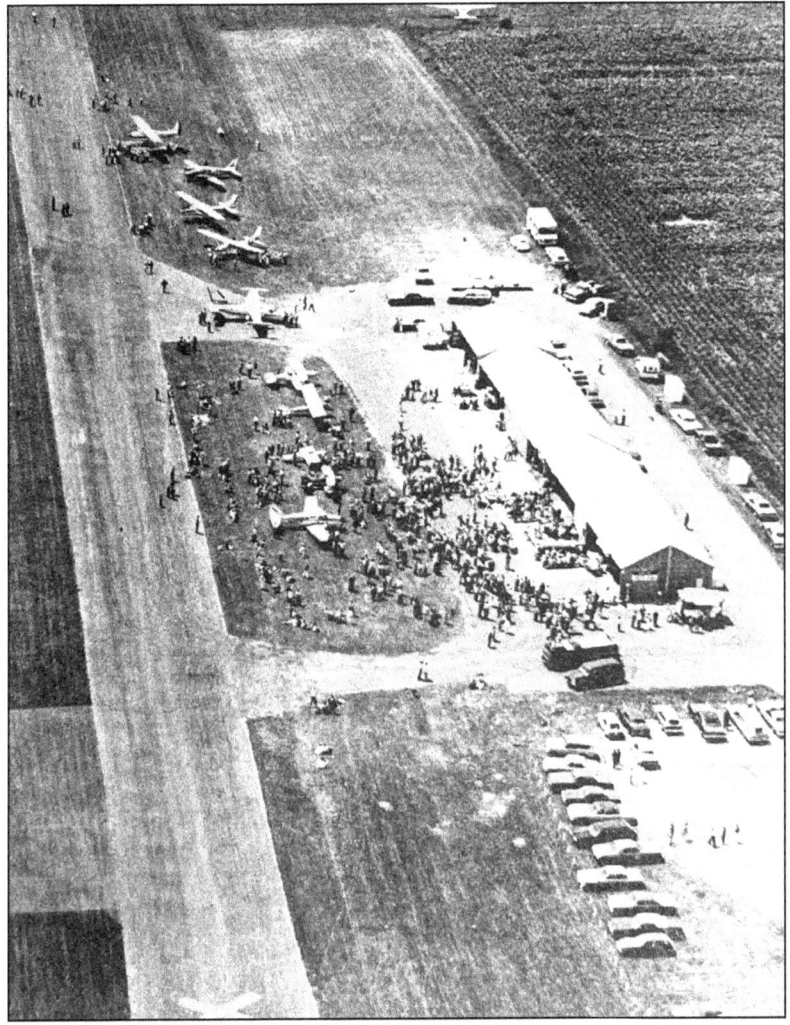

Figures 06.69. Aerial shot of Ellen Church Field on dedication day, 13 July 1975. Courtesy of Barbara Prochaska, Howard County Historical Society.

Two airline stewardesses, Barbara Links and Beverly Bloomer from Los Angeles, flew in to present the bronze Ellen Church memorial plaque United Airlines had furnished for the Field. The Minnesota Chapter of the Ninety-Nines joined the Iowa Chapter and held their July meeting following the dedication. [151]

Stunt flyer, Eldon McDaniels, performed upside-down flying, barrel rolls, and power-dives. Parachute jumpers demonstrated controlled spot-landings for the cheering crowd. [152]

Chapter Six

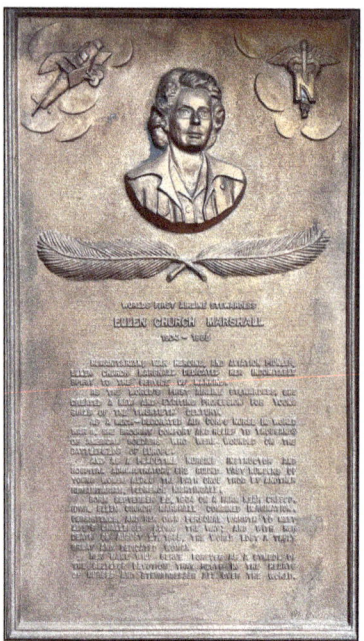 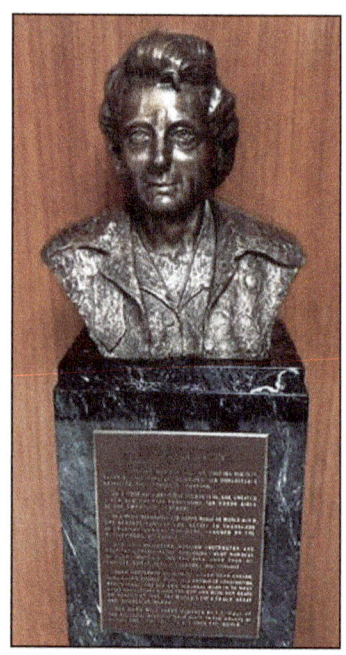

Figure 06.70. The United Airline memorial plaque created for the airport dedication, 1975. Photo by Barbara Prochaska. Figure 06.71. Ellen Church Memorial Statue at United Airlines Education and Training Center, 1966. Courtesy of Barbara Hanson, UAL. The inscriptions say:

> Humanitarian, war heroine, and aviation pioneer, Ellen Church Marshall dedicated her indomitable spirit to the service of mankind. As the world's first airline stewardess, she created a new and exciting profession for young girls of the twentieth century. As a much-decorated Air Corps Nurse in World War II, she brought comfort and relief to thousands of American soldiers who were wounded on the battlefields of Europe.
>
> As a nursing instructor and hospital administrator, she guided vast numbers of young women along the path once trod by another humanitarian, Florence Nightingale. Born September 22, 1904, on a farm near Cresco, Iowa, Ellen Church Marshall combined imagination, persistence, and her warmth, to meet life's challenges along the way, and with her death on August 22, 1965, the world lost a truly great and dedicated woman. Her name will serve forever as a symbol of selfless devotion that rests in the hearts of nurses and stewardesses all over the world.

Commanders
Margaret Mary Gudobba Killen, RN

Public Relations for Co. A-5; Flight Nurse

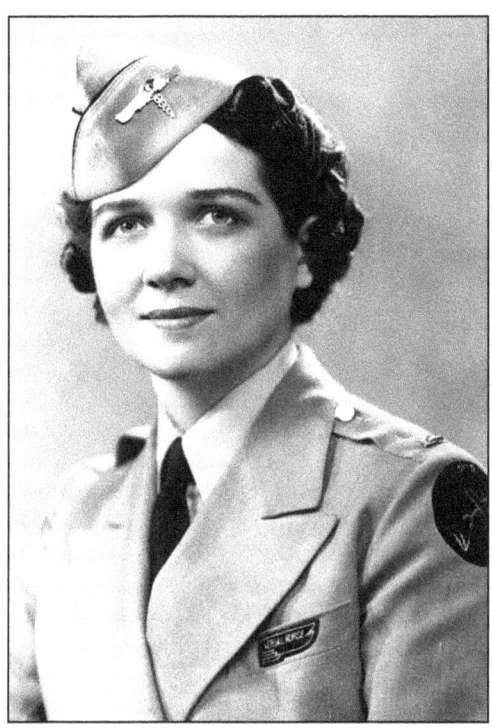

Figure 06.72. Margaret Gudobba, RN, 1939, wearing her ANCOA uniform. Born in October 1908 in Detroit, MI, she joined ANCOA on 9 December 1938 as recruit #170. Leora Stroup Papers, AMEDD.

Figure 06.73. A-5 ANCOA nurses, as salesgirls, during their yearly poppy sale for Disabled American Veterans. L to R, Margaret Gudobba, Ellen Cloke, Leora Stroup, and Eileen Newbeck, c. 1940.

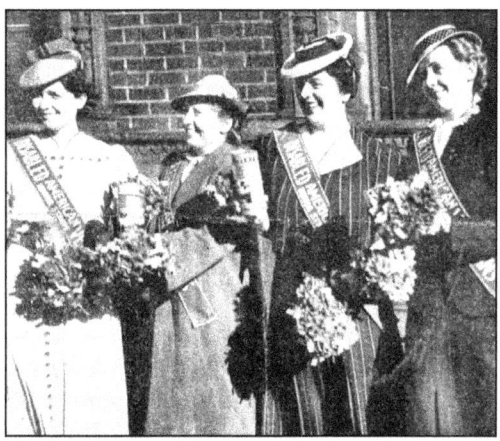

Red poppies are remembrance symbols for victims of war. After WWI, red poppy flowers bloomed on the scarred battle fields of Belgium and France.

Chapter Six

Gudobba joined the Army Nurse Corps in March 1941, before the attack on Pearl Harbor and before most other ANCOA nurses had joined. She was scheduled to leave on 19 April but postponed it because she was the General Chairman for the ANCOA dance at the Scarab Club; she felt responsible for its success. She told her friends Leora Stoup and Eileen Newbeck, "I wish you two were coming with me."

"Don't worry, we'll be seeing you," they told her. "The Army's going to need a lot of nurses before this show is over." [153] She left the next day for Fort Bragg in North Carolina.

She received her first leave in August 1942 from working in the hospital ward and headed for Detroit because she was homesick. She didn't want to waste 36 hours on a train; instead, she hitch-hiked on a parachute plane—the ideal view for her photography hobby. She tried to catch a mail plane but had to transfer to a cargo so old they called it "Lady Halitosis." Although she'd flown with the ANCOA on many trips, this was the first time she'd flown above the clouds.

She told the reporter she had hoped for a transfer to the Air Evac Nurse training, but if that didn't happen, she planned to ask for foreign service.

> I'd really like to feel like I was doing something to help. Not that working in the hospital isn't necessary. It's just I feel I can do more.

Her patients would probably have disagreed. During Christmas 1941, she noticed only two of her ward patients had a present for Christmas. She bought and wrapped gifts for all twenty-eight. They appreciated it so much they each gave her an insignia; she fixed them to blue velvet and hung them on her wall. "I can see the face of everybody who gave them to me," she said. [154]

Finally, in February of 1943, she received the long-awaited transfer to Bowman Field for Flight Nurse training. She met with her two ANCOA friends, Stroup and Newbeck, for a beautiful reunion. After training, the military assigned her to MAETS Squadron 806. She said of the work:

> No girl would hesitate to join if she knew what a thrill it is when they pin your gold wings. You work hard, unbelievably hard, but it's worth any amount of effort.

She couldn't understand why young women wouldn't enter the Army Nurse Corps. But she had to admit the Army was far from her previous life as an industrial nurse. [155]

Commanders
Mary Eileen Newbeck Christian, RN

Second Commander of Co. A-5; Flight Nurse

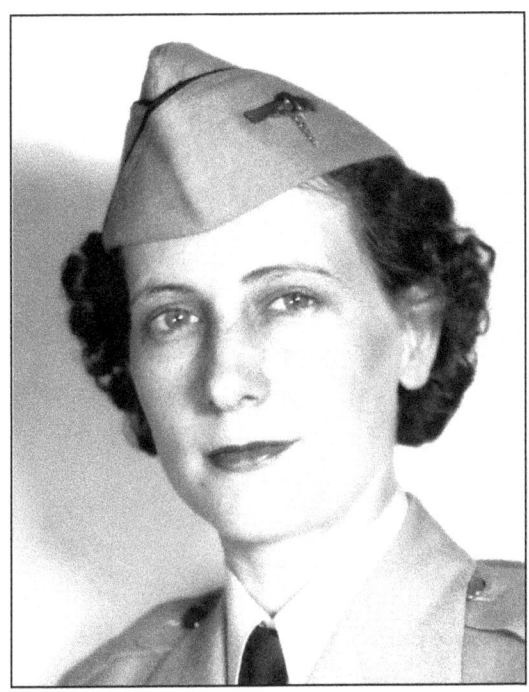

Figure 06.74. Eileen Newbeck, RN, in her ANCOA uniform, 1939. AMEDD.

Born in Canada on 27 January 1915, Newbeck was an American citizen because the Ford Motor Company in Walkerville employed her father. At eighteen-months of age, they moved to Detroit. She graduated from Providence Hospital School of Nursing in 1937 and worked as an industrial nurse, one of the most sought-after nursing positions then. [156-157]

She joined the ANCOA on 11 February 1939 as recruit #184. She assumed Commander role of A-5 when Schimmoler promoted Stroup to President in 1942. Her new position didn't last long—she soon joined the Army, and ANCOA friends Stroup and Gudobba, for Flight Nurse training at Bowman.

Newbeck joined the group of Flight Nurses graduating in February 1943, the 805th MAETS. For her first assignment, she and five other 805 nurses evacuated injured soldiers from a former training site in the desert in Thermal, California. Next, they assigned her to Alaska; she initially accompanied patients from Edmonton, Alaska, to Iowa on a train. [158]

Chapter Six

When the military finally assigned her to evacuation flights, they were primarily for government civilians injured while working on the Alaska Highway. She said the flight nurses' squadron numbers were inconsistent—they changed frequently, and nurses often had to scramble to catch their flight at the last minute.

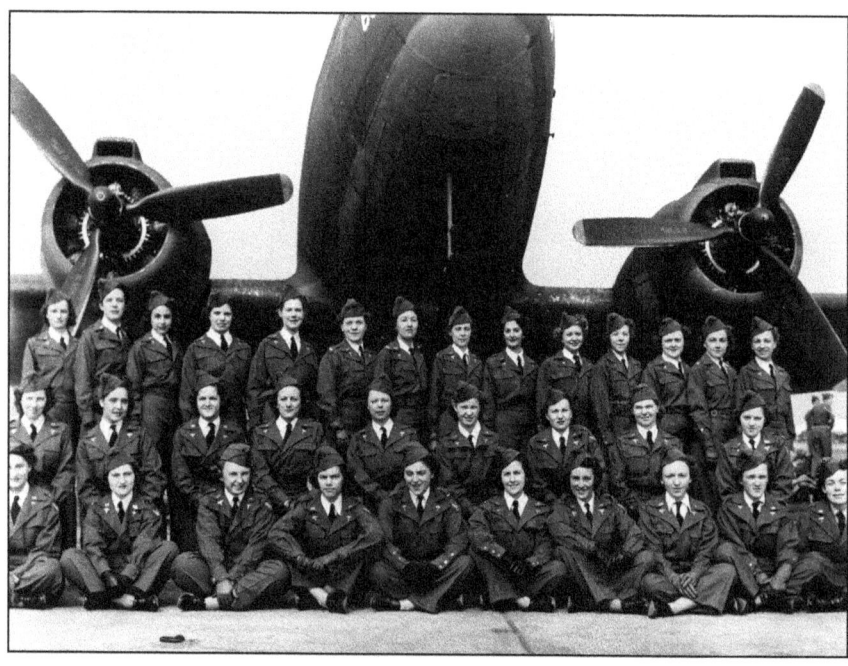

Figure 06.75. Eileen Newbeck, standing eight from left, and the 805th MAETS, 1943. Leora Stroup Papers, AMEDD. The military re-designated the name Medical Air Evacuation Transport Squadron (MAETS) to the Medical Air Evacuation Squadron (MAES) in July 1944.

The zero-degree flights stretched from Anchorage, Alaska, to Great Falls, Montana. Alaskan flights were notoriously dangerous—second only to those over the Himalayas, Newbeck learned.[159] One of her fellow nurses in the 805, Lt. Ruth M. Gardiner, was the first Flight Nurse killed in action when her plane crashed into the sea off Naknek, Alaska.[160]

Like the other flight nurses, she learned to adapt, improvise, and use her brain when the situation didn't fit the textbook. "Nothing is going to be textbook, period," she said. Although challenging, she enjoyed the work. Newbeck visited places she had always wanted to see in Alaska. And as a bonus, she met her husband, William Christian.[161]

Commanders

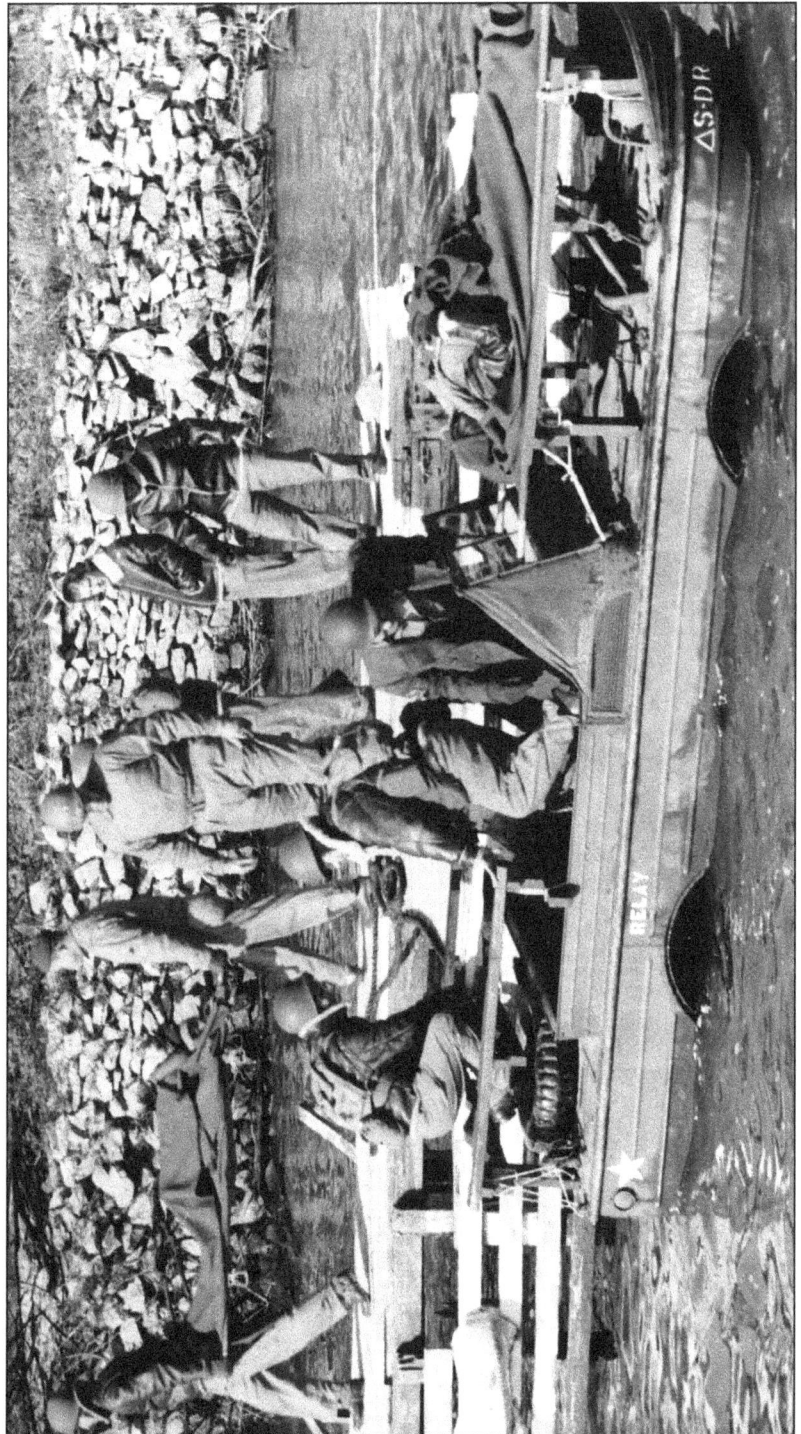

Figure 06.76. Leora Stroup and other Flight Nurses during a water rescue training exercise, 1944. Leora Stroup Papers, AMEDD.

Chapter Seven
Air Ambulance Histories

The United States in WWI

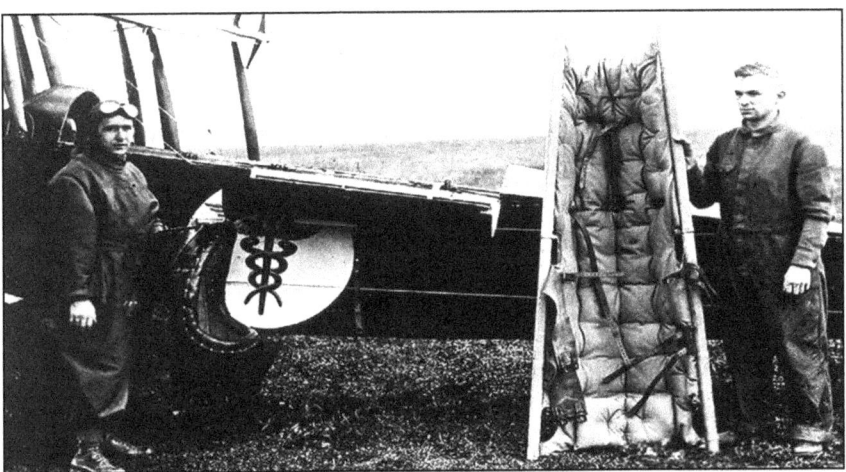

Figure 07.01. A converted Curtiss JN-4 "Jenny" used during World War I, 1918. Air Force Medical Service History Office photo.

During WWI, the United States converted old Curtiss JN-4 aircraft into air ambulances. They were costly to maintain, and the plane's set-up with the patient in the lower compartment behind the pilot would not allow anyone to attend to the patient during the flight. [1]

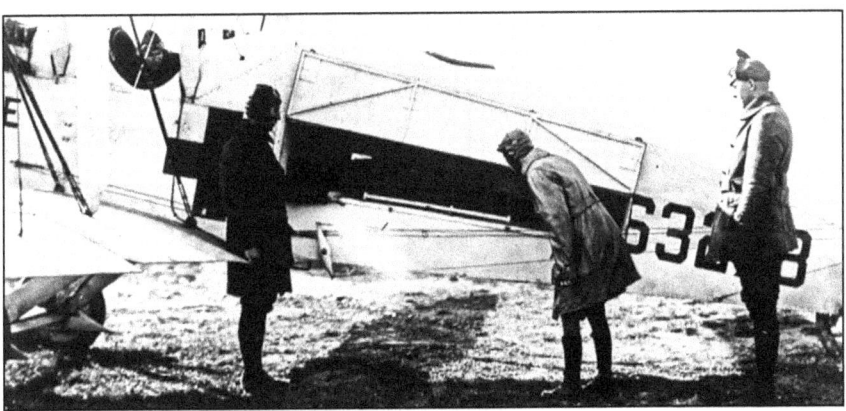

Figure 07.02. Patient compartment in a larger DH-4 airplane, 1918. NARA.

Figure 07.03. Fabric removed to show a patient's position inside the litter, 1918.

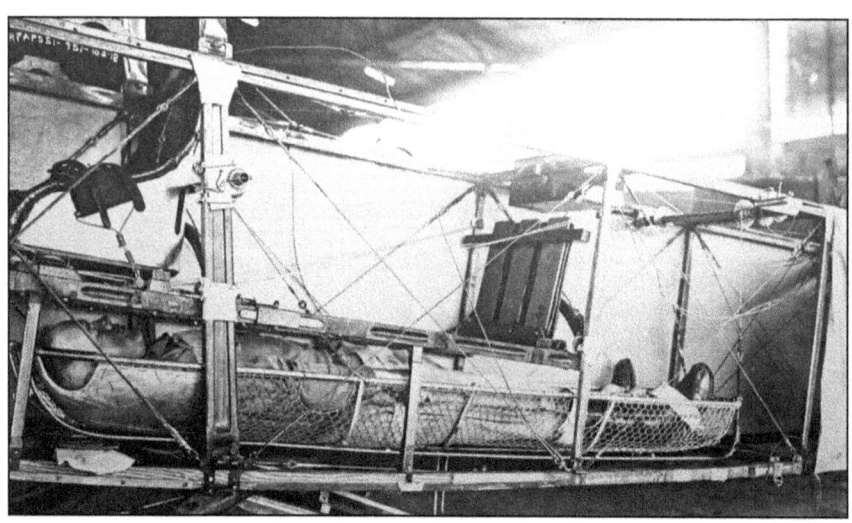

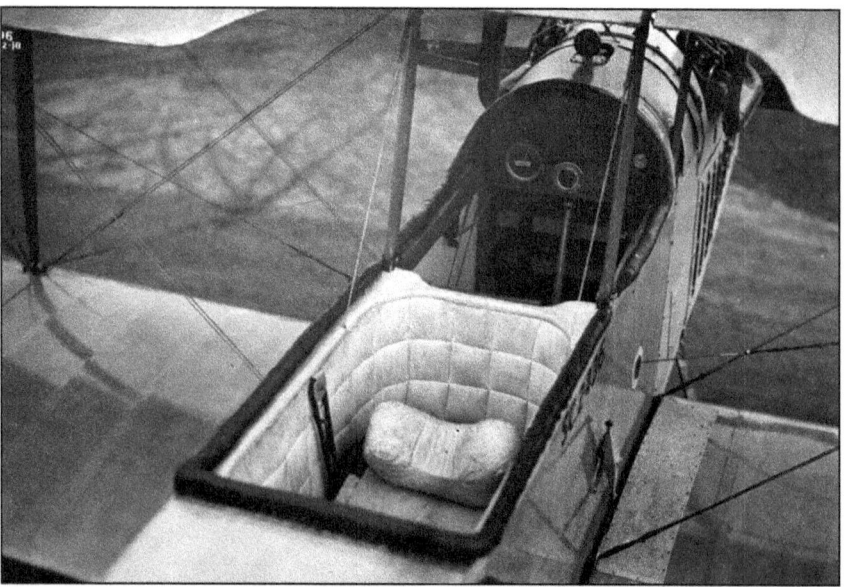

Figure 07.04. A view inside the patient transport area of a Curtis Jenny, 1918.

THE BRITISH MILITARY IN WWI

The first documented incident of an airplane for patient transport occurred in 1917 when British forces in Turkey used a biplane to transport a wounded soldier. Instead of the arduous three-day overland, the flight took 45 minutes. [2]

MARIE MARVINGT

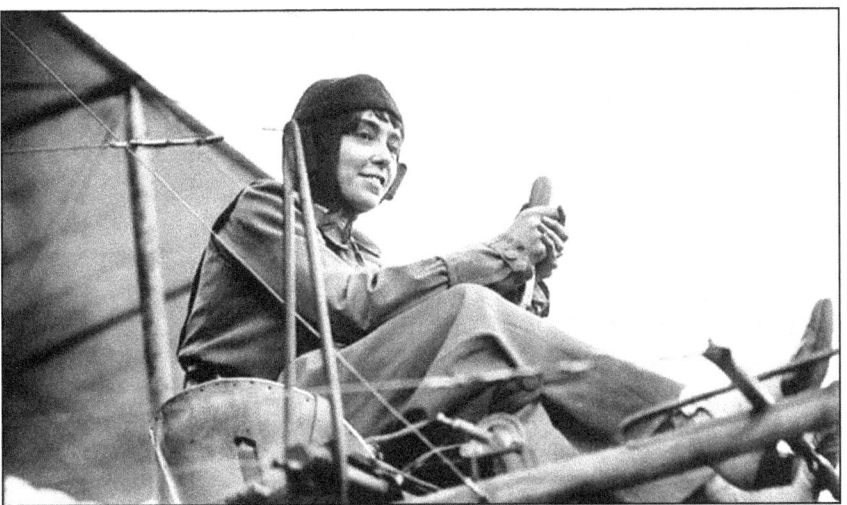

Figure 07.05. Marie Marvingt, 1912.

In 1907 French nurse Marie Marvingt, became the first woman to pilot a balloon from France to England over the English Channel. She obtained her fixed-wing pilot license in 1910. She served as a Red Cross Nurse, as a war correspondent in WWI, and was the first woman—in the world—to fly combat missions. She received a Croix de Guerre and multiple other awards.

After the war, Marvingt concentrated on her pre-war idea: aerial ambulance service. She gave 3,000 seminars on air ambulances and co-founded Friends of Medical Aviation (Les Amies De L'Aviation Sanitaire). In 1934, she started an air ambulance service in Morocco using skis she designed to land on the desert sand; the French Government awarded her the Medal of Peace of Morocco. In 1931 she created a contest, the Captain Écheman Challenge (Challenge Capitaine Écheman), with a prize for the best transformation of a civilian aircraft into an air ambulance.

Marvingt believed nurses should accompany patients in the air ambulance. Since no flight nurse training program existed then, she started her own— Nurses in Air (Infirmières de l'Air). In 1935 she became the first certified flight nurse.[3] By 1939, more than 500 nurses with at least ten hours of flying experience had trained with her and joined the Nurses in Air. When planes couldn't land, they would parachute into the area.[4]

She's listed as the only woman to hold four simultaneous pilot's licenses in 1955: balloon, fixed wing, hydroplane, and helicopter. The most decorated woman in France, she received thirty-four awards in wildly diverse fields.[5]

Chapter Seven

Australian Inland Mission Aerial Medical Service

In 1917 an injury in remote Western Australia, and an idea from medical student and pilot Lieutenant Clifford Peel, prompted Rev. John Flynn to plan the Australian Inland Mission Aerial Medical Service. In 1928 H.V. Mckay bequeathed Flynn a large donation and he was able to begin.

On 17 May 1928, pilot Arthur Affleck made the service's first flight with the first flying doctor, Dr. Kenyon St. Vincent Welch, from Cloncurry, Queensland, in a single engine bi-plane named "Victory." In 1955, they changed the business name to the Royal Flying Doctor Service (RFDS).

Robin Miller

Robin Miller was born in Subiaco, Australia, in 1940 to author Mary Durak and Horrie Miller—co-founder of MacRoberson Miller Airlines. Her father taught her to fly and immersed her in the aviation world from a young age. In 1962, she graduated from nurse's training at Royal Perth Hospital.

Miller obtained her pilot's license in 1965 and a commercial license in 1966, even though employment for female commercial pilots didn't exist. The polio epidemic would help Miller advance into the commercial flying field.

Dr. Albert Sabin created the oral polio vaccine in 1961, but distribution to remote areas of Australia was complex. Miller designed a solution: she would fly to settlements and administer the vaccine. She borrowed $12,500 to purchase a Cessna 182 airplane. She administered 37,000 doses of oral polio vaccine in sweet sugar cubes, after which she became known as "The Sugarbird Lady."

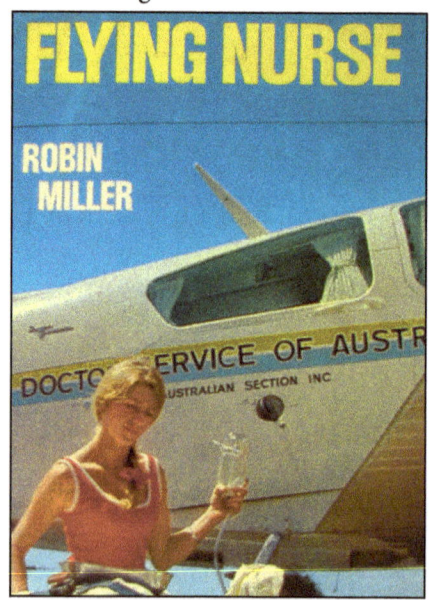

Next, Miller flew for the RFDS. She said a patient once went into labor while in the air; she shifted her plane into autopilot and delivered the baby. She published books based on her journals: *Flying Nurse* and *Sugarbird Lady*. Miller finished 6th in a 1973 transcontinental Powder Puff Derby air race. She died two years later, from cancer, at age 35.[6]

Figure 07.06. Robin Miller on the cover of her book *Flying Nurse*, 1971.

Nancy-Bird Walton

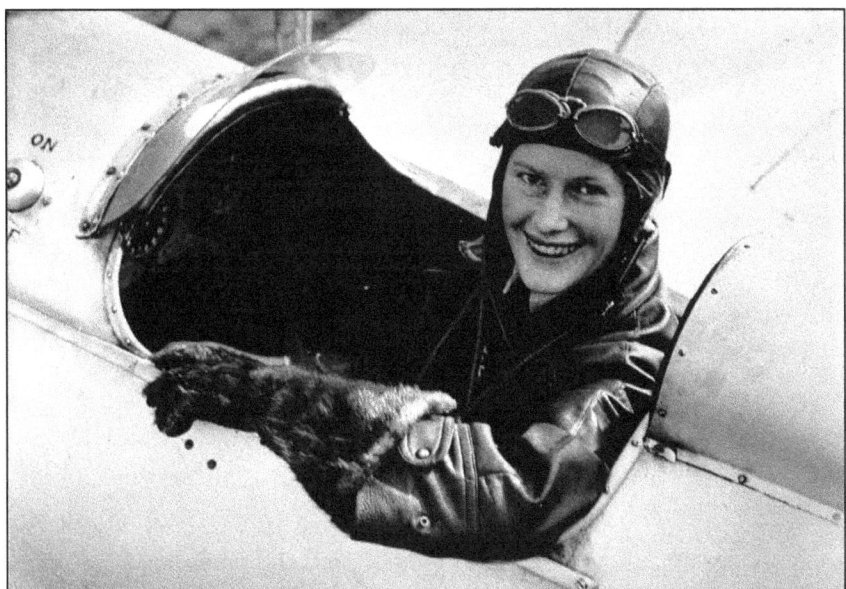

Figure 07.07. Nancy Bird in her Gipsy Moth plane at Kingford-Smith Flying School, 1933. Wikimedia.

In 1933, at the age of 18, Nancy Bird became Australia's youngest female commercial pilot—she'd only been flying for one year. She learned to fly from legendary aviator Charles Kingsford-Smith, who skippered the first plane across the Pacific (with three stops) in 1928. Bird joined his new flying school, one of his first students, and learned to fly in a Gipsy Moth airplane. [7]

She bought the same Gipsy Moth she had taken her first flight in, at 13, with money her great-aunt left to her. It was now a well-worn airplane. She called it Vincere, meaning to conquer. "I was determined to carve a place for myself in aviation," she said. Although other pilots told her barnstorming was dead, she decided to try it anyway.

In 1935 she teamed up with co-pilot Peggy McKillop, a friend who had trained with her. They formed the First Ladies Flying Tour. In 1936, she opened her first private aerial ambulance in Cunnamulla, Queensland; she flew 14,000 miles and carried 182 passengers. [8]

Rev. Stanley Drummond, the Superintendent of the Far West Children's Scheme, asked Bird to start a flying service for their baby clinic and to station her airplane (a brand new Leopard Moth) in the city of Bourke as an air ambulance. She intended to stay six months but remained for three

Chapter Seven

years as the only air ambulance pilot; she flew 20,000 miles and carried 275 passengers and patients. Later in life, people told her she had no idea the comfort it brought them to have a plane nearby that could fly them out in case they needed urgent medical treatment. [9]

After an educational aviation tour of Europe in 1938, she visited the U.S. and discovered the Ninety-Nines organization; she became a life member. She stopped in Los Angeles during this trip to visit Lauretta Schimmoler and the ANCOA.

She told the ANCOA nurses about her Australian air ambulance experience:

> In the inland or the "outback" are millions of acres of sheep and cattle stations. A large town is one with 2,000 people. The distances can be great between towns, often 200 miles apart. Families live 80 to 200 miles from a hospital. Many roads are only bush tracks; even a drop of rain makes miles of the county impassable.
>
> The homes we visited are not more than huts, mostly built of corrugated iron and wrought boards. These are the people the Scheme goes out to help. Our clinic trips of 400 miles took three days and would have taken over weeks by car. The mothers and children would be there to meet us. I always took lots of books and magazines which were looked forward to.
>
> While at Bourke, the air ambulance work was the most thrilling and worthwhile work I have ever done. I got great satisfaction being able to rush a patient to the nearest hospital when I knew he or she could not have been moved except by air. I always took a nurse or doctor with me to have someone to look after the patient while in the air. [10]

On the trip home from the U.S., Bird met Charles Walton on a ship. They married in 1939, and she took the name Nancy-Bird Walton, the nickname her husband used for her.

She received various national awards: an OBE (Order of the British Empire) in 1966, a Dame of the Knights of Malta in 1997, and an Order of Australia for outstanding achievement from the Australian government in 1990.

The new state-of-the-art Nancy-Bird Walton Airport (aka Western Sydney International Airport) in Badgers Creek, New South Wales, is under construction and is set to open in 2026.

Air Ambulance Histories

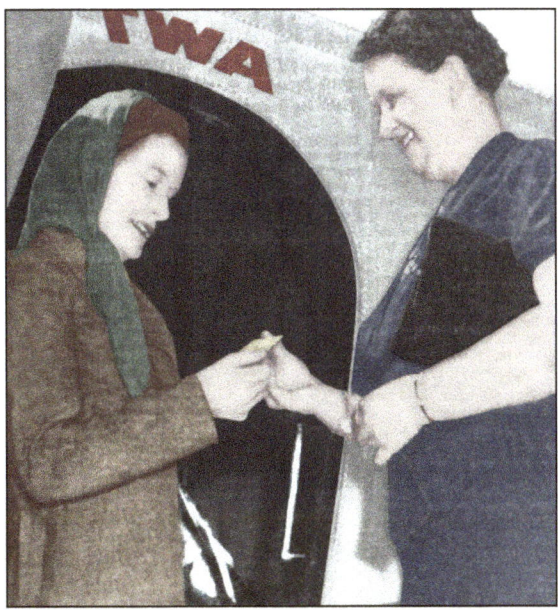

Figure 07.08. Lauretta Schimmoler presenting Nancy Bird with her honorary ANCOA membership card, 1938. Colorized clipping, BHS collection.

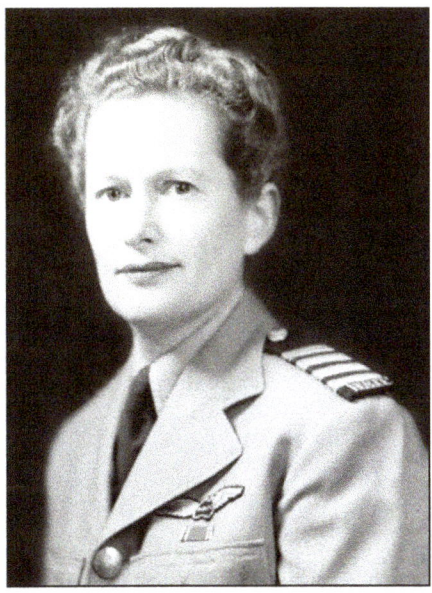

Figure 07.09. Walton's portrait, as Australian Commandant in the Women's Air Training Corps, during WWII. She joined the WATC in July 1942 and remained in the Corps until November 1944.

Chapter Seven

THE AMERICAN NURSES AVIATION SERVICE (ANAS)

In May 1932, Margaret Gilmartin, a New York pilot and nurse, began soliciting nurses and funds for the American Nurses Aviation Service with plans to train nurses for duties aboard aircraft. She believed nurses needed aerial training as most would become too airsick to help patients who needed emergency transport to a hospital by air. She also predicted:

> The next war will require nurses able to care for patients as they fly, and the service of nurses qualified for service aloft will be increasingly in demand in peace, as more and more ambulance service is required of airplanes. [11]

The *Journal of Aviation Medicine*, June 1932, published an article with the by-laws of the American Nurses Aviation Service, but it didn't mention Gilmartin's name. The service became famous for one mysterious event.

In September 1932, *Time* magazine listed the pilot Leon Martocci-Pisculli, MD, as the founder and director of ANAS. He bought a plane for them, the "Miss Veedol," a Bellanca CH-400—the first airplane to fly non-stop across the Pacific Ocean in 1931. He re-named it the American Nurse, painted it white with yellow wings, and scheduled the first flight. [12-13]

The Italian-born Piscilli hypothesized many pilots died on long-distance flights due to carbon monoxide buildup in the cabin. He planned to test his hypothesis on a flight from New York to Rome: Martocci-Pisculli would take blood specimens during the flight, and on arrival, he would perform basal metabolism tests. Finding a transport pilot wasn't difficult; he quickly located William Ulbrich, a young pilot with 3,800 hours of flying.

He had another novel idea: he wanted a nurse to parachute over Florence, Italy, dressed in a white riding habit, to pay honor to Florence Nightingale. Finding that crew member wasn't as easy. He wanted a nurse with a pilot's license and a parachute riggers license: he knew only two U.S. women who qualified in 1932. He asked the experienced Gladys Bramhal Wilner.

Nurse Wilner worked in Brooklyn and Manhattan. In 1931 she earned the first Parachute Rigger License ever awarded to a woman. She competed in air shows and air races, including the all-woman Annette Gipson Air Race, which she lost to Amelia Earhart. [14] Wilner was the perfect woman for the trip. At first, she expressed an interest; eventually, she declined.

Edna Newcomer from Williamsport, Pennsylvania, the other woman with the correct aerial licenses, was an undergraduate nurse. She accepted the challenge. Newcomer had been a showgirl with a reputation for "million dollar legs," which would add intrigue when she parachuted over Florence. An eclipse of the moon, and no light, was feared to cancel her jumping portion of the show. [15]

Martocci-Pisculli conscripted a fourth, albeit unwilling, crew member—a woodchuck named Tailwind. He believed woodchucks were more susceptible to carbon monoxide and would serve as a safety gauge. The plane left Floyd Bennet Field on 13 September 1932 about 6 a.m. The aircraft didn't have radios, so they carried a Dynamo light visible for 25 miles. [16] The Winnebago oil tanker spotted them mid-Atlantic. [17] A steamer ship, the Ashburton, sighted it 400 miles off Europe. The Ashburton sent a message by telegraph:

> The airplane circled the ship four times at a low altitude. It burned three green lights (a signal all is well). We signaled the pilot by blue flare. The engine was working smoothly. The plane disappeared in an east-by-southeast direction. [18]

That was the final confirmed sighting. Mussolini, the Prime Minister of Italy, ordered an intensive search for wreckage; his Chief of Aviation found nothing. They never located any remains. [19]

The ANAS attempted to re-organize the following year, but without the financial support from Martocci-Pisculli, they did not succeed.

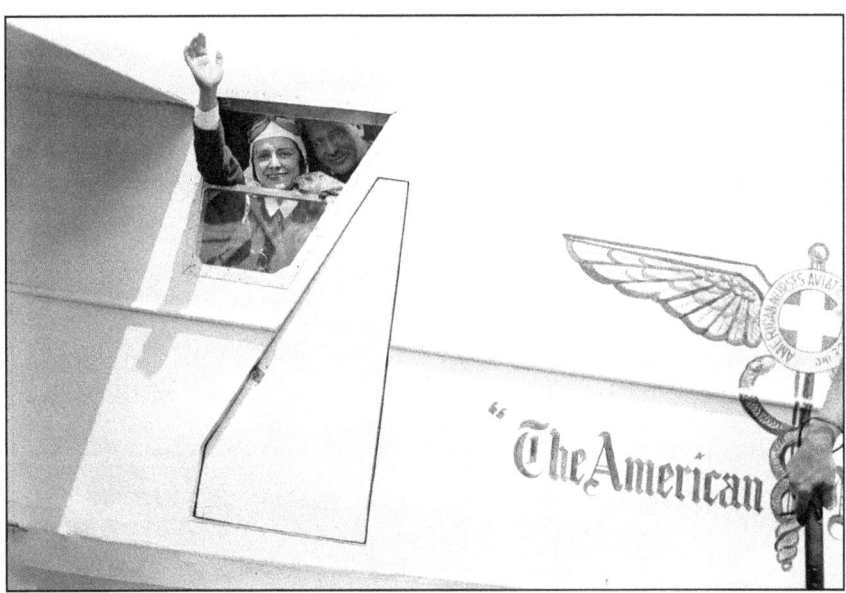

Figure 07.10. Edna Newcomer, Leon Martocci-Pisculli, and Tailwind, 1932. Courtesy of the Smithsonian National Air and Space Museum.

Chapter Seven

Relief Wings

Ruth Nichols soloed in 1924—the first woman in New York to complete this. She simultaneously held the women's world speed, altitude, and distance records for heavy landplanes in 1931. Her accomplishments and awards as a pilot could span pages. She founded an aviation club, an aviation magazine, was a charter member of the Ninety-Nines, and was the first female commercial airline pilot. Orville Wright, then-Chairman of the National Aeronautic Association, signed her NAA certificate in 1930.

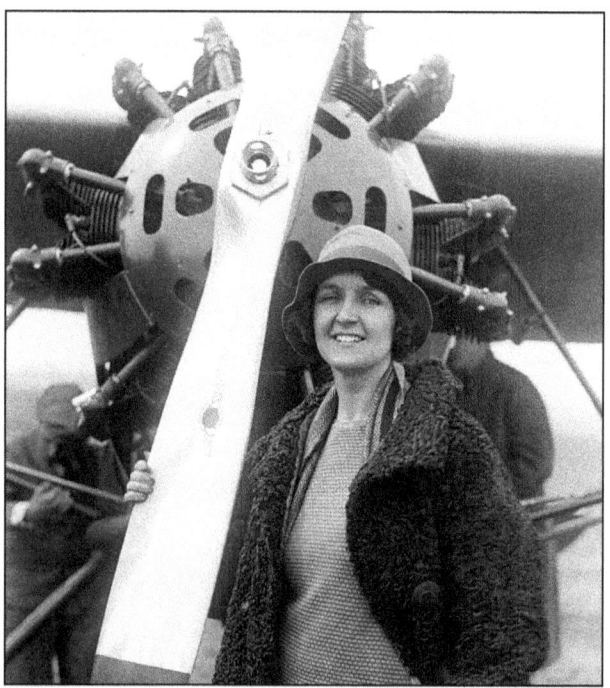

Figure 07.11. Ruth Nichols, 1929. Library of Congress.

Never enough for Nichols: she wanted to own an air ambulance service. She'd heard about the ANCOA. Their headquarters were on the West Coast; Nichols lived on the East. She thought she could cover her area. In 1939 she told her aunt:

> Ever since my crackup in St. Johns and my painful trip home in an ordinary plane, the idea of an air ambulance service had been in the back of my mind. [20]

On 7 July 1940, under Nichol's direction, one-hundred private planes from two organizations, Aircraft Owners and Pilots, and Relief Wings, staged a disaster drill for a hypothetical hurricane. The first of its kind. Two ANCOA nurses flew with Nichols: Matilda Grinevich and Juliann Sabatt. Grinevich was Commander of Company A-8 in New York and Sabatt a member. It's unclear if Schimmoler sanctioned this trip.

In December 1941, Nichols began a tour of the U.S. to raise money and organize her air ambulance. With Nichols' fame, she could attract more money and attention than Schimmoler. This idea couldn't have rested easily with Schimmoler, who'd been working on the concept since 1932.

Nichols told a New York reporter she'd just returned from California, where she'd launched a fundraising drive with aviation manufacturers and the Hollywood elite. She said:

> There's not one single twin-motored, specially equipped civilian ambulance plane in this county. We have sent hundreds of thousands of dollars to Great Britain and South America for ambulance planes, but we have none. [21]

She said she had established Relief Wings branches in Kansas City, New Mexico, and Los Angeles. Los Angeles? The national headquarters of the ANCOA? Perhaps this was a tipping point for Schimmoler. A letter to Schimmoler in Nichols' archive hinted at their conflict:

> Before announcing two years ago a project for a national air service to co-ordinate airplanes and other aviation facilities for civilian disaster relief, I wrote to you of our thinking and asked for your co-operation. You agreed the ANCOA would co-operate with Relief Wings, and we released a mutually acceptable newspaper story.

Nichols had no intention of training nurses. Instead, she planned to use "flight nurses from ex-stewardess, pilots, or members of the ANOCA... among the names were Grinevich and Sabatt." She said the nurses "would be run entirely under your control." Perhaps Schimmoler didn't believe this.[22]

Nichols also complained Schimmoler had since told the ANCOA New York and Florida nurses "not to have any relationship with us, that you considered us a commercial organization because we raise money from the public." But this disagreement quickly became irrelevant. Any rift would have died as WWII began that month, and private planes were grounded.

Nichol's archives mention she had organized chapters in thirty-six states. Perhaps the companies were only on paper—she didn't have enough time to form the groups before WWII started.[23]

Chapter Seven

Relief Wings, in its intended role, could no longer function. It's unclear if the organization transported any patients before WWII began. Nichols shifted her focus to working with the Civil Air Patrol. A July 1942 letter from Army Air Force Major Earl Johnson to CAP headquarters stated:

> Relief Wings, an organization by Miss Ruth Nichols, is a group of nurses who are anxious and willing to co-operate with the Civil Air Patrol whenever it is necessary...we are perfectly willing if you deem it so advisable for your Wing to co-operate with Relief Wings, however, CAP should not assume any financial responsibility for this organization. [24]

Nichols hadn't initially planned to train a cadre of nurses; now she did. She organized CAP nurses under her Relief Wings' banner and created a special lapel pin to distinguish them. They probably wore CAP uniforms. Nichols flew her plane with CAP and she received the CAP rank of Lieutenant Colonel. Her written details about Relief Wings and CAP are brief.

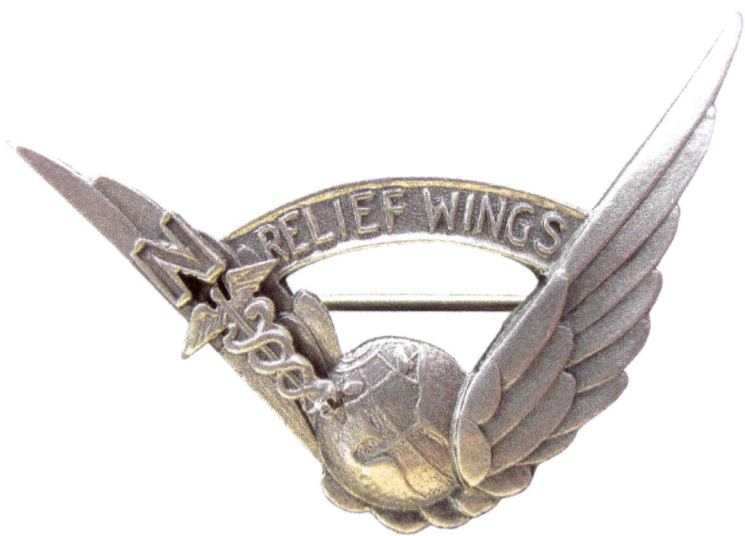

Figure 07.12. Relief Wings nurse's pin, 1943. Valkyrie wings, N for nurse, a caduceus, a globe, a Relief Wings banner. The Valkyries are mythological female Norse warriors who fly over battlefields and choose who can enter Valhalla—a sign of female power and prestige. Cliff Presley Collection.

Nichols created a second pin with Air Corps-style wings.[25] She wasn't a nurse so she probably wore that pin. Nichols continued after WWII with her life as an accomplished flyer, which she detailed in her 1957 autobiography, *Wings for Life*.

Air Ambulance Histories

Beryl Clutterbuck Markham

England-born in 1902 but raised in rural Kenya from age four, Beryl Markham lived a wild childhood learning to hunt, wrestle, and speak Swahili from the Nandi, Kikuyu, and Kipsigis tribes. She became the first female Kenyan bush pilot; she transported oxygen cylinders, medicines, doctors, and patients. Once when stricken with malaria, she learned a patient's experience of air transport. Her accounts speak to the need for medical accompaniment on evacuation flights. She said that blackwater malaria cases "nearly always die...if left alone in the back of the plane."[26]

Her piloting skills were legendary. In 1936, she became the first person to fly non-stop from Europe to the U.S. over the Atlantic Ocean "the hard way, against headwinds." She detailed her flying in the highly acclaimed book *West with the Night*. She lived in Los Angeles with Jacqueline Cochran while working on a movie as an aerial technical advisor; when WWII began she wanted to fly for CAP. They were interested, but it didn't work out.[27]

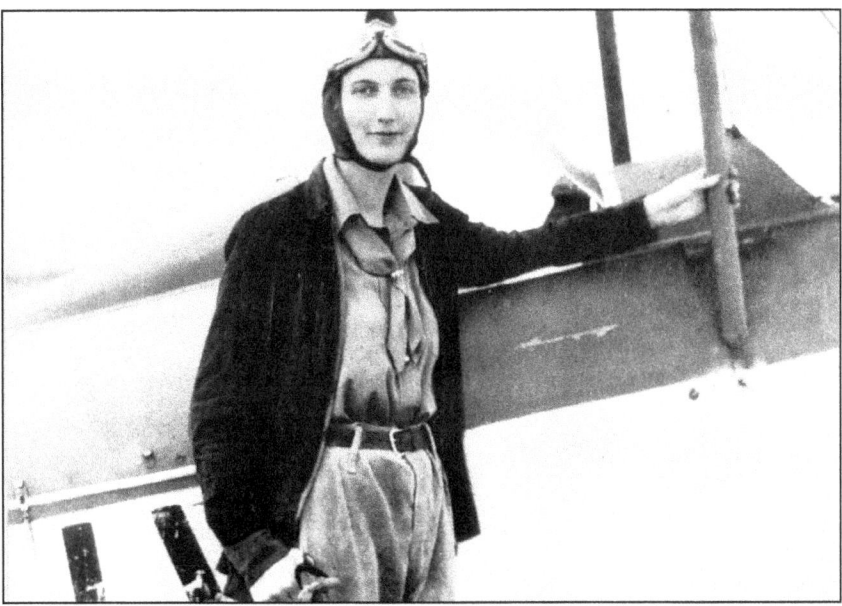

Figure 07.13. Beryl Markham posing with her Avro Avian IV, c. 1930s. Photo courtesy of Tekniska Museet.

In 1930, Veteran aviator and bush pilot Tom Campbell Black, taught Markham to fly. She learned in his de Havilland Gipsy Moth, then she bought a two-seater Avro Avian IV. She painted its registration letters (VP–KAN) silver-gold and its fuselage turquoise-blue—her horse-racing colors. She and her friends would henceforth refer to it as "Kan."

Chapter Seven

Individuals With Air Ambulances

In 1937 the *Los Angeles Times* reported on two nurse-pilots who operated air ambulances. Frances Kittredge, RN, called hers the first air hospital. She redesigned the stretcher and equipment, stocked a pharmacy, constructed a surgical and hospital room, and installed an oxygen tent for a single passenger. Although Kittredge was a pilot, she hired other pilots so she could attend to the patient. She also delivered oxygen tents, emergency serums, toxins, and iron lungs as needed. [28]

Donald Collins, MD, a physician-pilot, and Mrs. Joseph Washburn, RN, a nurse-pilot, operated an aerial hospital out of Los Angeles. Collins piloted the plane while Washburn cared for the patient and served as co-pilot. [29]

Certainly, these two groups of nurse-pilots and physician-pilots were not the only medical professionals in the U.S. in the 1930s to develop and fly a medically equipped airplane—the idea was in the air.

Organized Air Ambulance Services Begin

After WWII, the Canadian government established North American's first air ambulance service in Regina, Saskatchewan. Then, in 1947, a German immigrant, Walter Schaefer, founded the first service in the U.S. in Los Angeles—the Schaefer Air Service. The service later became the first FAA-certified air ambulance. Schaefer founded the largest ground ambulance service in 1932 and probably worked with the ANCOA. Both ground and air services closed in 2019 due to a changing financial climate. [30]

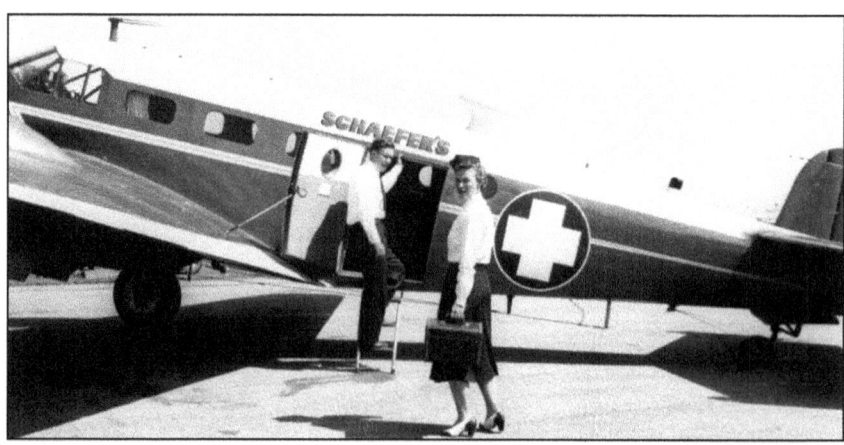

Figure 07.14. Pilot Ted Sanderson and Louella Schaefer, RN, holding a medical flight kit, board a Schaefer Air Service plane on 3 March 1956. Valley Times Photo Collection/Los Angeles Public Library.

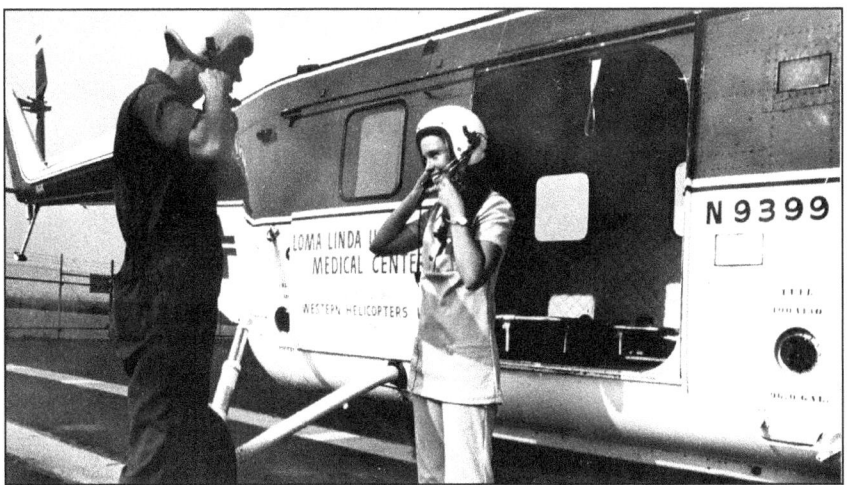

Figure 07.15. Dawn Graves, the first U.S. Helicopter Transport Nurse, suits up for a flight in a Sikorsky S55B (a rebuilt H-19D4 Chickasaw), c. 1972. Archives and Special Coll., Loma Linda Univ. Libraries, Loma Linda, CA.

The Hospital of Harlaching, Munich, Germany, flew the first civilian helicopter ambulance in 1970 called the Chistoph 1. In 1972, two U.S. hospitals began helicopter ambulance services: California's Loma Linda University Medical Center in June, and St. Anthony Central Hospital in Denver, Colorado, in October.[31-32] The time was ripe for helicopters to enter the U.S. medical evacuation field—the decades-long Vietnam War had created experienced helicopter rescue pilots.

Helicopters, or rotor wings, improve rescues for short distances between hospitals and for emergencies when transport time is crucial. They can land and take off in most locations, preferably on a flat space free of debris with a minimum area of 100 feet by 100 feet.

Medical transport companies use fixed-wing airplanes when the patient is stable and for distances of 100 miles or more. Potential adverse effects prevent the use of helicopters in certain situations: medical conditions requiring a pressurized aircraft, excess patient weight, inclement weather, and financial concerns—a fixed-wing aircraft costs significantly less to fly than a helicopter for medical transport.[33]

Providers transport about 640,000 critical cases in the U.S. annually: 300,000 rotor wing, 40,000 fixed-wing, and 230,000 ground transports.[34] When a fixed or rotor wing takes off on a medical evac, a highly skilled Flight Nurse with multiple certifications always accompanies the patient. The dreams of Lauretta Schimmoler and Leora Stroup became a reality.

Notes

Chapter 1

1. Skinner, R. E. "Roots of Flight Nursing, *Aviation Space and Environmental Medicine* 55, (1) 72-77, 1984.
2. Postcard from the Judy Wieging Collection, Fort Jennings, Ohio.
3. "Marriage Record," Ohio, County Marriages 1789-2013, 322.
4. "Schimmoler Papers," n.d., Bucyrus Historical Society (BHS).
5. Watts, Cindy, "Aviatrix Spends Early Life in Sycamore," unnamed newspaper clipping, n.d., BHS.
6. www.nationalmuseum.af.mil/Visit/Museum-Exhibits/Fact-Sheets/Display/Article/197387/flights-to-high-altitude, accessed 10 Oct 2017.
7. "Schimmoler Papers."
8. Skinner, R. E. "Roots of Flight Nursing."
9. Crain, M.A., "Lauretta Schimmoler," *Flashes*, Apr 1940.
10. *The Gregg Writer: A Magazine for Secretaries, Stenographers and Typists*, Volume XXXII, No. 3, Nov 1929 (Gregg Publishing Company).
11. Crain, M.A., "Lauretta Schimmoler"
12. Letter of Recommendation from W.J. Schwenck to Martin L. Sweeny, 27 Jan 1933.
13. "Schimmoler Papers."
14. Crain, M.A., "Lauretta Schimmoler"
15. "Schimmoler Papers."
16. "Foster Ends Exciting Airplane, Missile Career," *Martin Marietta News* (Denver, CO), 25 Jan 1974, 3.
17. Department of Commerce, Aeronautics Branch, 10 Aug 1929.
18. "Bucyrus woman named advertising manager." *Toledo Ohio Blade*, 19 Oct 1929.
19. "Schimmoler Papers."
20. "Aviators Log Book," (unpublished, 14 Aug 1929), BHS.
21. Ibid.
22. Watts, Cindy, "Aviatrix Spends Early Life in Sycamore."
23. Crain, M.A., "Lauretta Schimmoler."
24. Studer, Clara, "Despite a Mere Mayor" *Ninety-Nine*, 15 Feb 1933, www.ninety-nines.org/pdf/newsmagazine/193301.pdf.
25. "Bucyrus Wants Port," *The Journal News*, 23 Aug 1929.
26. "Only Ohio Woman is Also a Fighter," *Plain Dealer Special*, n.d.
27. Kane, Joseph, *Famous First Facts and Records*, (Ace Books, 1975).
28. "Airport Manager-Woman," *Aviation Airport*, (page 1021, Schimmoler, Lauretta, *Guinness Book of Records*, 28 May 1932, 72), BHS.
29. "Air Stunts Today at Culver City," *Los Angeles Times*, 9 May 1930.
30. Drennen, Margaret, "Milady Adopts the Airport," *Los Angeles Times*, 27 July 1930, J4.
31. web.archive.org/web/20070819111903fw_/http://www.ameshistoricalsociety.org/exhibits/snook4.htm, accessed 11 Aug 2023.

32. "Miss Schimmoler named Governor of 99s" unnamed newspaper clipping, 9 May 1931.
33. "Aviators Log Book."
34. Schimmoler, Lauretta, "And They Said it Wouldn't Be Done," (unpublished manuscript, 1966).
35. "News of the Schools," *Aero Digest*, Nov 1933, 40.
36. "Aviators Log Book."
37. "State Office Probes Fire," *The Star*, 20 Aug 1930.
38. Ibid.
39. "City Port Not Probable," *The Star*, 20 Aug 1930.
40. "Mayor Hits at Airport Price," *Marion Star*, 3 Dec 1930, 9.
41. "Council Overrides Mayor's Veto," *The Star*, 12 June 1931.
42. "Override Veto to Buy Airport," *News-Messenger,* (Fremont Ohio), 22 June 1931, 3.
43. "Council Paves Way to Airport Purchase", *The Marion Star,* 22 June 1931.
44. "Chamber of Commerce Negotiates for New Aircraft factories," *The Marion Star,* 24 Feb 1931,10.
45. "Start Work on New Hanger," *The Marion Star*, 12 Apr 1931, 12.
46. Watts, Cindy, "Aviatrix Spends Early Life in Sycamore."
47. "Lands at Field," *The Marion Star,* 27 Apr 1931, 10.
48. "Learn to Fly," *News-Journal,* 30 July 1931, 13.
49. "Start Work on New Hanger," *The Marion Star,* 2 Apr 1931, 12.
50. "Crestline Club Moves Equipment to Bucyrus," *News-Journal,* 18 May 1931, 5.
51. "Schimmoler Papers."
52. "Start Work on New Hanger," *The Marion Star,* 2 Apr 1931, 12.
53. Ibid.
54. "Override Veto to Buy Airport," *The News-Messenger*, Fremont, Ohio, 22 June 1931, 3.
55. "Bucyrus Airport Dedicated Sunday," *Capital New Bureau,* Columbus, Ohio, 20 July 1931.
56. "At the Airports," *Aero Digest*, 1932, 8.
57. "10,000 Attend Airport Event," *Marion Star,* 20 July 1931, 10.
58. *The Illustrated Encyclopedia of Aircraft*, Aerospace Publishing.
59. "Bucyrus Port Dedicated by Ohio Birdmen," *Mansfield Ohio Journal*, 20 July 1931.
60. Ibid.
61. *Illustrated Encyclopedia of Aircraft*, Aerospace Publishing.
62. "Bucyrus Port Dedicated by Ohio Birdmen," *Mansfield Ohio Journal*, 20 July 1931.
63. "Make Airport Available," *News-Journal,* 19 July 1931, 12.
64. McColl, Jeanette, "Silhouettes," *Detroit Free Press,* 15 Apr 1932.
65. "Glider's Club Members Pass," *New-Journal,* 26 July 1931, 11.
66. "Will Mark Port," *The Marion Star,* 5 Aug 1931, 8.

67. Mola, Rodger, "Show Me The Way to Go Home," https://www.smithsonianmag.com/air-space-magazine/show-me-the-way-to-go-home-9723795/, accessed 20 Oct 2020.
68. Smith, Fred, "Air Marking in Ohio" *Journal of Law and Commerce*, Vol. 4, 1933.
69. "Airway Bulletin of Commerce Department Commends Local Port," unnamed newspaper, 26 Aug 1932, BHS.
70. Mola, Rodger, "Show Me The Way to Go Home."
71. "Believe Air Marker Story Press Agent's Hoax," *Evening Independent*, Massillon, Ohio, 11 Aug 1942, 2.
72. "They Deserved to Go," *Coshocton Tribune*, 20 Sep 1942, 2.
73. Mola, Rodger, "Show Me The Way to Go Home."
74. "Woman Flyer is Spark Plug To Get U.S. Airways Properly Marked," *Newark Advocate*, 29 July 1948, 4.
75. "Air Markers for 100 Cities Planned," *Daily Times*, 12 Oct 1956.
76. Crain, M.A., "Lauretta Schimmoler"
77. "Delivers Chicks By Air," unnamed clipping, 17 May 1932.
78. "Silhouettes," *The Detroit Free Press*, 16 June 1932.
79. "Paves Way to Airport Purchase", *Marion Star*, 22 June 1931.
80. "No Bids Are Received To Lease Port," (Bucyrus, OH), *Telegraph-Forum*, 8 Apr 1932.
81. "Port Bucyrus Is Closed By City Officials," Bucyrus, OH, *Telegraph-Forum*, 20 Apr 1932.
82. "Padlock Threat Initiates Move To Preserve Bucyrus Field," *News-Journal*, Mansfield, OH, 17 Apr 1932.
83. Ibid.
84. Ibid.
85. Ibid.
86. "Port Bucyrus Is Closed By City Officials," (Bucyrus, OH), *Telegraph-Forum*, 20 Apr 1932.
87. "Council Will Re-Advertise For Port Bids," (Bucyrus, OH), *Telegraph-Forum*, 20 April 1932.
88. "Airport Will Re-Open Today," *Telegraph-Forum*, 22 Apr 1932.
89. "Municipal Airport Leased," *Marion Star*, 31 May 1932.
90. "Schimmoler's Pilots Log," BHS.
91. "Visit in Cleveland," unnamed clipping, 3 Mar 1932, BHS.
92. "Only Ohio Woman Airport Manager Is Also a Fighter."
93. terrellmuseum.info/news/150709, accessed 20 Oct 2020.
94. "Local Aviatrix Greets Amelia" unnamed clipping, 24 June 1932.
95. "Woman Pilots Stay at Westlake" *Rocky River Ohio*, 11 Aug 1932.
96. "Bucyrus Only Aviatrix Will Be Manager of City's New Airport," unnamed newspaper clipping, 17 April 1931. BHS Collection.
97. Letter from Opal Kunz to President Kennedy, John F. Kennedy Library, Boston, White House Central Name File, Box 1532, Folder: KUNZ. 14 Apr 1961.

98. "Want Akronites To Enter Glider Meet," *Akron Beacon Journal*, 30 June 1932, 10.
99. "Michigan Gliders Take Meet Honors," *Akron Beacon Journal*, 8 Aug 1932, 13.
100. "Franklin Texaco Eaglet," Smithsonian National Air and Space Museum, www.si.edu/object/nasm_A19310039000.
101. "Michigan Gliders Take Meet Honors," *Akron Beacon Journal*, 8 Aug 1932, 13.
102. "Glider Meet Draws Throngs to Bucyrus," *Mansfield Journal*, 8 Aug 1932, 1.
103. "Port Bucyrus Head Lauds Loomis Record," *Mansfield Journal* 20 Aug 1932, 9.
104. terrellmuseum.info/news/150709
105. "Hopes to Endurance Hop," *Mansfield Journal* 20 Aug 1932, 9.
106. Non-titled clipping, *Mansfield Journal*, 31 Aug 1932, 1, BHS.
107. terrellmuseum.info/news/150709
108. "Woman Flyer Stays Aloft for Eight Hours," *New York Times*, 21 Dec 1928, 22.
109. North Carolina State Archives, accessed 20 Oct 2018.
110. "Air Show Opens at Bucyrus," *News-Journal*, 11 Sep 1932.
111. "Boudoir Flyer Bucyrus Guest," *Sandusky Register*, 9 Sep 1932.
112. Skinner, R. E. "Roots of Flight Nursing," *Aviation Space and Environmental Medicine* 55, 1984, 72-77.
113. Studer, Clara, "Despite a Mere Mayor."
114. ninety-nines.org/our-history.htm, accessed 20 Oct 2018.
115. "All-Ohio Chapter History," *99 News*, Sep 1976,
116. "Local Aviatrix Honored by 99s," *Telegraph-Forum*, n.d.
117. "Bucyrus Aviatrix Wants Women Flyers At Cleveland Port" *News-Journal*, 2 Nov 1932, 16.
118. Emerson, F.W., "The Most Recent Emergency Unit," *The Guardians of Peace and Prosperity*, 1938.
119. Planck, C., *Women With Wings*, (Harper & Brothers, 1942) 186.
120. Schimmoler, Lauretta, "And They Said it Wouldn't Be Done,"
121. Emerson, F.W., "The Most Recent Emergency Unit."
122. Schimmoler, Lauretta, "And They Said it Wouldn't Be Done."
123. Ibid.
124. Ibid.
125. Cooper, Margaret, "99 Notice," *Ninety-Nines*, July 1993.
126. "National Air Races, 1933," *The Ninety-Niner*, 15 July 1933.
127. Schimmoler, Lauretta, "And They Said it Wouldn't Be Done."
128. "Application for Membership in Ninety-Nines," 29 Mar 1939.
129. Email from Parks, Dennis, "My best guess for manufactures designation," curator of the Museum of Flight, Seattle, WA.
130. "Southwestern-The Los Angeles Chapter," *News Letter* (the Ninety-Nines) Aug 1936.

131. "News of the Schools," *Aero Digest*, Nov 1933, 40.
132. Kessler, Lauren, *The Happy Bottom Riding Club: The Life and Times of Poncho Barnes*, (Random House, 2010).
133. Letter Depart. of Commerce, Aeronautics Branch, 10 Aug 1929
134. Pope, Nancy, "1934 Airmail Scandal," March 2009, accessed 7 Nov 2017.
135. Frisbee, John, "Valor: AACMO—Fiasco or Victory?" *Air Force Magazine*, Mar 1995.
136. www.postalmuseum.si.edu, accessed 7 Nov 2017.
137. Baker, Ira C. Letter to Lauretta Schimmoler "Commendation for Exceptional Work Done on Air Mail," 9 May 1934.
138. "May We Present," *The Pilot*, May 1937, 13.
139. "Throngs See War Games," *Los Angeles Times*, 5 Apr 1936
140. "Flying Medical Corps of Women's Air Reserve Display Emergency Methods for Disasters," *Los Angeles Times*, 2 July 1935.
141. "Aircraft Show Throngs Crowd 100,000 Mark," *Los Angeles Times*, 9 Feb 1936.
142. "Southwestern," *The 99er*, 2 Feb 1934.
143. "Friendly Competition," *The 99er*, 2 Jan 1934.
144. Schimmoler Papers, BHS Colection.
145. "Santa Barbara Aviatrix Wins San Diego Air Race," *Los Angeles Times*, 21 Oct 1935, 3.
146. www.rafmuseum.org.uk/blog/posts-from-the-archive-evelyn-hudson-and-ata, accessed 1 Feb 2013.
147. "Air Stunts Give Thrill to 10,000: Bomb Dropping Simulated and Feminine Trio Fly in Formation at Air Show," Unnamed clipping, 6 July 1936, BHS.
148. "The Mirror of the Sky," *Popular Aviation*, Sep 1935,164.
149. Schimmoler, Lauretta, "And They Said it Wouldn't Be Done."
150. Smith, Fred, "Letter to Lauretta Schimmoler," 30 June 1936.
151. www.alphaetarho.org/history.html, accessed July 8, 2020.

Chapter 2

1. uahf.org/ua_flight_attendants_founders.asp, accessed 24 Nov 2017.
2. "Southwestern Section," *99 News Letter*, March 1937.
3. "History of the Cleveland National Air Races"clevelandairshow.com/about-us/national-air-racing-history, accessed 1 Dec, 2017.
4. www.usinflationcalculator.com, accessed 2 July 2020.
5. "Troops Police Race Grounds," *Los Angeles Times*, (Los Angeles, CA, 8 Sep1936), 6.
6. "Air Racers Guard Plans," *Los Angeles Times,* (Los Angeles, CA, 17 Aug 1936), A2.
7. "Dare-Devil Pilot Here for Races," *Los Angeles Times*, (Los Angeles, CA, 22 Aug 1936), A3.

8. "Races Lure Foreigners," *Los Angeles Times,* (Los Angeles, CA, 23 Aug 1936), A2.

9. "National Air Race Program," 1936.

10. Thaden, Louise, *High, Wide, and Frightened*, (New York, Stackpole Sons, 1938).

11. "Dare-Devil Pilot Here for Races," *The Los Angeles Times*, 22 Aug 1936, A3.

12. "Film Player Send Invitation for Air Races," *Los Angeles Times*, 15 Aug 1936, A12.

13. "Leaders of Latin America Will Depart Today," *Los Angeles Times*, 18 Sep 1936, 6.

14. "Film Player Send Invitation for Air Races," *Los Angeles Times*, 15 Aug 1936, A12.

15. "Ace Offered Parade," *Los Angeles Times*, 28 Aug 1936, page A3.

16. "Pilots Set for Races," *Los Angeles Times*, 2 Sep 1936), A3.

17. "America's Women Flyers Flock To Air Races Today," *Los Angeles Times*, 4 Sep 1936, 9.

18. "National Air Race Program," 1936.

19. "Thrills of Air Races Billed for Dialers," *Los Angeles Times*, 4 Sep 1936, A18.

20. "Ace Offered Parade Post," *Los Angeles Times*, 28 Aug 1936, A3.

21. *The Sportswoman*, Vol.12, issue 1, 8, accessed 17 Apr 2017.

22. "Women in Air Racing," https://www.ninety-nines.org/women-in-air-racing.htm, accessed 16 Dec 2017.

23. Thaden, Louise, *High, Wide, and Frightened*, (Stackpole Sons, New York, New York, 1938).

24. Ibid.

25. "Throngs Awed Aerial Spectators," *Los Angeles Times*, 6 Sep 1936, 6.

26. Meyer, J.H. "The 1936 National Air Races," *Popular Aviation, Aeronautical*, Nov 1936.

27. *1936 Air Races R-1, Suzy Crash*, https://youtu.be/8tbn2dJ44mM, accessed 30 Dec 2017.

28. "Four Planes in Crashes at Air Races," *Los Angeles Times*, 6 Sep 1936, 1.

29. Schimmoler, Lauretta, "And They Said it Wouldn't Be Done," (unpublished manuscript), BHS.

30. Sternberg, Rose Marie, "1st Division News," *Flashes*, July 1937, 3.

31. Meyer, J.H. "The 1936 National Air Races."

32. "America's Women Flyers Flock To Air Races Today," *Los Angeles Times*, 4 Sep 1936, 9.

33. "National Air Race Program," 1936.

34. "High Spectacle Ends Races: Frenchman Wins Final," *Los Angeles Times*, 8 Sep 1936, 1.

35. "Hats Autographed by Noted Pilots; Seen As New Fad," *Los Angeles Times*, 8 Sep 1936, 6.

36. Schimmoler, Lauretta, *ANCOA Regulations Manual*, (Burbank, CA, 1940).
37. Ibid.
38. Crein, M.,"Lauretta Schimmoler," *Flashes*, 1940.
39. Pearce, Carol A, "Amelia Earhart," *Facts on File*, (New York, 1988).
40. "Flying Hospitals," *American Aviation*, 1 June 1937, 11.
41. "Flying Ambulances Vision of Air Nurses Organizer," *Akron Beacon Journal*, 9 Sep 1937.
42. Schimmoler, Lauretta, *ANCOA Regulations Manual*.
43. Ibid.
44. Wakeman, Ruth, *99 Newsletter,* Sep 1937, 3.
45. "Miss Schimmoler Here En Route to Nat'l Air Races," unnamed newspaper clipping, n.d., accessed 17 Apr 2017.
46. "Orders from Headquarters," *Flashes*, 3 Mar 1938.
47. "Aerial Nurse Corps," pamphlet, 1940.
48. Speck, Jane, "Help Wanted—Nurses Needed," *The Red Cross Courier*, accessed 17 Apr 2017.
49. Schimmoler, Lauretta, *ANCOA Regulations Manual*.
50. Letter, Lauretta M. Schimmoler to Clara D. Noyes, American Red Cross, 9 Jan 1933.
51. Letter, Clara D. Noyes, National Director, Nursing Service, ARC, to Lauretta M. Schimmoler, 13 Jan 1933.
52. Letter, Ida F. Butler to Mrs. Maynard L. Carter, 30 Aug 1937.
53. Letter, Ida F. Butler to Gladys L. Badger, 3 Sep 1937.
54. Letter, Ida F. Butler to Maynard Carter, 17 Sep 1937.
55. Ibid.
56. Letter, Ida F. Butler, to Gladyce L. Badger, 3 Sep 1937.
57. Letter, Cary T. Grayson to Charles R. Reynolds, 25 Oct 1937.
58. Letter, Charles R. Reynolds to Cary T. Grayson, 29 Oct 1937.
59. Ibid.
60. "General Henry H. Arnold," http://www.af.mil/About-Us/Biographies/Display/Article/107811/general-henry-h-arnold, 7 Jan 2018.
61. "Schimmoler, Lauretta, "And They Said it Wouldn't Be Done."
62. Link, M.M and Coleman, H. A. *Medical Support of the Army Air Forces In World War II*, Office of the Surgeon General, 1955.
63. Letter, Gen. H. H. Arnold to Lauretta M. Schimmoler, 10 Nov 1937, written by Col. M. C. Grow.
64. Link, M.M and Coleman, H. A. *Medical Support of the Army Air Forces In World War II*, Office of the Surgeon General, 1955.
65. Ibid.
66. Letter, Schimmoler, L. M. to Flikke, J.O., 23 Apr 1938.
67. Letter, Flikke J.O. to Schimmoler, L. M., 28 Apr 1938.
68. Letter, Ida F. Butler, to Julia O. Flikke, 28 May 1938.
69. www.smithsonianmag.com/history/the-man-who-wrote-the-pledge-of-allegiance-93907224, accessed 4 May 2018.

70. Bintliff, Douglas, "Aerial Nurse Corps," *Air Trails*, (Street and Smith Publications, New York, NY, Nov 1940).

71. Sternberg, Rose Marie, "1st Division News," *Flashes*, July 1937.

72. "Giving Wings to Nursing," *National Aeronautics*, (Washington D.C., June 1938), 12.

73. Ibid, 11.

74. "May We Present," *The Pilot*, May 1937.

75. Emerson, E. W., "The Most Recent Emergency Unit of the Los Angeles County Sheriff's Department," *The Guardians of Peace and Property*, (Los Angeles, CA, 1939), 10.

76. Lackner, Hilda, "Ohio Air News," *Flashes*, Feb 1940, 4.

77. "Stewardess," *Flashes,* Vol.1 No. 3 Feb 1938.

78. "A Colonel Inspecting Air Nurses," *Detroit Times*, 2 Feb 1939.

79. "Sheriff's Aero Squadron Shows its Efficiency for Emergencies," *Los Angeles Times*, 5 Mar 1934, A1.

80. "First Airplane Detail In the Nation," *Your Sheriff's Department*, Los Angeles, CA, 6 Mar 1999, 55.

81. www.shq.lasdnews.net, accessed 17 Feb 2018.

82. "Co. A 1st Div. News," *Flashes*, Oct 1939, 2.

83. Bintliff, Douglas, "Aerial Nurse Corps."

84. "The Roots of Flight Nursing," *Aviation, Space and Environmental Medicine*, Jan 1984, 74.

85. "Aerial Nurse Corps Affiliates," *National Aeronautics*, Feb 1939.

86. *Flashes*, Mar 1938, 3.

87. Schimmoler, Lauretta, "And They Said it Wouldn't be Done.

88. Ibid.

89. Schimmoler, Lauretta, "General Headquarters Activities," *Flashes*, Apr 1939.

90. Schimmoler, Lauretta, "Prospectus," 1940.

91. "Angeles," *The American Magazine*, (Crowell-Collier Publishing Co., Nov 1941), 93.

92. Bintliff, Douglas, "Aerial Nurse Corps." *Air Trails*, (Street and Smith Publications, New York, NY., Nov 1940).

93. "Fifteen From Orphans Home Given Their First Sky Ride," *Los Angeles Times*, 31 July 1939, A10.

94. Skinner RE. "The making of the air surgeon: the early life and career of David N. Grant," *Aviation Space Environ Med.*, Jan 1983, 75-82.

95. Ibid.

96. Sternberg, R.M., "Editorial," *Flashes*, Apr 1939, 1.

97. Bolch, Ruby, *Flashes,* Apr 1939, 2.

98. "Angels," *The American*, Nov 1941, 93.

99. www.usinflationcalculator.com, accessed 17 Apr 2023.

100. *Flashes*, Jan 1939, 6.

101. www.engineer-exchange.com/8-historical/53-radio-licenses, accessed 5 May 2018.

102. "Safety-Procedures," *National Aeronautics*, (National Aeronautics Assm. Dec 1939).

103. Memo, Lt. Col. R. J. Platt to Supt., Army Nurses Corps, SGO, 18 Feb 1939.

104. Letter, Mary Beard to Mr. Hughes, 31 Mar 1939.

105. Letter, Mary Beard to Mr. Hughes, 1 May 1939.

106. Letter, Virginia M. Dunbar to Mary Beard, 1 June 1939.

107. Letter, Mary Beard to Lauretta M. Schimmoler, 7 July 1939.

108. "Major Strommes's Paper," *Flashes*, Dec 1939, 1.

109. Letter, Gill Robb Wilson to Mary Beard, 16 Apr 1940.

110. Ruth G. Mitchell, "The Aerial Nurse Corps of America," speech given at Meeting of Delegates of the California State Nurses Association, San Francisco, 15 Aug 1939.

111. Mary Beard, "Aerial Nurse Corps of America, Inc.," 23 Jan 1940.

112. "Report of the Committee of C.S.N.A.-Advisory Council for A.N.C.O.A.," 14 Oct 1940.

113. Ibid.

114. Letter, Gladyce L. Badger to Mary Beard, 30 Oct 1940.

115. Letter, Lauretta Schimmoler to Gladyce L. Badger, 28 Oct 1940.

116. Letter, Gladyce L. Badger to Mary Beard, 30 Oct 1940.

117. Eck, Emily K., "Outline for Aviation Nursing," 3 May 1941.

118. Dunbar, Virginia M., "Notes on the meeting of Aerial Nurse Corps," 3 May 1941."

119. Letter, Mary R. Beard to Edna L. Hedenberg, 17 Sep 1940.

120. "Special Committee of the ANA to Confer with the Aerial Nurse Corps of America Report," 16 May 1941.

121. Ibid.

122. Leora Stroup Papers, U.S. Army Medical Dept. Museum.

123. Letter, Nichols to Harriet Fleming, "Tentative Reorganization Plans, Aerial Nurse Corps of America," 16 Feb 1942.

124. "Nurses Mobilize for Air Duties in New Home Defense Service," *Los Angeles Times*, 23 Mar 1941.

125. Ibid.

126. "Aerial Nurse Women Patriots," *Los Angeles Times*, 10 Sep 1941.

Chapter 3

1. Letter, Reed G Landis to Lauretta Schimmoler, 16 Nov 1941.

2. gocivilairpatrol.com/about/history-of-civil-air-patrol, accessed 28 June 2020.

3. "City's Airfields Blacked Out," *Los Angeles Times*, 8 Dec 1941, 1E.

4. "Private Planes Except Airliners Are Grounded," *Washington Evening Star*, 8 Dec 1941.

5. "Duty Roster Personnel, Grand Central Air Terminal," 11 Jan 1942.

6. "Civil Air Patrol Wants Flyers," *Los Angeles Times*, 5 Feb 1942.

7. "Fund for Air Nurses," *Los Angeles Times*, 25 Feb 1942.
8. "Aerial Nurses Volunteer," *California Wing Tips*, May 1942.
9. capchistoryproject.org/shoulder-patches.html, accessed 2 June 2020.
10. Letter, Schimmoler, Lauretta to Stroup, Leora, 7 Feb 1942.
11. capchistoryproject.org/uniforms.html, accessed 2 June 2020.
12. "Aerial Nurses Wing Way Into Service of Their Country," *Sunday Journal Herald Spotlight,* 18 Oct 1942.
13. Letter, John G. Slevin to Leora Stroup, 16 Jan 1941.
14. "Airfield Notes," unnamed newspaper clipping, n.d.
15. Letter, Stroup to Schimmoler, 24 Feb 1942.
16. www.airzoo.org/enshrinees, accessed 3 March 2023.
17. https://iwasm.omeka.net/items/show/1405, accessed 3 Mar 2023.
18. Letter, Lauretta Schimmoler to Leora B. Stroup, 26 Jun 1942.
19. Letter, Lauretta Schimmoler to David N.W. Grant, 24 Jul 1942.
20. "Air Ambulance Passes Its Test," *Detroit News,* 15 Oct 1940.
21. Letter, David N. W. Grant to Lauretta Schimmoler, 3 Aug 1942.
22. "I Was There," Bob Hope, July 1995.
23. Rian, James, "Revised final draft of screenplay," *Parachute Nurse,* (Columbia Pictures, 6 Mar 1942).
24. *Parachute Nurse,* (Columbia Pictures, May 1942).
25. "Dedication of the Movie," *Parachute Nurse.*
26. "Parachute Nurses?" *RN: A Journal for Nurses,* 5 Feb 1942, 56.
27. "Ex-Bucyrus Airport Manager Turns to Movies," *Mansfield News-Journal,* 16 Aug 1942.
28. "WGN Bouquet of Honor Goes to Two Women," *Chicago Tribune,* 15 Nov 1942.
29. Planck, C.E., *Women with Wings,* (Harper & Brothers 1942).
30. www.scott.af.mil/News/Article-Display/Article/160389/scott-airman-awarded-by-air-force-association, 18 July 2020.
31. Letter, Lauretta Schimmoler to Leora B. Stroup, 26 Jun 1942.
32. army.mil/women/history/wac.html, accessed 8 July 2020.
33. usinflationcalculator.com, accessed 7 July 2023.
34. Letter, Lauretta Schimmoler to Colonel Ether Kovach, 8 July 1966.
35. npr.org/2010/03/09/123773525/female-wwii-pilots-the-original-fly-girls, accessed 7 July 2020.
36. Schimmoler, Lauretta "And They Said it Wouldn't Be Done."
37. Ibid.
38. "BURBANK: Aerospace Plant Near Airport to Close," *Los Angeles Times,* 2 Aug 1994, 2 A.
39. "Earhart Legion Post Gets Oil Portrait of Aviatrix," *Valley Times,* 24 Oct 1946.
40. "Women's Post Named for Amelia Earhart," *National Legionnaire,* 20 May 1946.
41. "Legion Has 144 Women Posts; 83 of War II Vets," *News Service, the American Legion,* No. 50, n.d.

42. "Famed Flyer Painted by Lockheed," *Lockheed Star*, 1 Nov 1946.
43. "Earhart Portrait to Post," *National Legionnaire*, Dec 1946.
44. "Famed Flyer Painted by Lockheed," *Lockheed Star*.
45. airandspace.si.edu/collection/id/nasm_A19500112000, accessed 17 July 2020.
46. "Wisconsin Chapter," *99 News*, Vol. 2 No. 2, May/June 1974.
47. airandspace.si.edu/collection-objects/jacket-suit-flying-civilian-ninety-nines/nasm_A19550103000, accessed 17 July 2020.
48. twentyandfour.org/, accessed 17 July 2020.
49. "Legion Revives Annual Aerial Membership Roundup, June 2," *American Legion Magazine*, July 1946.
50. Ibid.
51. "Founder Aerial Nurse Corps California Legionnaire," unnamed newspaper clipping, Nov 1975, BHS.
52. Stickel, John, "Lauretta Schimmoler," 11 May 2012.
53. Letter, H.A. Coleman to Lauretta Schimmoler, 8 Mar 1945.
54. Letter, Lauretta Schimmoler to H.A. Coleman, 22 Mar 1945.
55. Ibid.
56. La Vriha, Jack, "Heads Training of Aviation Nurses," unnamed newapaper clipping, n.d., Forsyth Library Collections, FHSU.
57. Letter, Lauretta Schimmoler to Leora B. Stroup, 26 Jun 1942
58. Letter, H. A. Coleman to Pvt. L.M Schimmoler, 28 Mar 1945.
59. Schimmoler, Lauretta, "And They Said it Wouldn't Be Done."
60. Letter, Col. Stromme to Lt. Col. M.D. Grenevich, 23 Mar 1966.
61. Letter, Agnes Arrington to Matilda Grinevich, 15 Sep 1965.
62. army.mil/article/33680/william_billy_mitchell_the_father_of_the_united_states_air_force. 14 July 2020.
63. Letter, Agnes Arrington to Matilda Grinevich, 15 Sep 1965.
64. "Miss Schimmoler Awarded Honorary Flight Nurse Certificate and Wings," *Aerospace Medicine*, July 1966.
65. "Lauretta Honored," *The Beam*, Post #678, 10 May 1966.
66. "Honorary Flight Nurse Flies Again," *Marion Star*, 13 Jan 1968.
67. Letter, Schimmoler L., to Bucyrus Hist. Society, 9 June 1970.
68. Schimmoler, L., "Upon my departure to Post Everlasting," BHS.
69. Letter, Mickie Grinevich to Robert Skinner, 4 Feb 1982.
70. "Schimmoler, Lauretta" *Bucyrus Telegraph-Forum*, 24 Jan 1981.
71. "Monument Dedicated for Schimmoler," *Bucyrus Telegraph-Forum*, 7 Sep 2014.
72. Letter, Roberta Steinbacher to Alberta Brown, 1 Nov 1985.

Chapter 4

1. Preston, D., "Nursing School's Founder was Pilot, Army Nurse," unnamed newspaper clipping, 13 Feb 1985.
2. "Detroiter Receives Ideal Job," unnamed clipping, 6 Oct 1942.

3. Document from Ellis Historical Society exhibit, 2017.
4. Knight, G. Alan, "Leora B. Stroup," *On Point: The Journal of Army History*, Vol.16 No.1, 2010.
5. "Leora B. Stroup, RN," *Personal Resume*, 1956, FHSU.
6. Ibid.
7. "More Notes on Miss Leora B. Stroup," 25 Apr 1958, Forsyth Library Collections, FHSU.
8. Crain, M. Aileen, "Leora B. Stroup, RN," *Flashes*, 1939.
9. Spangler, Robert J., "News From Fort Hays," Stroup Interview, 15 Apr 1958, Forsyth Library Collections, FHSU.
10. "More Notes on Miss Leora B. Stroup."
11. "New Member," *Airwoman*, Mar 1935.
12. "N. Central, Cleveland," *News Letter, Ninety-Nines*, June 1936.
13. "Leora B. Stroup, RN," Personal Resume.
14. "Training Center for Nurses Will Be Opened Wednesday," *Detroit Free Press*, 31 Oct 1937, 5.
15. "Flying Nurse," *Montana Butte Standard*, 13 Feb 1938, 58.
16. Interview with Olive Hay, "Leora B. Stroup: A Legacy Lives On," 16 Oct 1966., Forsyth Library Collections, FHSU.
17. "Aerial Nurse Corps Head to Speak Here," *Lansing State Journal*, 28 Jan 1942, 9.
18. "Colonel Inspecting Air Nurses," *Detroit Times*, 2 Feb 1939.
19. "To Tell Nurse Role," *Lansing State Journal*, 3 Feb 1942, 2.
20. "CWVS Board Pans Tea to Consider Defense," *Detroit Free Press*, 18 Jan 1942.
21. "Three Aerial Nurse Pioneers Reunited at Bowman Field," *The Courier-Journal*, 2 Mar 1943.
22. "Ex-Clevelander Foresaw Air Evacuation Need," non-dated, unnamed news clipping, FHSU.
23. Spangler, Robert J., "News From Fort Hays."
24. "2 Flying Grandmothers Lead Detroit Flight Here," *The Courier-Journal*, 9 Jul 1944, 1.
25. www.ncbi.nlm.nih.gov/pmc/articles/PMC5651504/, accessed 27 Aug 2020.
26. "Detroiter is Only Nurse Teaching Air Evacuation," *Detroit Free Press*, 2 Apr 1943.
27. "Unique Reunion Planned Today at KC Honoring Leora Stoup," *The Hays Daily News*, 07 Oct 1962,1.
28. Spangler, Robert J., "News From Fort Hays."
29. Murphy, Clara Morrey, "Air Evacuation—World War II—African-European Theater," First unabridged draft of speech, 12 Nov 1992.
30. Stroup, L.B. "Aero-Medical Nursing," *American Journal of Nursing*, Vol. 4. No. 6, June 1944, 575-577.
31. Ibid.
32. "Pioneer Flight Nurses Returns," *Courier-Journal*, 28 Aug 1944.

33. Knight, G. Alan, "Leora B. Stroup," *On Point, Journal for Army History*, Vol.16 No.1, 2010.
34. "Unique Reunion Planned Today at KC Honoring Leora Stoup."
35. "30 Pair of Eyes Follow Nurse Across the Ocean," *New York World-Telegram*, 11 May 1945.
36. "Miss Leora Stroup First Civilian Nurse in Korea," untitled newspaper clipping, n.d., Forsyth Library Collections, FHSU.
37. "She Recalls Another Hostage Release," *The Hays Daily News*, 22 Jan 1981, 3.
38. Stroup, Leora, "Untitled handwritten account of her air evacuation escort of the POW nurses in 1945," n.d., AMEDD.
39. "After Helping to Organize Original Flight Nurses," *Great Bend Tribune*, 16 Oct 1966.
40. "Former Flight Nurse Has Led Exciting Life Here and Abroad," *Lansing State Journal*, 30 Dec 1954, 9.
41 "Trumball Woman Heads Nurses Doing Air Evacuation of Pacific Wounded," *Ohio Nurse Review*, Oct 1945.
42. Ibid.
43. "Miss Leora Stroup First Civilian Nurse in Korea," unnamed newspaper clipping, n.d., Forsyth Library Collections, FHSU
44. Ibid.
45. "Cleveland Nurse Wins Air Medal," *News*, 13 May 1947, Forsyth Library Collections, FHSU.
46. "More Notes on Miss Leora B. Stroup."
47. "Leora B. Stroup, RN," Personal Resume.
48. Letter, Stroup to Dear All, 15 Nov 1952, Forsyth Library Collections, FHSU.
49. "Leora B. Stroup, RN," Personal Resume.
50. "Preston, D., "Nursing School's Founder was Pilot, Army Nurse."
51. "Large Gift Will Finance FHS Faculty Chair," *Salina Journal*, 27 Mar 1968.
52. "Leora Stroup Builds With Firm Hand."
53. "Purely Personal," *Hays Daily*, 28 July 1961, Forsyth Library Collections, FHSU.
54. "Taking Time Out Between Performances," *Great Bend Daily Tribune*, 02 July 1967.
56. "Nurses Elect Hays Woman," *Salina Journal*, 14 Sep 1959.
57. "Leora B. Stroup, RN," Personal Resume.
58. "Nursing School's Founder was Pilot, Army Nurse."
59. Letter, Stroup to Dear All.
60. "Profile of Leora Belle Stroup," 20 Apr 1978, Forsyth Library Collections, FHSU.
61. "Unique Reunion Planned Today at KC Honoring Leora Stoup," *The Hays Daily News*, 7 Oct 1962, 1.
62. Letter from Leora Stroup to Agnes Arrington, 20 Feb 1968.

63. Rodgers, Katherine, Untitled paper, 1 Nov 1968, FHSU.
64. "Record Number of Men Nursing Students at Hays," *Salina Journal*, 10 Sep 1970.
65. "Program Aids Doctor-less Towns," *Salina Journal*, 16 Sep 1970.
66. Kohler, Scott, "The Development of the Nurse Practitioner and Physician Assistant Professions" *The Commonwealth Fund*, Robert Wood Johnson Foundation, and Carnegie Corporation of New York, 1965.
67. *The 1956 Reville of Fort Hays Kansas State College*," 1956, 136.
68. "Army Flight Nurse to Tell Her Story at Rotary Ladies Night," *Coopersville Observer*, Vol. 71, n.d.
69. "Funerals," *Great Bend Tribune*, 12 Feb 1973.
70. Document from Ellis Historical Society Exhibit, 2017.
71. "Activities center requested," *The Salina Journal*, 4 Dec 1974, 2.
72. "Area Aging Agencies Honor Leora Stroup," *The Hays Daily News*, 30 May 1975, 5.
73. "Heads Together," *The Hays Daily News*, 06 Feb 1976, 5.
74. "Ecarta," *The Hays Daily News*, 8 Feb 1977, 5.
75. "Meals program set for NWK senior citizens," *The Salina Journal*, 20 Dec 1973, 23.
76. "Hays Woman Cited for Senior Citizen Service," *The Hays Daily News*, 28 May 1975, 3.
77. Leora Stroup Papers, AMEDD.
78. "Art Department believes in value...," 7 Nov 1966, http://bigcat.fhsu.edu/currentevents/display_event.php?id=2913, accessed 2 May 2020.
79. Fleming, L. "Selections from the Leora Stoup Collection," unpublished thesis, Dec 2005, (Oklahoma State University).
80. Notes from the Exhibition, Kakemono of Japan, Leora Stroup Papers, 1983, Forsyth Library Collections, FHSU.
81. "Korean Pottery to Hays Museum," *The Salina Journal*, 22 Aug 1960, 15.
82. "Korean Ceramics of the Koryo and Yi Dynasties, " Information card, Stroup Archive, Forsyth Library Collections. Source unidentified.
83. "YMCA Members Model Kimonos," unnamed clipping, n.d.
84. Spangler, Robert J., "News From Fort Hays."
85. Ibid.
86. Rodgers, Katherine, "Leora Left her Mark on Hays," unnamed newspaper clipping, 2 Feb 1985.

Chapter 5

1. *Aerial Nurse Corps*, 1940.
2. *Company Commander's Handbook*, 2 July 1938.
3. Ibid.
4. "Prospectus" *Aerial Nurse Corps of America*.
5. Ibid.

6. "Aerial Nurse Corps Prepares," *Flashes,* 1940.
7. "Unit of Aerial Nurses Formed by Local Young Woman," unnamed newspaper clipping, n.d., MMM.
8. "Flying Nurses Train," *Detroit Evening News,* 2 Feb 1939.
9. "Great Lakes Breezes," *Flashes,* July 1939.
10. Ibid.
11. Non-titled, unnamed newspaper clipping, 3 Sep 1938, MMM.
12. https://.airman.dodlive.mil/2018/05/03/icon-of-airmanship.html, accessed 12 Aug 2018.
13. "Stewardess," *Flashes,* Feb 1938.
14. *Aerial Age Weekly,* Vol XV, No. 1, 13 Mar 1922, 417.
15. Ibid.
16. "Air Nurses Train for Flights of Mercy," *Journal-Herald Spotlight,* 9 July 1939.
17. Ibid.
18. Ibid.
19. Hamilton-Patterson, James, *Marked for Death,* (Pegasus Books, May 2015).
20. Ibid.
21. www.dayton.com/news/special-reports/what-store-for-downtown-dayton-fidelity-building/XPfbMxtAds1sJ5Du5O8gZL/, 22 July 2018.
22. Unnamed clipping, MMM scrapbook, 25 Sep 1938.
23. "Ford to Dine with Wright," unnamed clip, n.d., MMM.
24. "Progress," *Flashes,* Nov 1938, 2.
25. Ibid.

Chapter 6

1. "Merle McGriff, RN," *Flashes,* 1938.
2. Ibid.
3. "Aerial Nurses Given Flying Instructions," unnamed clip, n.d., BHS.
4. Letter from Merle McGriff McAfee to Judy McAfee Johnson, n.d.
5. "Named to Hospital Staff," *Evening Independent,* n.d.
6. United States Census, 1920.
7. "General Headquarters," *Flashes,* Apr 1938.
8. Norman, Elizabeth, *We Band of Angels,* (Random House, 1999).
9. Monahan, Evelyn, *All This Hell,* (Univ. Press of Kentucky, 2003).
10. www.ancestery.com, accessed 26 Sep 2022.
11. www.corregidorisland.com.ph, accessed 26 Sep 2022.
12. "Ruth G. Mitchell" *Flashes,* Feb 1940.
13. Ibid.
14. Jezierski, M., "Mickie Grinevich: Air evac nurse in World War II and in Korea," *Journal of Emergency Nursing,* Aug 1995, 365.
15. Ibid.
16. Ibid.

17. Skinner, Robert, "The Roots of Flight Nursing: Lauretta Schimmoler and The Aerial Nurse Corps of America," *Aviation, Space and Environmental Medicine*, Jan 1984.
18. *The Story of Air Evacuation 1942-1989*, (WWII Flight Nurses Assoc., 1989), 137.
19. Jezierski, M., "Mickie Grinevich: Air evac nurse in World War II and in Korea."
20. *The Story of Air Evacuation 1942-1989*.
21. Ibid.
22. "MacLauchlan is Named to Lead Nurses," *Decatur Daily Review*, 19 Dec 1942, 10.
23. "Vital Advice by an Oregon Nurse," *Albany Democrat-Herald*, 27 Jun 1959, 6.
24. "Moody Wins State Fair Air Tour," *The Pantagraph*, 9 Aug 1940.
25. "15 Decatur Girls Form Aerial Nurse Corps Unit," *The Decatur Herald*, 7 Oct 1940.
26. "New Chapters," *Ninety Nine Newsletter*, Mar 1940.
27. "Miss Waples, Lewis to Represent Decatur," *The Decatur Daily Review*, 13 Aug 1940.
28. "Two Nurses Buy Airplane," *Decatur Daily Review*, 5 Sep 1940.
29. "Clovers for Luck," *Decatur Daily Review*, 7 Jun 1941, 10.
30. "MacLauchlan is Named to Lead Nurses."
31. "State Nurses, District Nine, to Meet Here Next Saturday," *The Decatur Herald*, 26 Feb 1941.
32. "Brief Stays Urged On Hospital Patients," *Decatur Daily Review*, 22 Jan 1943, 28.
33. "Nurse Shortage Nearing Crisis Stage Here," *Decatur Daily Review*, 4 Apr 1943, 3.
34. "Nursing Class Exams," *Decatur Daily Review*, 28 Dec 1943.
35. "D.M.C.H. Seeks Student Nurses for Fall Classes," *Decatur Herald* 26 Jul 1943.
36. "Presented a Permanent Patient," *Decatur Herald*, 26 Jul 1943.
37. "Nurse Shortage Called Critical," *Decatur Herald*, 26 Jul 1943, 3.
38. *University of Oregon Medical School Catalog*, 1945-1948, OR.
39. *Thesis and Dissertations, 1943-1959*, Oregon State College, OR.
40. "Eugene Nurses Hear of Program, Flight Training," *Eugene Guard*, 27 May 1948, 11.
41. Ibid.
42. "Flying Nurse Served Here," *Decatur Daily Review*, 15 Nov 1948.
43. "Oregon Chapter," *Ninety-Nines Newsletter*, 15 Feb 1948.
44. Ibid.
45. "Oregon Chapter," *Ninety-Nines Newsletter*, 15 Feb 1948.
46. "Air Markers for 100 Cities," *Daily Times*, 12 Oct 1956, 12.
47. "Roster as of Dec 31 1948," *Ninety-Nines Newsletter*, Jan 1949.
48. "Oregon Chapter," *Ninety-Nines Newsletter*, 15 Apr 1949.

49. Waples Smith, G., *Care of the Patient with a Stroke*, (New York, Springer Publishing Co. Inc, Mar 1959).
50. "Vital Advice by an Oregon Nurse," *Albany Democrat-Herald*, 27 Jun 1959, 6.
51. Waples Smith, G., *Care of the Patient with a Stroke*.
52. "Interesting people here for convention of ONA," *Bend Bulletin*, 1 Oct 1959, 6.
53. "Nurses Receive Diplomas," *Milwaukee Journal*, 27 Aug 1936.
54. "Mother in Auto," *Chicago Tribune*, 7 Sep 1938.
55. "Aerial Nurse Corps Being Organized Here," *Milwaukee Sentinel*, 10 July 1940.
56. "Nurses Will Study Effects of War Gas," *Milwaukee Sentinel*, 13 Apr 1941, A-7.
57. "Confer with Director," *Milwaukee Sentinel*, 30 Jan 1941.
58. www.legendsofflightnurses.org, accessed 21 Jun 2021.
59. "New Officers Named by Jane Delano Post," *Milwaukee Journal*, 12 June 1947.
60. www.emke.uwm.edu/entry/veterans, accessed 30 Jan 2021.
61. "Yippee! 103 Planes Round Up 46,000 New Legion Members," *Milwaukee Sentinel*, 12 Nov 1947.
62. "MATS Makes Mercy Flight," *Sunday Light*, San Antonio, Texas, 30 Oct 1949.
63. "Air Unit Plans an Open House."
64. "Woman's Way," *Montgomery Adviser*, 2 Aug 1959.
65. "Social Events Take Place at Eglin AFB," *Pensacola News Journal*, 23 Nov 1960.
66. "Poise for Flight," *Montgomery Advertiser*, 25 Jul 1963.
67. "Air Forces Flying Nurses," *Milwaukee Sentinel*, 2 Feb 1968.
68. "Flyers Visit Manitowoc," *Manitowoc Herald Times* 7 Mar 1970.
69. "Women Pilots Meet Here," *La Crosse Tribune*, 16 Aug 1970.
70. "Wisconsin Chapter," *99 News*, May/June 1974.
71. Thomasson, W. "Wife, Mother, Nurse and Pilot," *Southern Flight*, Oct 1938.
72. United States Federal Census, 1910.
73. bratenahlhistorical.org/index.php/school-year-1908-09, accessed 7 Nov 2020.
74. Barille, Ann, "Sketch of Florence Boswell," *Ninety Nine Newsletter*, Sep 1939.
75. Ibid.
76. "Personal Mention," *Cleveland Plain Dealer*, 22 Apr 1934, 2.
77. "Modern Mother Uses Plane for Busy Week's Engagement," *Cleveland Plain Dealer*, 17 Jul 1939.
78. *Report of the Second Annual Meeting of the National Association of Nurse Anesthetists*, Nat. Assoc. of Nurse Anesthetists, 25-27 Sep 1934.
79. Barille, Ann, "Sketch of Florence H. Boswell."

80. "New Assignments," *Flashes*, May 1938.
81. "Roster of Personnel, Aerial Nurse Corps of America," n.d.
82. "Good Will Planes Today," *Cleveland Plain Dealer* 26 Aug 1938.
83. Don Patrick, letter to Edythe Maxim, 24 June 1979.
84. "New Assignments," *Flashes*, May 1938.
85. "Lightening Bolt Hit Plane," unnamed clipping, n.d., BHS.
86. "Cleveland Woman Plane Hit by Lightning," *Flashes*, May 1938.
87. "Women's History in Northeast Ohio," www.wrhs.org, accessed 20 Oct 2018.
88. "All-Ohio Chapter," *Ninety Nine Newsletter*, Sep 1939.
89. "News from the Sections," *News 99 Letter*, Apr 1937.
90. "Heard Over Teacups," *Cleveland Plain Dealer*, 11 May 1941.
91. "Wins Air Prize," *Cleveland Plain Dealer*, 7 Mar 1941.
92. Barille, Ann, "Sketch of Florence H. Boswell."
93. Ibid.
94. Ibid.
95. "Judges Named for $100 Air Quiz," *Plain Dealer*, 3 Mar 1940.
96. "Heard Over Teacups," *Cleveland Plain Dealer*, 2 Feb 1941.
97. "United States Women in Aviation 1930-1939," (Smithsonian Institution Press 1985).
98. "Calls Ohio Women to Defense Work," *Cleveland Plain Dealer* 26 Mar 1941.
99. "Calls Women to Join Defense Unit," *Plain Dealer*, 24 Jun 1941.
100. www.twudigital.contentdm.oclc.org/digital/collection/p214coll2/id/4141/, accessed 3 Jun 2021.
101. "They Share Top Honors With Service Men," *Cleveland Plain Dealer*, 26 Sept 1942, 12.
102. "Achievements of Florence Boswell," International Womens Air & Space Museum.
103. Ibid.
104. Ohio Sterberegister, 1938-2018.
105. *Fort Lauderdale News*, unnamed news clipping, 20 Aug, 1941.
106. "The Leaf Fan," *Fort Lauderdale News*, 27 Feb 1941.
107. "Ft. Lauderdale Woman Fliers," *Miami News*, 26 Sep 1944.
108. "Major Mayes Awarded Medal for Gallantry," *Fort Lauderdale News*, 18 Oct 1945.
109. "Fay Mayes, Author, Pilot," *Fort Lauderdale News*, 17 Dec 1975.
110. www.nrotc.org/blue.star.mem.hwy.htm, accessed 28 Jan 2021.
111. "Fay Mayes, Author, Pilot," *Fort Lauderdale News*.
112. "Roster of Personnel, Aerial Nurse Corps of America," n.d.
113. Schafroth, Grace, *Flashes*, June 1939.
114. "Student Decorum Approved," *San Diego Union*, 21 Nov 1939.
115. Gans, Eric Lawrence, *Carole Landis: A Most Beautiful Girl*, (Univ. Press of Mississippi, 2008).
116. Ibid.

117. *Tampa Bay Times*, 1943, 11.
118. Ibid.
119. "Landis in War," untitled magazine, 12 May 1942, BHS.
120. "Stars Help Set the Pace for Civilian War Work," *Joplin News Herald*, 29 Apr 1942, 3.
121. Ibid.
122. www.worthpoint.com/worthopedia/bundles-britain-bluejackets-america-127309536, accessed 22 Sep 2022.
123. Gans, Eric Lawrence, *Carole Landis: A Most Beautiful Girl*.
124. "Record Breaking Crowd," *The National Legionnaire*, Oct 1941, 3.
125. Flemings, E.J., *Hollywood Death and Scandal Sites*, (McFarland and Company, North Carolina, 2015), 269.
126. Landis, C., *Four Jills in a Jeep*, (Random House, NY, 1944).
127. www.rtv2-production-2-6.rottentomatoes.com/m/four_jills_in_a_jeep, accessed 22 Sep 2022.
128. www.carolelandis.net/2012/11/carole-and-tommys-wedding.html, accessed 22 Sep 2022.
129. www.en.wikipedia.org/wiki/Carole_Landis, 22 Sep 2022.
130. Fleming, E. J., *Carole Landis: A Tragic Life in Hollywood*, (McFarland and Company, North Carolina, 2005).
131. www.projects.latimes.com/hollywood/star-walk/carole-landis/index.html, accessed 22 Sep 2022.
132. www.walkoffame.com/carole-landis, accessed 22 Sep 2022.
133. Oral History Office, Columbia University, *Reminiscence of Ellen Church*, 1960.
134. Ibid.
135. www.iowapbs.org/iowapathways/mypath/2493/ellen-church-nurse.
136. Steve Stimpson at the 25th Anniv. Stewardess Luncheon, UAL.
137. First Airline Stewardess is Pioneer Flight Nurse," *Esu Claire Leader*, 24 Mar 1945, 4.
138. "Aerial Nurses Will Study Sky Ambulance," *Milwaukee Sentinel*, 19 Oct 1940, 7.
139. "Louisville Director of Nurses Originated Air Hostess Idea," *Courier-Journal*, 9 July 1041, 11.
140. "Kitties Also Have Their Ups and Downs In Life," *Courier-Journal*, 20 July 1942, 68.
141. Ibid.
142, "History of 802nd MAES", *The Story of Air Evacuation 1942-1989*, 1989,71.
143. "Airline Stewardess Dean Back Form Combat Areas," *Tampa Bay Times*, 8 Apr 1945, 16.
144. www.thisdayinaviation.com/tag/ellen-church-marshall.
145. Sarkar, Dipa, "Church Flew to New Heights," *Tribune-Star*, n.d.
146. Bennet, Mark, "Discarded tribute rekindles memories of aviation pioneer," *Tribune-Star*, 29 Sep 2019.

147. Sarkar, Dipa, "Church Flew to New Heights."
148. www.flyingmuseum.com/hall-of-fame, accessed 13 Jan 2023.
149. www.aircharterserviceusa.com, accessed 13 Jan 2023.
150. "Airport Dedication," *Lime Springs Herald,* 17 Jul 1975.
151. "Iowa Chapter," *Ninety-Nine News,* Jul 1975.
152. "Airport Dedication at Cresco," *Lime Spring Herald.*
153. "Three Aerial Nurse Pioneers Reunited at Bowman Field," *The Courier-Journal,* 2 Mar 1943.
154. "Army Nurse Hitch-Hikes Home by Plane," *Detroit Free Press,* 17 Aug 1942, 9.
155. "Army Nurse Sprouts Wings in the Air Evacuation Unit," *Detroit Free Press,* 23 May 1943, 50.
156. Interview by Judith Barger with Mary Christian, 21 May 1966, accessed 3 Mar 2023.
157. Author interview with Bev Giffin, 3 Mar 2023.
158. Barger, Judith, *Beyond the Call of Duty,* (Kent State University Press, Kent, Ohio, 2013).
159. Ibid.
160. *The Story of Air Evacuation, 1942-1989.*
161. Barger, Judith, *Beyond the Call of Duty.*

Chapter 7

1. www.aneskey.com, accessed 21 Feb 2021.
2. Dolev, Eran, "The First Recorded Aeromedical Evacuation in the British Army," *J R Army Med Corps,* 1986, 34-36.
3. www.sps-aviation.com/ story/?id=1359, accessed 21 Jan, 2023.
4. "Airwomans Flying Ambulance," *Sydney Herald,* 6 Nov 1939.
5. www.wanderwomenproject.com/women/marie-marvingt, accessed 21 Jan 2023.
6.. https://www.flyingdoctor.org.au/news/sugar-bird-lady, accessed 21 Feb 2021.
7. www.ninety-nines.org/userfiles/file/Nancy_Bird_Walton.pdf.
8. Kolp, Jimmie, "Ninety-Nine Newsletter," June 1939.
9. www.royalfarwest.org.au/about-us/our-history, 21 Jan 2023.
10. *Flashes,* July 1939.
11. Heath, L., "Women's Activities," *Popular Aviation,* May 1932, 308.
12. "Aeronautics: Jumping Nurse," *Time,* 23 Sep 1932.
13. www.historynet.com/clyde-pangborn-and-hugh-herndon-jr-first-to-fly-nonstop-across-the-pacific, accessed 21 Jan 2023.
14. https://aerospaceblog.wordpress.com/2011/05/29/gladys-bramhall-wilner, accessed 3 Mar 2023.
15. https://susquehannavalley.blogspot.com/2022/06, 3 Mar 2023.
16. "Edna Newcomer and the American Nurse Plane," *Pittsburgh Press,* 15 Dec 1934.

17. "The Latest Atlantic Flight," *Flight Magazine*, 16 Sep 1932, 874.
18. www.forgottenstories.net/2014/08/10/tailwind, 21 Feb 2021.
19. Ibid.
20. Nichols, Ruth, *Wings for Life*, (J.P. Lippincott, 1 Jan 1957), 267.
21. "Ambulance Planes for Civilians," *New York Times*, 22 Dec 1941.
22. Letter from Nichols to Schimmoler, 5 Dec 1941.
23. Ruth Nichols Collection, IWASM.
24. Letter from Major Earl Johnson to Office of the Civilian Defense, 20 July 1940.
25. Ruth Nichols Collection, IWASM.
26. Markham, Beryl, *West with the Night*, (Houghton Mifflin Company, Boston, MA, 1942).
27. Lovell, Mary S., *Straight on Till Morning: The Life of Beryl Markham*, (St. Martins Press, New York, NY, 1987).
28. "Pilot-Nurse Operates First Air Hospital Service," *Los Angeles Times*, 14 Apr 1937, part II.
29. "Plane as Ambulance," *Los Angeles Times*, 8 Dec 1937, part I.
30. https://sas-amb.com/aboutus.html, accessed 9 Jun 2023.
31. "Dawn Graves First Nurse," *Loma Linda Nurse*, Fall 2022, 30.
32. www.mercyflight.org/history-of-ems, accessed 13 Jul 2023.
33. www.csiaviation.com, accessed 13 Jul 2023.
34. www.airmedicaljournal.com, accessed 15 Jul 2023.

BIBLIOGRAPHY

Barger, Judith, Beyond the Call of Duty, Kent State University Press, Kent, OH, 2013.
Fleming, E. J., Carole Landis: A Tragic Life in Hollywood, McFarland and Company, Jefferson, NC, 2005.
Flemings, E.J., Hollywood Death and Scandal Sites, McFarland and Company, Jefferson, NC, 2015.
Gans, Eric Lawrence, Carole Landis: A Most Beautiful Girl, University Press of Mississippi, MS, 2008.
Kane, Joseph, Famous First Facts and Records, Ace Books, 1975.
Kessler, Lauren, The Happy Bottom Riding Club: The Life and Times of Poncho Barnes, Random House, NY, 2010.
Landis, Carole., Four Jills in a Jeep, Random House, NY, 1944.
Link, M.M and Coleman, H. A. Medical Support of the Army Air Forces In World War II, Office of the Surgeon General, 1955.
Lovell, Mary S., Straight on Till Morning: The Life of Beryl Markham, St. Martins Press, New York, NY, 1987.
Markham, Beryl, West with the Night, Houghton Mifflin Company, Boston, MA, 1942.
Mayes, Fay McWhorter, Public Relations and Publicity Pointers, National Council of State Garden Clubs, 1963.
Miller Robin, Flying Nurse, Rigby Publishing, AU, 1971.
Miller, Robin, Sugarbird Lady, Landsdown, Sidney, AU, 1979.
Monahan, Evelyn, All This Hell, University Press of Kentucky, KY, 2003.
Nichols, Ruth, Wings for Life, J.P. Lippincott, Philadelphia, PA, 1957.
Norman, Elizabeth, We Band of Angels, Random House, NY, 1999.
Pearce, Carol A, Amelia Earhart, Facts on File, NY, 1988.
Snook, Neta, I Taught Amelia Earhart to Fly, Vantage Press, NY, 1973.
Schimmoler, Lauretta, ANCOA Regulations Manual, Burbank, CA, 1940.
Planck, Charles E. Women with Wings, Harper & Brothers, NY, 1942.
Rufus, Maude Squire, Flying Grandma or Going Like Sixty, University Lithoprinters, Ann Arbor, MI, 1942.
Thaden, Louise, High, Wide, and Frightened, Stackpole Sons, NY, 1938.
Waples Smith, G., Care of the Patient with a Stroke, Springer Publishing, NY, 1959.
Whyte, Edna Gardner, Rising Above It: An Autobiography, Crown Publishing Group, NY, 1991.
WWII Flight Nurses Assoc, The Story of Air Evacuation 1942-1989, 1989.

INDEX

1st Division, 49, 58, 71, 192
1st Wing, 71, 192
2nd Division, 58, 71, 204
2nd Wing, 71, 232
3rd Division, 58, 71, 204
3rd Wing, 71, 204, 232
4th Division, 58, 71, 204
5th Division, 58, 71-72, 156, 158, 206, 276
6th Division, 58, 71, 232
7th Division, 58, 71, 232
8th Division, 58, 71, 232
9th Division, 58, 71
25th Anniversary, Flight Nursing, 117, 144, 177-179
40et8, 210
50th Anniversary, School of Aerospace Medicine, 144, 177
349th Air Evacuation Group, 158, 166
801st MAETS, 252, 262
802nd MAETS, 291, 262
805th MAETS, 299-300
806th MAETS, 298
814th MAETS, 266
828th MAES, 178
1453rd MATS, 254

A

Act first-then talk, vi, 78, 143
actors, 43, 49, 122-125, 284-285
ad/per aspera ad astra 231
aerial message bombs, 77
Aeronca airplane, 29, 115-117, 225, 262
Aerial Roundup, 135, 267
Aerospace Nursing/Medicine, 140-141, 144
Aero Squadron, Sheriff's, 76-78, 106, 111, 126, 113-114
air ambulances, 30, 34, 40, 52, 64, 68, 71, 79, 81-82, 90, 93-94, 121, 128-129, 137, 142-143, 158, 221, 260, 303-317
Air Congresses, 79
Aircraft Owners and Pilots, 312
Air Evacuation School, 189
Air Force, United States, 44, 61, 79, 112, 121, 126-128, 136, 138-139-144, 158, 162, 177, 219, 233, 252-256, 260, 262, 266-268, 275, 280, 285, 303
Air Mail, 31-32, 143

airmarkers, 17-18, 263,
air meets, 24, 28, 64, 78, 93, 235
airports/flying fields, 6-11, 16-20, 23-28, 32-33, 40-47, 50, 59, 70-71, 79, 84, 104, 115-119, 126, 135, 147, 152-153, 168-170, 209, 220-227, 143, 263, 271, 293-296, 308
airport manager, 6-8, 110
air races/air shows, 13-17, 21-24, 28, 30, 33-34, 39, 41-49, 55, 64, 72, 74, 81, 119, 136, 153, 216-217, 226-230, 238-240, 271, 274, 310,
Air Raid Warden, 284
Air Transport, 12, 31, 40-42, 52, 58-63, 68-71, 76, 80, 95, 100, 115, 129, 139, 155-161, 165, 170, 210, 220-221, 233, 253, 266-268, 271, 276, 288-191, 300, 303-317
Alaska, 267, 299-300
Alpha Eta Rho (AHP), 37
Allison, Captain, 210-211
American Legion, 78, 84, 131-135, 145-146, 187, 210, 267, 284
American Nurses Association (ANA), 58-60, 99, 103, 121, 176, 266, 277
American Nurses Aviation Service, 310-311
American Women's Voluntary Services, 274, 276
ANC (Army Nurse Corps), 55, 58-64, 95-98, 120-121, 140, 169, 179, 246, 252, 266, 280, 298
ANCOA Board of Governors, 58, 75
ANCOA car, 227-228,
ANCOA chevrons, 56-57
ANCOA flag, 109, 190, 120, 122-123, 207
ANCOA General Headquarters (GHQ)/National Headquarters, 51-52, 59, 65, 67, 70-71, 90, 235-236
ANCOA mascots/logos, 191, 194, 198-201, 206-207, 215, 231
ANCOA National Theme Song, 190-191
ANCOA *Regulations Manual*, 54, 57, 6,
Annette Gipson Air Race, 310
Army Air Force, United States, 121, 128, 136, 138, 162, 252, 262, 266
Arrington, Lt. Colonel, Agnes M. 139-140, 177
Arnold, Brigadier General Henry (Hap) 61, 136, 139, 141, 233, 253
Australian air ambulances, 306-309
Australian Inland Mission Aerial Medical Service, 306
Aviation Ball, 229
Aviation Emergency Corps, National, 104-107, 110, 122-123, 281-282
Aviation First Aid Duty Manual, 85
Aviation Medicine, 90, 158, 162, 310
awards, 73, 113, 126, 130, 132, 135, 141, 148, 173, 181, 255, 258, 268, 276 293, 305, 308, 310, 312

B

Badger, Gladyce L., 99-100
Bal des Avions, 196-197
Baran, Lt. Anne, 161
Barnes, Poncho, 30, 33
Barran, Captain Nancy, 144
Bataan, Phillipines, 246-248
Beard, Mary, 95-101
Bellanca CH-400 airplane, Miss Veedol/American Nurse, 310
Bendix Race, 42-47, 51
Betsey Ross Flying Corps, 21
Bird, Nancy, 307-309
blanket flying permit, 262
blind flying and radio-beam flying, 271
blood plasma, 159-160, 162
Blue Star Memorial Program, 278
Boeing Air Transport, 12, 40, 118, 219, 288-289
Bohannon, Colonel, 140-141
Bomber airplanes, 127, 211, 213, 219
Boswell, Florence, 214, 239, 269-277
Bowman Filed, 157-166, 177, 253, 298
Brown Derby Restaurant, 124
Bucyrus Institute of Aviation, 11, 14, 20-21
Bucyrus, Ohio, 2-28, 55, 145-148
Bundles for Blue Jackets, 283
Burbank, California, 30, 50-52, 70-71, 74, 126-127, 130, 236
Butler, Ida F., 59-61, 64, 95

C

C-54 airplane, 128-129, 136, 255
Cadet Nurse Program, 260-261
California State Nurses Association (CSNA), 60, 67, 97-102
call to the colors, 115, 280,
Case Western Reserve University, 152
cat elevator/Cap and Mittens, 290
certificates, 73-74, 181-182, 240-241,
Cessna airplane, 181, 269, 272-273, 276, 306
Chagrin Harbor Airport Ground School, 271
chemical irritants and chemical warfare, gases, 85-86, 119, 162, 265
Chicago, Illinois, 45, 71, 126, 174, 204, 265, 287, 293
chickens, 4, 18-19, 24, 146
Chief Nurse, 140, 161, 166, 168, 254-255, 268, 280
Chief of Staff, 97, 235-236, 245, 249
China, 166
Church, Ellen, 40, 137, 204, 287-296

Civil Aeronautics Administration, 126
Civil Air Patrol (CAP), 109-120, 126, 157, 159, 181.
Civil Defense, 112-113, 126, 136, 182, 194
civilian planes grounded in WWII, 110, 313
Cleveland, Ohio, 8, 14, 21, 23-30, 41, 55, 71-72, 102, 152-153, 183, 206, 214-217, 228, 238-239, 242, 269-277
Cleveland Institute of Aviation, 152-153
Cochran, Jacqueline, 153, 271, 315
Coleman, Hubert H., x, 136-138
College Women's Volunteer Service, 157
commercial airlines, 40, 110, 156, 209, 288
Company A-1, 39, 49, 58, 80, 88-89, 192-196, 236
Company B-1, 198
Company C-1, 199
Company D-1 200, 236
Company K-1, 201-201, 236
Company A-2, 204, 236
Company A-3, 204, 236
Company A-4, 204, 236
Company B-4, 204-205, 236, 265
Company C-4, 205, 236, 257
Company A-5, 151, 156, 206-213, 231, 236, 279
Company B-5, 214, 230, 236, 269
Company C-5, 88, 215-230, 236-237, 240
Company D-5, 231, 236, 240
Company E-5, 231
Company A-6, 232, 236
Company B-6, 232, 236
Company A-7, 232, 236
Company A-8, 232-233, 236, 251
Company Commanders, 55, 58, 78, 93, 189, 235-300
contests, 68, 84, 227, 258
Cooper, Margaret Perry, 7
Corns, Edith, 50, 192-193, 245-248
Corregidor Island, 168, 247248
crash wagons, 222-223
Cub/Piper Cub airplanes, 155, 243, 257, 259, 263
Curtiss airplanes, 12, 24, 211, 213, 220, 303

D

Dayton, Ohio, 3, 56, 71-72, 84 86-87, 106-107, 115, 189, 196, 206, 215-231, 236-244
Dayton Tri-Flyers Club, 229
Decatur, Illinois, 71, 205, 236, 257-261

degrees, academic, 152-153, 173, 175, 180, 183, 185, 250, 254, 257, 268, 270, 287
Defense, national/home/civilian, 63, 99, 102-106, 109-113, 118, 123, 126, 136, 157, 182, 274, 276
Delano, Jane, 267
Denver, Colorado 71, 79, 174, 176, 204, 276, 317
Department of Defense, 171
Department of Nursing, 182-183
detective, 135, 138
Detroit, Michigan, 71, 72, 84, 102, 119-120, 137, 151, 153, 156, 159, 150, 181, 206-213, 231, 236, 238, 279, 297-299
Douglas Airplanes, 104, 189, 211-213

E

Earhart, Amelia, vi, 7, 21, 23, 25-26, 30, 42-47, 51-52, 131-133, 135, 143, 147, 153, 268, 271, 310
Eggen, Raymond, 180-181, 187
Ruth, 30, 33
Ellen Church Field, 293-295
Emergency Flight Corps 27, 40, 59
expansion of air or gas in the body, 162

F

Fairfield-Suisun Air Force Base, 128
female Norse warriors, 314
Fill, Wanda, 51, 200, 236, 279-280
Fintak, Florence, 133, 137, 178, 204-205, 236, 265-268
first aid, 33, 41, 47, 50, 53, 60, 62, 68-69, 72, 77-78, 81, 85, 87-88, 90, 104-106, 110, 113, 115, 118-119, 152-157, 190-191, 195, 205, 214-217, 221, 227, 235, 237, 239-240, 274, 276, 282
First Ladies Flying Tour, 307
First Reserve of ARC, 58-60, 95, 100, 118
Fixed-wing, 305, 317
Flashes, 65-67, 71, 74, 81, 84, 88, 90, 92, 97, 126, 193-207, 215, 231-233, 258, 271, 274, 279
flight nurse, 127-128, 136-144, 157-158, 161-162, 166-168, 177-180, 235, 251-255, 260, 262, 266-268, 280, 297-301, 305, 313, 317
flight suit, Amelia Earhart, 131, 268
flight training, 18, 166, 224
Flikke, Major Julia, 61-64, 157
float, parade, 28, 44, 47, 183, 284
float, plane, 155

Florence H. Boswell's Flying Service, Inc., 272
Flying Boudoir, 23-24
flying clubs (see also Ninety-Nines), 12, 16, 20-21, 229, 312
flying grandmothers, 159
Flying Health Nurse, 262
fly-in (American Legion Roundup), 135, 267
flying lessons, 16, 152, 224-225, 243, 271, 287-288,
Fort Hays State College/University, 173-176, 180, 182-183, 185-186
Fort Lauderdale, Florida, 71, 232, 278
Four Horseman, 178
Four Jills in a Jeep, 284-285
Four Meaningful Events, 145
foxholes, 292

G

Gentry, Viola, 23
glider planes, 10, 12, 16, 22-24, 47, 255
Gregg Artists, Order of, 3-4
Grand Central Air Terminal, 35, 69, 110
Grand Marshall, homecoming, 183
Grant, Brigadier General David N.W., 121
Grinevich, Matilda "Mickie," 137-139, 142, 146, 232, 236, 251-256, 313
Guadalcanal, 170
Gudobba, Margaret, 137, 158, 206-208, 211, 228-229, 279, 297-298

H

Hammond, Alice, 119, 159
Hartung, Howard, 209
Hay, Olive, 152, 155, 164, 177, 187
headstones/gravesite, 147, 187, 244, 248, 256, 268, 277, 280, 286
Hickam Field, 166-169, 247-248, 254
Hollywood Walk of Fame, 286
Honolulu, Hawaii, (also see Hickam Field), 35, 110, 167, 170, 181, 263
honors and prizes 3, 22, 42, 55, 119, 126, 132, 134, 135, 138, 140-141, 148, 153, 177, 181-183, 196, 207, 248, 278, 309,
Hudson, Evelyn, 34-35, 44
Hurst, Lucille, 58, 71, 83-84, 198

I

incorporated, 74
industrial nurse, 238, 250, 254, 298, 299
iron lungs transport, 316

J

Japan/Japanese, 110, 167-168, 170, 172, 183, 185-186, 246-247, 276
Jenny (Curtiss JN) airplane, 7, 303-304
Johnstown, Pennsylvania, 71, 232, 236

K

Kakemono Scrolls, 183-185
Kansas, 3, 24, 25, 47, 173-176, 181-182, 313
Kentucky, 157, 231, 272, 290
kimonos, 183, 186
kits, first aid & flight 50, 69, 77, 191, 193, 221, 316
Kitchen Cabinet Orchestra, 79
Kittredge, Frances, air hospital 316
Klingensmith, Florence, 45
Korea/Korean, 171-173, 180, 183, 185-186, 252, 254-255, 267-268, 280
Kovach, Colonel, 127, 140
Kwajalein Island, 168, 170

L

La Cross Flyers Association, 268
La Jolla, California, 71, 192, 200,
Landis, Carole, 281-286
Las Vegas, Nevada, 139-142, 255
Law, Ruth, 287
Leopard Moth/Gypsy Moth airplane, 307-308, 315
Leyte Island, Philippines, 168, 247-248
Licensed Pilots, 13, 16, 21, 22-26, 28-35, 43, 45, 48, 117, 119, 127, 133, 154-155, 159, 209, 221, 224-225, 237, 257, 269, 278, 287, 305, 307, 310, 312, 315, 316
litters/stretchers, 68-69, 71, 79-80, 129, 160-161, 168, 220, 268, 291, 316
Lockheed Aircraft Corp., 34, 36, 40, 47, 70, 104, 131-132, 143, 211, 213
Loma Linda Helicopter Ambulance Service/Graves, Dawn, 317
Los Angeles, California, 7, 28, 30, 34-37, 39-48, 49, 70-71, 76-78, 84, 104-105, 111-113, 123-126, 138, 192-197, 245, 266, 282, 295, 308, 313, 315, 316
New Orleans, Louisiana, 44, 79, 250

M

Macready, Lt. John, 3
MAETS to MAES, 300
Markham, Beryl, 315

male nurses, 179-180
Mantz, Paul, 47, 51-52, 69,
Marsalis, Frances Harrell, 23-24
Martocci-Pisculli, Leon, 310-311
Marvingt, Marie, 305
Mayes McWhorter, Fay, 236, 278
McArthur, General, 171
McGriff McAfee, Merle, 75, 87, 93, 95, 106-107, 115, 189, 204, 206, 215-217-233, 236-244,
McLaglen, Victor, 40, 48-49, 122
medals, 113, 130, 173, 253, 255, 268, 292, 305, 308
Medical Aspects of Chemical Irritants, 85, 162
Medical Support of the Army Air Forces in World War II, xii, 138, 341
Memphis Belle airplane, 219
Miller, Robin, 306
Milwaukee, Wisconsin, 71, 204-205, 236, 265, 268, 287
Mines Field, Los Angeles, 28, 41-42, 44
Mitchell, Billy, 121, 139, 141-142, 267
Mitchell, Ruth G., 97, 236, 249-250,
model airplanes, gas & rubber-powered, 68, 84, 226, 227
Morgan, Captain Claude, 76, 113
Morgan, Captain Jane, (see also *Parachute Nurse*), 122-125
Morgan, Captain Robert, 218-219
mottos/logos 93, 133, 190, 194, 199-201, 206-207, 215, 231,
movies, 60, 64, 130, 132, 134-137, 202
movie stars, 43, 48-49, 122, 281
Musselman, Tim, 147

N

National Advisory Committee for Air Progress, 47, 76-77, 84, 227,
National Aerographic Academy, 73
National Aeronautic Association (NAA)/ Aero Club of America, 56, 74, 97, 237, 242, 273, 276-277, 312
National Air Races, 21-24, 28, 30, 33, 39, 41-48, 55, 72, 74, 81, 136, 216-217, 226, 229, 238-239, 271
National Korean Nurses Association, 172
National League of American Pen Women, 110, 277
National League of Nursing, 101
Navy Bureau of Aeronautics, 126, 130
Newbeck, Eileen, 137, 158, 206-207, 228, 297-300
Newcomer, Edna, 310311
New York, New York, 23-24, 42, 45, 59, 71, 95, 138, 170, 173, 209, 232-233, 236, 251-252, 254, 265-266, 310, 312-313
Nichols, Ruth (also see Relief Wings), 137, 312-314

Ninety-Nines/99s, 7, 17-18, 21, 25, 28, 30, 34, 48, 119, 132-133, 153, 258,
    261, 263-264, 267-268, 273, 276-278, 295, 308, 312
Non-Scheduled Instrument Rating, 271
Normandy during WWII, 268
Noyes, Blanche, 15, 18, 45-46, 153
Noyes, Clara, 59
nurse anesthetists, 270, 276
nurse-pilots, 93, 235, 237, 239, 257, 265, 269, 278, 287, 305, 306, 310, 316
nurse practitioner program, 180
Nurses' Aeronautical Digest, 67

O

Oak Leaf Cluster, 248, 253, 255
O'Brien, Adelade, 258
Office of the Surgeon General, 149-150
Ohio Women's Hall of Fame, 126, 148-149
O.J. Whitney, Inc, 71
Okinawa, 166, 170
One-Take Schimmoler, 125
Oregon State Nurses Association (OSNA), 261-261
original eight air hostesses (also see United Airline Stewardess), 287-289
Orphans Home Society, 84
Owen, Bessie, 34-35
oxygen, 3, 50, 87, 162, 315-316

P

Pacific Ocean area, 17, 34, 131, 161, 170, 254-255, 307, 310
Pacific Airmotive Corporation, 130, 135
paper airport flags, 170
parachutes, 23-24, 45, 47-48, 77-78, 110, 112, 122-124, 178, 217, 226,
    295, 298, 305, 310-311
Parachute Nurse, 123-125
parliamentary law, 278
Pasadena, California, 49, 71, 192-193, 198
Pearl Harbor, 110, 169-170, 246, 276, 280, 282, 298
Permanent Patient, 261
Philippines, 168, 246-248
Phoenix, Arizona, 44, 71, 192, 199
Pietenpol Air Camper airplane, 60 horsepower Corvair car engine, 294
pins/badges/patches, 1, 26, 37, 40, 49-50, 53-56, 92, 105-106, 111-114,
    118, 122-123, 129-130, 133-135, 141-142, 144, 151, 180, 237, 245,
    249, 268, 274-275, 281, 298, 283, 314
platoons, 123

Pope Air Force Base, 254-256
poppy sale for Disabled American Veterans, 297
Port Bucyrus/Bucyrus Municipal Airport, 6-24, 26, 37
Post #43, American Legion, Hollywood, 284
Post #181, American Legion, Colonel Crawford, 148
Post #127, American Legion, Glendale, 135
Post #408, American Legion, Jane Delano, 267
Post #678, American Legion, Amelia Earhart, 131-133, 143, 268
Post #674, American Legion, Windham, 187
POW nurses (prisoner of war), 168-170, 246-248
practical nurses, 120, 153
Presidents, 8, 25, 31-32, 51, 59, 72, 74, 97, 101-103, 119-120, 136, 140, 151, 157, 176, 181, 238, 249, 268, 270, 273, 276, 278, 293, 299
Put-in-Bay, 274

R

Radio Telephone Operator License, 91
raffle, round-trip flight, 209-210
Red Cross, 95-101, 110, 118-119, 121, 136, 141, 143, 152, 159, 260, 305
Relief Wings (see also Nichols, Ruth), 137, 232, 312-314
retired, 138, 180, 256, 268, 292
Rifle Auxiliary, 113
Rin Tin Tin, 155
Ripley's Believe It or Not! 170
Roundup, American Legion, (fly-in), 135, 267
Royal Flying Doctor Service, 306
Ruptured Duck, 130, 187
Ruth Chatterton Trophy 41-42

S

Saskatchewan, Regina, 316
San Diego, California, 34-35, 44, 52, 71, 192, 200, 236, 279
San Francisco, California, 71, 97, 168-169, 192, 249, 287-288
Sansone, Josephene, 137, 291
Santa Monica, California, 28, 49, 106, 192-193, 199, 236, 284
Sarasota, Florida 118, 232, 236
Schaefer, Louella/Schaefer Air Service, 316
Schimmoler, Lauretta, 1-37, 39-41, 48-51, 54-55, 61-64, 68-69, 73-81, 90, 94, 100, 102-106, 109-113, 119-121, 153, 155, 162, 177-178, 233
Scroggs House Museum/Bucyrus Historical Society 145-148
Seattle, Washington, 71, 118, 192, 201-203, 236
Selfridge Field, 211-213
Semper Paratus, 66

Senior Center, Hays, 181
Seversky airplane, 211
Sheriff, Los Angeles, (also see Aero Squadron) 76-78, 106, 111, 126, 113-114, 135, 138
Sikorsky helicopter, 317
Skinner, Robert E., ix, 252
Smith Waples, Genevieve, 118, 236, 257-264
Snook, Neta, 7
Snow White Airplane, 220-222, 242
solo flying, 6, 11, 51, 154, 243, 288
Southern California Aviation Medical Advisory Board, 52
Speed-O-Print machine, 65
Spitz Flight Recorder, 36, 82
Spoils Conferences, 31-32
Springfield Airport and Flying School, 224-225
Squadrons, 76-78, 110, 114, 115-117, 119, 159-160, 171, 189, 193, 198-199, 252-253, 266-267, 276, 285, 291, 298-299
stewardess/air hostess/Sky Girls, 40, 74, 196, 209, 219, 287-289, 291, 293, 296-297
Star Trek, 231
Stimpson, Steve, 288-289
Stinson family, 132-133, 207
Stinson airplanes, 29, 133, 271
stretchers/litters, 40, 68-69, 80, 115-117, 129, 160-161, 220-221, 252, 316
stroke (cerebrovascular accident), 146, 263-264
Stromme, Major J.L., 138-140
Stroup, Leora, 75, 91, 93, 102-103, 111, 118-120, 136-137, 151-187, 231, 209-212, 266, 271, 273, 279, 298-299, 301
Stroup, Leora B., Nursing Scholarship, 183
struck by lightning in a plane, Boswell, 272
stunt flyers, 30, 35, 47, 51-52, 133, 226-227, 238, 295,
Superintendents, 61, 95, 260, 263, 289

T

Temple, Shirley, 48-49
Thaden, Louise, 23, 25, 44-46,
The Angeles of Bataan and Corregidor, 247-248
They said it wouldn't be done, 129
Third-Class Radio license, 78, 91, 203
Tokyo, Japan, 167, 170-171
Tommy Drum Saloon, 176
Traffic Controller, 126
transport/evacuation plane, 63, 161-162, 165, 170
tricycle landing gear, 81

Turkey, first airplane for patient transport, 304
Twenty and Four, 134

U

uniforms, 33, 40, 49, 76, 92-93, 104, 111-112, 114, 119, 122, 127, 157, 159
    165, 169, 180, 193, 208, 219, 220, 228, 238-239, 275
Union Air Terminal, Burbank, 36, 51-52, 70-71, 79, 80, 104, 143
Union Hospital, Terra Haute, Indiana, 293
United Airlines Stewardess/Boeing, 287-289, 293
United Service Organization (USO), 284-285
United States Navy Bureau of Aeronautics, 126

V

Vi-Air-Ways, 8, 25-27, 102
Victory Caravan, 122
Victory Medal, 255, 268, 292
Vietnam War, 252, 254, 280
Von Hagenburg, Count Otto Heinrich, 238
VJ Day, 166-167

W

Waco airplanes, 4, 8, 10, 12, 29, 220
Walter Reed General Hospital, 157
War Operations, 126
Washington D.C., 232
watermanship and ditching, 267
Weskiva Youth Camp Fund, 278
Wilner, Gladys Bramhal, 310
Windham, Ohio, 152, 187
Wolfram, La Verne, 34-35
Woman of the Year Award, 181
Woman's Air Reserve (WAR), (also see Pancho Barnes), 33
Women's Air Force Service Pilots (WASP), 127, 260, 275
Women's Army Corps (WAC), 126-127
Women's Aviation Aeronautical Association, 78
Women's CAP Squadron, 119, 159
Women's Past Commanders Club, 134
Woodchuck named Tailwind, 311
World's Fair, 209-210
Wright Brothers & Wright Field, 24, 12, 61, 84, 141, 196, 219-222, 242-
    243, 312
Wright-Patterson Air Force Museum, 219

WWI, 133, 152, 210, 287, 297,
WWII, 68, 74, 110, 135-138, 159, 168, 173, 187, 219, 229, 244, 246, 251-254, 258, 260, 263, 265-266, 276, 278, 280, 282, 291-292, 309, 313-315

Z

Zip n' Zephyr, 259, 263

Archives utilized and their abbreviations

- Bucyrus Historical Society=BHS
- International Women's Air & Space Museum=IWASM
- Ellis County Historical Society
- Forsyth Library University Archives, Fort Hays State University=FHSU
- U.S. Army Heritage and Education Center
- Army Medical Education Department, Center of History & Heritage=AMEDD
- Special Collections & Archives, Wright State University.
- National Museum of the United States Air Force=NMUSAF
- Merle McGriff McAfee Scrapbooks=MMM
- The Smithsonian National Air and Space Museum

The author illustrated the re-created drawings and colorized clippings. The colors are not historically correct due to lack of historical color information.

Cynthia Broze began her life surrounded by hundreds of books on her mother's and aunt's shelves. "Reading is like breathing," they told her. She developed a love for books at the age of four. But, like many children, history didn't interest her until much later.

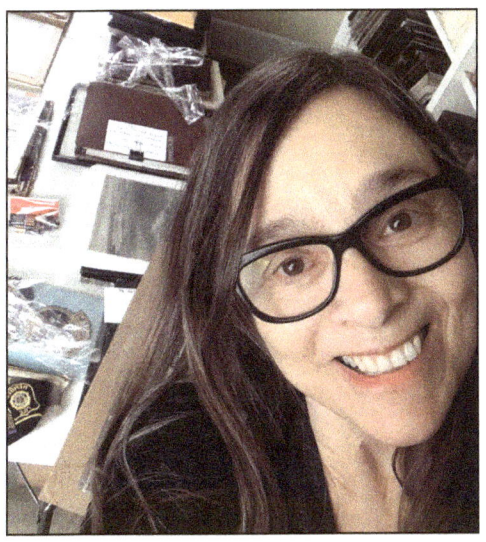

She became a nurse at 18 and continued until she completed a Nurse Practitioner program, with a Master of Science and studies in design and history along the way. She worked in various nursing specialties, including seven years as a Neonatal Intensive Care Nurse and twenty-six as a Nurse Practitioner.

She wanted to write the stories circling in her head, especially when she returned from the Peace Corps in the Philippines. She pivoted to a position at a famous medical center where she wrote educational articles and drew illustrations for the company's website. To improve her writing skills, she completed the Master Novel Writing Program at UCLA in 2003.

She stumbled into writing history when she wondered who started the first school for nurses in Los Angeles. A few had claimed that status. She answered the question when she published *Nurses of Los Angeles: Uncapping the Mystery* in 2010. She found the fascinating story of the Aerial Nurse Corps of America during that research. She knew they would be her second book. Although she never became a pilot or flight nurse, she developed an interest in airplanes—notably the dangerous old planes covered in fabric and the courageous women who flew them.

Her style of history/biography book includes hundreds of old photographs because they help tell the story and people always like them. She enjoys publishing photos of pins, patches, and the ephemera hidden in archived collections as that type of art is disappearing.

The photo above is Broze at Bucyrus Historical Society, sorting through Schimmoler's archive inside the Scroggs House Museum in 2017. Several of the items she photographed are on the table in the background.

For additional information about her books, visit cynthiabroze.com.

www.ingramcontent.com/pod-product-compliance
Lightning Source LLC
Chambersburg PA
CBHW040551010526
44110CB00054B/2604